Organ Transplantation

A book from the Park Ridge Center for the Study of Health, Faith, and Ethics

Organ Transplantation

Meanings and Realities

Edited by
Stuart J. Youngner,
Renée C. Fox,
and
Laurence J. O'Connell

The University of Wisconsin Press

The University of Wisconsin Press
114 North Murray Street
Madison, Wisconsin 53715

3 Henrietta Street
London WC2E 8LU, England

Printed in the United States of America

Library of Congress Cataloging-in-Publication Data
Organ transplantation : meanings and realities / edited by Stuart J. Youngner,
  Renée C. Fox, and Laurence J. O'Connell.
      298 pp.   cm.
  Includes bibliographical references and index.
      ISBN 0-299-14960-9 (alk. paper).   ISBN 0-299-14964-1 (pbk. alk. paper)
      1. Transplantation of organs, tissues, etc.—Social aspects.   2. Transplantation of or-
gans, tissues, etc.—Psychological aspects.   3. Transplantation of organs, tissues, etc.—
Moral and ethical aspects.   4. Transplantation of organs, tissues, etc.—Religious as-
pects.   I. Youngner, Stuart J., 1944–   .   II. Fox, Renée C. (Renée Claire), 1928–   .
III. O'Connell, Laurence J.
RD120.7.M38   1996
617.9'.5—dc20   95-29995

Contents

Acknowledgments

The editors would like to thank the Park Ridge Center, whose commitment and support made this project possible; the participating scholars for their dedication and collegiality; and Alan Weisbard, who helped give the project form and substance.

Organ Transplantation

1 *Renée C. Fox, Laurence J. O'Connell, and Stuart J. Youngner*

Introduction

This book grows out of a project sponsored by the Park Ridge Center for the Study of Health, Faith, and Ethics in Chicago. The project involved the convening of an exceptionally broad and dynamic interdisciplinary group of scholars, who met periodically over the course of two years (1991–93) to explore the phenomenological reality of organ transplantation and examine its human and cultural meaning. This group—in which the book's authors participated—spanned the fields of art, literature, history, religion, philosophy, anthropology, folklore, sociology, psychology, psychiatry, and surgery. Within these fields, the authors brought knowledge of many historical periods; a wide range of cultural traditions (American, British, Canadian, Indian, Japanese, and ancient Greek and Roman) and religious traditions (Jewish, Catholic, Protestant, Buddhist, Confucian, Hindu, and Shinto); and some of the distinctive subcultures of modern medicine, especially those of transplant surgeons, psychiatrists, internists, and nurses.

At the inception of the project, we had different kinds and degrees of knowledge about organ transplantation, and varying contacts with it. It was part of the everyday, operating-room reality of transplant surgeon Barry Kahan, for example; it was psychodynamically familiar to Stuart Youngner through his experience conducting psychiatric evaluations of prospective heart- and liver-transplant candidates; and it was central

3

to the firsthand medical, sociological research in which Renée Fox had engaged for forty years.

In contrast, Ruth Richardson approached this subject through the historical past and her immersion in the "popular culture of death and the history of anatomical training and experiment" in seventeenth- to nineteenth-century Britain. Literary critic and teacher of English Leslie Fiedler averred that the closest he had previously come to "[thinking] very much about organ transplantation at all" was through the medium of science fiction. And Leonard Barkan, scholar of the literature and art of antiquity and the Renaissance, described himself as "an alien visitor to the world of those who have studied the history of medicine, the ethics of modern technology, and the clinical or sociological practices of transplant in the modern hospital." Margaret Lock traveled to the universe of transplantation by way of her long involvement in "matters relating to the body in health and illness" in Japan; Wendy Doniger, out of the realm of myths; Laurence O'Connell and Elliot Dorff, from the spheres of philosophy and religion; and Thomas Murray, through his interest in the gift relationship, "gifts of the body," and "the needs of strangers."

Although we did not have a fixed conceptual framework, from the outset we were united in our reasons for undertaking this joint exploration; and we shared certain convictions about what organ transplantation entails, what it stands for, what it evokes, and how best to ponder and express its deepest and widest import. It was not primarily the biomedical, psychosocial, or bioethical parameters and implications of organ transplantation that drew us toward the topic. Rather, it was our recognition that organ transplantation—through which the living parts of a person, offered in life or death to known or unknown others, are implanted in the bodies and existences of individuals in the end stages of serious diseases—is intrinsically and profoundly connected with experiences and questions concerning the human condition that are at once elemental, transcendent, and fraught with ambiguity and mystery. These are matters concerning life and death, immortality and finitude, body and mind, psyche and soul, self and other, egoism and altruism, and the primordial bonds, particularistic ties, and universalistic links out of which human identity and solidarity are forged. In our view, these constituent elements of transplantation have the transformative power to carry those involved in it beyond what the philosopher Alfred Schütz terms "the paramount reality of everyday life" into other domains of existence and meaning, providing that one is willing to undergo the "shock" and make the "leap" that the voyage calls for.[1]

The group was both willing and able to make such a leap. Whether physician, social scientist, religionist, or humanist, all members were attuned to these provinces of being and reality through their intellectual work and by personal inclination. They moved with competence and ease in the terrains of the unconscious and preconscious, feelings and dreams, symbols and rituals, images and metaphors, myths and magic, folklore and legend, the spiritual and the miraculous. What is more, they saw the relevance—even the necessity—of looking into their own conceptions and misconceptions, beliefs and sentiments, and life experiences pertaining to organ transplantation while they undertook their explorations in the group. The decision to preface each chapter with an autobiographical statement about the author's personal relationship to transplantation grew out of this common perspective.

Ours was not a research project in the conventional sense. But, individually and collectively, we did seek to penetrate more deeply what Laurence O'Connell refers to in his chapter as the "curious" and "disquieting" presence of organ transplantation, and the issues that "shadow" it. We studied and discussed whatever articles and books about organ transplantation members of our group had previously published, along with the manuscripts that they prepared explicitly for our meetings. We reviewed the vast corpus of medical and psychiatric literature about transplantation that has been generated since the first successful human kidney transplants were performed in the mid-1950s, concentrating on writings that contained primary, qualitative data on the reactions of donors, recipients, their families, and the members of transplant teams to what is involved in giving, obtaining, and receiving organs, and in transposing them from one person's body to another.

The humanists in our group took us into fictive and folkloric, religious and historical texts, and into the visual representations of paintings, to contemplate analogous phenomena. Together, we examined relevant legal and public-policy documents and reflected on the persistent and salient attention that the print and electronic media have accorded transplantation for decades. We watched a three-hour Japanese television program about brain death and organ transplants,[2] and the famous early *Frankenstein* movie (starring Boris Karloff), later engaging in a lively content analysis of both. We also arranged to have a transplant coordinator talk to us about the process and problems of procuring organs, and we interviewed him about his macabre lifesaving work and the way he thinks and feels about it.

The biomedical status of transplantation in the early 1990s, the availability of donated organs, and the system of allocating them, particularly in the United States, provided the context for our reflection. Although the U.S. organ transplantation situation was our baseline in this regard, we did not assume, as Margaret Lock put it, that it should be "taken as the gold standard for what is natural and inevitable" with regard to the transplanting of human organs.

Our meetings occurred in what might be described as the cyclosporine era of transplantation, when this immunosuppressive drug, discovered in the 1970s and developed in the 1980s, was considered the most potent and efficacious agent available to prevent graft failure caused by the rejection of transplanted organs. The rejection-reaction phenomenon, due to "the innate and unrelenting intolerance of individuals to grafts of other people's tissues and organs,"[3] remains the most critical source of medical uncertainty and limitation regarding the outcome of organ transplants. Nevertheless, the superior ability of cyclosporine over previous immunosuppressive drugs to forestall the body's immune system from rejecting tissue and organ transplants has played a major role in emboldening physicians and transplant centers to enter the field.

At the time we were convening, the types of solid organ transplants being performed included cadaveric, living related, and living nonrelated kidney, heart, liver, pancreas, and lung transplants, singly and in various combinations and clusters, as first transplants and as retransplants. By November 1993, these procedures were taking place in 275 transplantation centers across the United States, within 798 programs approved by the United Network for Organ Sharing.[4] As many as 8,886 kidneys, 2,160 livers, 412 pancreases, 89 lungs, and 70 hearts in combination with lungs were transplanted in the United States during 1989.[5] However, both despite and partly because of the expansion of organ transplantation, an estimated 30,000 patients were awaiting transplants in the United States that year.[6] Nationally, the number of cadaveric donors in 1990 was no more than 4,152, and has remained almost constant since then.[7]

Medical and public enthusiasm about the progress that had been made in the quality and duration of life after transplantation was high. However, while the waiting lists for transplants grew longer, concern about the scarcity of organs, their procurement, and their allocation mounted. During 1991–93, new ways of obtaining more organs were being set forth and debated—among them: the use of so-called non-heart-beating cadaver donors and of organs from "nonideal donors (as defined by age, disease, or mode of death)";[8] financial incentives and rewards for organ donation; and the passage of "presumed-consent" (for organ donation) legislation. Only occasionally was it suggested that perhaps "the growth of transplant centers [had] been excessive"[9] and, even more rarely, that the "ultimate prize of transplantation would be for the basic principles learned to facilitate the prevention of the disease that necessitates transplantation in the first place."[10] These scientific, clinical, and atmospheric features played an integral role in our analysis of organ transplantation.

Our reflections on the larger significance of organ transplantation centered around metaconceptions and metameanings of the human body and the human person, of death, of the gift and the gift relationship, of individuality and community, of the market and the allocation of scarce material and nonmaterial resources, and of self-interest, generosity, and compassion. Our searching discussions took place in what Laurence O'Connell characterizes as an implicitly phenomenological framework of "common understanding" that allowed for "widely divergent interpretations" and "many layers of meaning." A key aspect of our common understanding was our nonpositivist approach to scientific interpretation. It allowed us to suspend hyperrationality when we entered the worlds of feelings, beliefs, dreams, and myths, and also the recesses of science, where assumptions and phenomena that are not in themselves scientific coexist with those that are, to make what philosopher Jean Ladrière calls the "scientificness" of a science.[11]

Some of the images and metaphors that are coded into the medical language of organ transplantation were particularly important in giving us entrée to these latent levels of science. We were struck, for example, by the at-once military and anthropomorphic nature of all the immunological references to the "invasion" of the body by "foreign" tissue, its capacity to "recognize" such tissue as "nonself," and to the confrontation between "killer" cells and "helper" cells that this defensive recognition evokes. Equally notable was how frequently transplant teams use the phrase "harvesting organs" when they write or speak of the process of surgically extracting them from a donor's body. As Ruth Richardson points out, harvesting is a euphemistic term that "exudes pastorality" and "fertility"; suggests "natural ripeness" and an abundant crop; and is also tinged with gallows-humor-like allusions to "Death, the Grim Reaper."

Still another facet of our shared perspective was our sense that, no matter how surgically and medically commonplace organ transplantation might become over time, the feelings and experiences that lie below its surface will not be dispelled. Nor will they merge with the "taken-for-granted reality of everyday life." In our view, as Stuart Youngner states, the "inherent nature of transplantation provides both a stimulus and rich material" for what Sigmund Freud identified as unconscious or preconscious "primary-process" thinking. This is true for several reasons: because "in order for some to live and benefit from transplantation, others must die"; because "conventional boundaries between persons are violated" when organs are transplanted; and because it entails the "mutilation" of the bodies of the newly dead persons from whom the organs are taken.

Despite our acceptance of the concept and reality of both individual and collective primary-process thinking, not everyone in our group subscribed to the Freudian assumption that it is a more primitive and infantile form of thought, less organized and less rational than so-called secondary-process, conscious thinking. And some of us were more impressed than others by the role that cultural and historical factors, as well as personality factors, can play in shaping the content and imagery of unconscious or preconscious thinking. For example, during the spring of 1994, while we were still meeting periodically, we read newspaper reports about two American women, traveling as tourists in the Mayan highlands of Guatemala, who were attacked by mobs because they were suspected of kidnapping children and shipping them to the United States to be killed so that their organs could be sold and used for transplantation. Stories of this genre, chiefly involving victims in Third World countries, have appeared recurrently in the press. But in this case, a few of us were impressed by the antiquity and cultural specificity of the fears that seemed to underlie these incidents, and their historical association with the beliefs held by Mayan mothers in the sixteenth century that the pale-skinned, blond Spanish conquistadores who invaded the Guatemalan highlands needed the blood of brown-skinned babies to cure their anemia.[12]

Within the framework of our common angle of vision, perhaps the greatest divergence between us concerned our differing views on what kinds of parallels can be drawn between the past and the present, and between various societies and cultures; and if illuminating parallels were to be discovered, in the words of Leonard Barkan, "through what systems of interpretation and translation" should we operate when we "visit" times and countries "of which we are not natives"? How legitimate is it, for example, to make analogies between "an ancient myth about exchanging bodies or a nineteenth-century fiction about a monster fabricated in a laboratory" and the modern medical and cultural actualities of organ transplantation?

Wendy Doniger articulates and espouses the most transhistorical and transcultural position on these questions. In her view, "certain myths have a universal human meaning . . . that transcends and supplements the local, cultural meanings. . . . Just as it is possible to transplant an organ from one body to another, so it is possible to transplant a myth from one culture to another." In contrast, Leonard Barkan expresses the greatest wariness about the "potential danger . . . in bridging the gap be-tween modern transplant and the history of culture," arguing that "each cultural representation is embedded in the language, the hermeneutics, the aesthetics, and the social and political conditions of its own historical moment and its own past." These "nuanced particularities" of history and culture, he contends, must interrogate "our methods as much as our methods interrogate [them]."

Margaret Lock's perspective falls somewhere between the Doniger and Barkan poles. As an anthropologist who has conducted research in Japan for twenty years, she is expertly mindful of how the "particularities" of Japanese history, culture, and society affect the so-called brain-death problem and its relationship to transplantation in contemporary Japan. But, like most anthropologists today, she says, she is very "sensitive about how we represent the 'exotic other.'" The "goal of anthropology," she affirms, "should be not only to represent how others differ from us but also to use this knowledge to interrogate ourselves" and to search for "the basis of our shared humanity." What Laurence O'Connell describes as the "free play of a plurality of voices and viewpoints" took place within our group on this issue (and on others), without disrupting the "unity-in-diversity" of the whole organ transplantation project. The essays brought together in this volume reflect both that unity and diversity.

The initial chapter, by Laurence O'Connell, "The Realities of Organ Transplantation," introduces the project and describes and analyzes its phenomenological framework of reflection. It proceeds to apply this outlook and method to the ways in which developments in the field of organ transplantation are compelling us to reconsider haunting questions about discerning when a person is dead and about what death and being *really* dead" mean.

In his evocatively titled chapter, "Some Must Die," Stuart Youngner pursues the relationship between death, organ procurement, and transplantation, particularly what he terms the "controlled death" that transplantation entails, and the impact that the notion of brain death has had on health professionals, patients, the public, and popular culture. He draws on a thematic analysis of the way that organ transplantation is presented in the media, films, and science fiction, and on his clinical experience as a psychiatrist working with transplant patients, their families, and the nurses and physicians who care for them. In the process, he explores what he regards as a central paradox of organ transplantation in the United States—a societywide ambivalence about the uplifting and lifesaving meaning of *giving* organs, on the one hand, and resistance to *taking* organs from the bodies of former loved ones, patients, or our imagined dead selves on the other. Examining the resistance leads Youngner to compare the phenomenon of organ transplantation with both "survival and ritual cannibalism." Here, the predominantly Freudian framework within which his chapter is cast, with its emphasis on the powerful subterranean role that "primary-process thinking" plays in individual and collective reactions to transplanting organs, comes dramatically to the fore.

Leslie Fiedler's chapter, "Why Organ Transplant Programs Do Not Succeed," delves deeply into the same ambivalence about transplantation that Youngner identifies. Fiedler investigates what he calls the "profound contradiction" between our "conscious acceptance" of transplantation and the "unconscious repulsion" that it arouses in us, calling on four popular novels from the nineteenth century to do so. There are *Frankenstein, Dracula, Dr. Jekyll and Mr. Hyde,* and *The Island of Dr. Moreau,* which in reprint, and through their translation into plays, films, television shows, and comic strips, still attract a mass audience. These mythic tales, he contends, "try to frighten us with . . . the new horrors . . . created by modern science and technology, particularly in the field of medicine." Like organ transplantation, these tales depict vivisection, blood transfusions, psychochemistry, and plastic surgery that threaten our "primal notions" about the meaning of life and death and the sanctity and integrity of the human body. On the basis of his examination of these tales and what he considers to be their bearing on organ transplantation, Fiedler concludes that it is the "dark side" of our "quest for immortality," implicit in organ transplantation, that underlies the deepest doubts and fears it elicits. Although Fiedler's approach is highly compatible with Youngner's psychoanalytic perspective, it challenges Leonard Barkan's reservations about using "imaginative modes of analogy" to declare a nineteenth-century gothic tale about a monster made in a laboratory relevant to twentieth-century organ transplantation.

The burning question at the center of Ruth Richardson's chapter is posed by the title: "Fearful Symmetry: Corpses for Anatomy, Organs for Transplantation?" Richardson comes to this subject after many years of research on the history of anatomical training and experimentation and on the popular culture of death in Britain from the Renaissance to the present day. Her chapter concentrates on the "historical affinities" she has discovered between the difficulties past practitioners of anatomy experienced in obtaining human bodies for dissection and the current difficulties of physicians in obtaining human organs for transplantation. The chief parallel she identifies is the "constant refrain of shortage"—of corpses for dissection, on the one hand, and of organs for transplant, on the other. Like Youngner and Fiedler, she associates this shortage with deep-seated psychological and cultural fears about mutilating the bodies of individuals, removing parts from them, inflicting pain upon the dead or "the sentient corpse," and facing "retribution from the grave." But unlike them, she argues that "much of the fear may not, in fact, be irrational" because, in her view, disquieting "symmetries" exist between measures that today's transplanters are considering to increase the supply of organs, such as financial inducement and so-called presumed consent, and the means British anatomists resorted to 150 years ago to obtain sufficient corpses. On historical grounds, she warns, trying to push the pace of "cultural change in this tender area of human consciousness" in such ways may carry us morally to the edge of a very slippery slope. She reminds us that using financial inducement in the past to procure corpses for dissection led to body-snatching thefts and serial murders, and legislation that appropriated the bodies of the poor without their consent so negatively affected the public that people were unwilling to donate their bodies for scientific and medical use for more than a century.

Ruth Richardson's admonitions provide a historical context for the next chapter, by Thomas Murray, titled "Organ Vendors, Families, and the Gift of Life." In detail and depth, Murray considers three proposals that have recently been set forth in the United States to deal with the shortage of organs for transplantation. All three proposals—creating a futures market in organs, giving discounts on health insurance to prospective donors, and offering money to families of donors to be used for funeral expenses—employ financial means to induce people to allow their own or their relative's organs to be used for transplanta-tion. Murray critically examines the economically deterministic, market-driven, supply-side premises on which these proposals are based, and he finds them empirically dubious. He seriously questions their implicit suppositions that human organs are no different from other commodi-ties, either substantively or representationally; that financial incentives will operate in this sphere as they do with other commodities in the market; and that money has the supreme motivating power to overcome whatever sentiments and beliefs people may hold that incline them to act in "nonrational" ways. The ideological worldview from which these assumptions stem, Murray points out, fails to account for why so many people donate organs under the "gift of life" system that now exists in the United States. It also disregards the meaning of the human body and human relationships (with strangers, a well as with family members and friends), and the significance of human death. What is more, it negates the role that caring, generosity, compassion, and love can and do play in the decision to donate human organs, and in human existence more generally. Because, in Murray's view, such a narrowly economic outlook is flawed in these ways, attempts to increase the supply of organs through financial enticements are unlikely to work and may very well backfire. But even if they were to reduce the organ shortage, Murray believes, strong social, moral, and spiritual reasons justify a gift-based rather than a market-oriented system of obtaining organs. "Markets are principally about goods and money," he states. "Gifts are about human relationships," and in the deepest sense, this is what organ transplantation is about, too.

It is from within the universe of transplant surgeons that surgeon-immunologist Barry Kahan discusses what he regards as some of the critical scientific, moral, and policy issues that currently surround organ transplantation. His chapter, "Organ Donation and Transplantation—A Surgeon's View," is structured around the complex set of phenomena triggered by the development of the immunosuppressive drug cyclosporine, and the resulting improvement in handling the body's rejection of transplanted tissue. The introduction of cyclosporine in 1983, he writes, "represented the greatest boon to clinical transplantation since the introduction of azathioprine in 1964," and it "brought transplant surgeons out of the cave and into the daylight."

"Boon" though cyclosporine may be, in Kahan's opinion, it "took a few years for our eyes to adjust and to see the long-term limitations intrinsic to the therapy." It led transplant surgeons into what Kahan considers overly optimistic and insufficiently rigorous clinical and research behavior. Because "rejection processes remain multifaceted and unpredictable" and "frequently vitiate technical efforts," Kahan avers, transplantation should be approached as an immunology-centered "investigative endeavor," not just as a surgical treatment. Furthermore, he argues, the continuing scientific and clinical uncertainties surrounding rejection after "three decades of intensive inquiry" into it should act as a constraint on organ transplantation.

Instead, Kahan finds it both ironic and distressing that the discovery of cyclosporine and the increased success of transplantation accompanying it have led to the flourishing of a surgical "cult." In contrast with the scientific expertise in immunology that characterized the surgeons who entered the field of transplantation at its inception, Kahan contends, these cult members deny the need to understand rejection; are reluctant to employ randomized clinical trials; emphasize quantity over quality in the transplants that are performed; and play down limitations and imperfections, including the inexorable nature of the rejection reaction and the side effects of cyclosporine. In his opinion, "the aura of 'good science'" that formerly prevailed in the field of transplantation has been "exchanged for the halo of publicized 'success.'" This pattern

has been augmented by what Kahan describes as a "synergistic relation" involving the transplant surgeon, media, public, and government,
which has brought the transplant process to the point where the "only
constraints" upon it are "organ-donor availability and payment for the
procedure."

Kahan insists that a "gatekeeper" is urgently needed in this situation to moderate professional behavior, to establish more responsible
medical criteria for screening potential organ recipients, and to restore
equilibrium between the "extreme demand" for organs and their "limited supply." While acknowledging the drawbacks of self-regulation,
he concludes that probably only the medical community has the professional competence to fill such a gatekeeping role.

In "Deadly Disputes: Ideologies and Brain Death in Japan," Margaret
Lock transports us to contemporary Japan to reflect on a national debate
that has taken place there over the past twenty-five years. This debate
revolves around what the Japanese call the brain-death problem. It
entails continuous controversy about whether to alter the conception
and definition of death to include brain death as the end of life. To date,
the "remaking of death" in this way has not taken place in Japan. As a
consequence, the types of organ transplants that require a brain-dead
donor (heart transplants, for example) are considered unacceptable in
Japanese medical practice and are not performed. Although this state
of affairs has persisted over time, it is the focus of unending, quite
passionate, political and legal discussion among the public and the
medical profession, with the mass media as vigorous and theatrical
participants and with continuous soundings of public opinion through
recurrent polls.

For Lock, this phenomenon "provides one of the best lenses through
which to view contemporary Japanese culture and society while it
struggles with the search for a cultural identity in late modernity."
Given the scientific, medical, technological, economic, and educational
sophistication of Japan, Lock reasons, the resistance to brain death
and to brain-dead donors is most likely attributable to some other
variable. And, she is convinced, it is primarily culture that is at work
here—an assumption that is reinforced when she compares the Japanese
situation with the widespread and relatively quiet acceptance of brain
death in Canada and the United States and the thousands of heart
transplants that have been performed in these countries. Public furor
about biomedical technologies in these Western societies, she contends,
centers on abortion, *in vitro* fertilization, and genetic engineering at the
beginning of life, rather than on dying, on brain-dead bodies, and on
their dismemberment in the context of organ transplantation.

Lock develops her analysis of the origins, dynamics, and significance of Japan's death-focused disputes within a comparative framework. She does so not only to sharpen her insights into the Japanese condition but also to stimulate self-interrogation among Americans and Canadians about why they approach the beginning and end of life and the role of modern medicine in the birth and death of persons the way they do. Her primary data are Japanese media materials; medical, legal, and popular documents; and public poll results. She concludes that Japan's brain-death–organ-transplantation debate is "overtly about scientific progress, the legitimation of scientific knowledge, the status of the medical profession, and patient well-being." But it is also concerned with "Japan's self-image as an advanced society, with what the outside world thinks of Japan," with the relationship between Japan and the West, and with "the question of continuity and the value of tradition" in the face of modernity.

Elliot N. Dorff writes about the manifest and latent influence of a particular religious tradition on attitudes toward transplantation. In "Choosing Life: Aspects of Judaism Affecting Organ Transplantation," he draws on his scholarly, philosophical, and religious background, and on his experiences as a Conservative rabbi teaching and counseling both observant and nonobservant Jewish persons. Dorff examines biblical, rabbinic, legal, literary, folkloric, and psychological aspects of Judaism that affect what Jews think, believe, and feel about transplantation, and how willing they are to donate organs for that purpose. He also identifies a number of legal and theological principles that have spurred most contemporary rabbis to permit, and even encourage, Jews to donate organs for transplantation, without obliging them to do so. The same concepts and features of Judaism that shape the rabbis' outlook and rulings, Dorff states, also deeply penetrate the Jewish psyche in ways that predispose Jews to think seriously about donating organs.

Undergirding all reasons that prompt Jews to contribute organs for transplantation is the obligation to save people's lives. It is a tenet, Dorff declares, that takes precedence over all other commandments, except the proscriptions against murder, idolatry, and illicit sex. Because saving a person's life is such a sacred value in Judaism, Dorff explains, even though a cadaveric donation involves mutilating the body (God's creation and property after death, as in life), it is considered "an honor to the deceased person . . . to use his or her bodily parts in [this] way." In addition, Dorff argues, Judaism's laws that require Jews to help others and generously give to those in need, as a duty to God and their fellow human beings, are part of the psychological background that impels them to consider donating organs and that infuses such gifts of life with high moral and spiritual meaning.

Dorff also reviews aspects of Jewish tradition that deter Jews from donating organs or make them feel anxiously reluctant about it, even though almost all rabbis writing on the subject have urged them to do so. He cites such factors as official and popular beliefs concerning the stages that the process of dying and leaving life entails, and the ambiguity about precisely when the moment of death occurs; folk beliefs in spirits who live on and who "look like the embodied people they were in life"; and both rabbinic and folk beliefs in the possibility of bodily resurrection after death.

In conclusion, Dorff maintains that the "imperative to save lives," the "biblical command not to stand idly by the blood of one's neighbor," and the Jewish conception of sharing and giving "as acts of justice, not charity" supersede these misgivings, fears, and uncertainties, and also the "normal prohibitions against invading the integrity of the corpse." "The clear mandate of the Jewish tradition," he affirms, "is that if organ donation can be done, both medically and financially, Jews must lend a hand in seeing to it that it is done."

Of all the contributions to this volume, Wendy Doniger's chapter, "Transplanting Myths of Organ Transplants," has the widest historical and cultural sweep. It encompasses themes in a number of centuries-old mythic traditions, themes that she considers relevant to organ donation and transplantation, with particular but not exclusive focus on South Asia, especially the mythologies of India, with which she is most familiar. In Doniger's view, for many centuries mythological texts have provided "a kind of virtual reality testing ground" for organ transplants, long before such operations became surgically possible. Some of these myths, she claims, anticipate "deep, often very dark, feelings" about transplanting part of one person's body into another person's body. On the "brighter side," she asserts, other myths offer "positive images of organ donation."

Doniger begins with Sanskrit texts dealing with the dismemberment of gods and humans at their death, starting in around 1000 B.C.E., with a *Rig Veda* funeral hymn in which the dead man gives his eye back to the sun. She goes on to texts about living human donors who give parts of their body, such as eyes (so that others can see, as recounted in Buddhist and Hindu texts); legs (involving two sets of twin brothers, the Greek Castor and Pollux, and the Christian saints Cosmas and Damian); hearts (the crocodile's wife who wanted a monkey's heart, narrated in Sanskrit and Persian texts); and heads (the Brahmin woman whose head was traded with that of an Untouchable woman, told in an ancient Indian story). Some of these myths, Doniger comments, speak of the power to restore youth. Problems of race and class also arise in "mythological organ donation."

Doniger then discusses what she terms "the great transference"—
the Hindu doctrine of the transfer of karma at death and during life—
and its implications for organ transplant. "Hindus believe that their
souls and their bodies are changed by any intense contact with another
person," she explains, "particularly those involving food and sex."
Karma is "encoded in both the body and the soul," and within the
context of this karma theory, in a very real sense, any gift given or
received is "a gift of a part of one's own body." This leads Doniger
to question whether transplants would be less threatening in societies
where people are raised with "the idea of karmic transfer and, hence,
with the idea of sharing other people's bodies," or in Western societies,
with their conception of a sharply defined and bounded, autonomously
individual self.

Throughout the chapter and in a final section, Doniger comments on
more modern myths, such as those explored by Leslie Fiedler, and on
myths and quasi myths created by the media, drawing certain parallels
between them and the ancient South Asian myths. She concludes her
chapter with a "personal postscript" about an organ transplantation that
unexpectedly took place in her family, and what it revealed to her about
her own unconscious ideas concerning death and transplants.

In sharp contrast with Wendy Doniger, Leonard Barkan focuses on
only one story in his chapter, "Cosmas and Damian: Of Medicine,
Miracles, and the Economies of the Body." He takes a strong stand
against assimilating "this remarkable story . . . to either a transhistorical
or an ahistorical world of analogy." And he does not attempt to place
it in the "universal matrices" of folklore about lost and regained parts
of the body. Rather, he seeks only to draw conclusions from historically
specific questions raised in the verbal and visual representations of this
story, which was first recounted in the Middle Ages and had a lively
existence in narration and painting through the early modern period.

Barkan begins by citing several versions of a miracle performed by
Cosmas and Damian, the twin-brother saints and patrons of medicine.
When a devotee of theirs in Rome was losing a leg to gangrene, they
effected a transplant from the healthy leg of a deceased African man;
in turn, the gangrenous leg was miraculously grafted onto the corpse.
Barkan tries to place himself inside the narrative, paying particular
attention to the details that vary from one version of the story to another, because these are the places, he says, which "one might call the
fault lines of the story . . . where successive tale-tellers have revealed
themselves and their own narrative needs." Through this kind of study
(which Barkan acknowledges is significantly influenced by the structuralist view of myth), he engages in three sets of interrogations: first, a

discussion of the interrelations between the medical and the miraculous; second, an analysis of the ways in which Christian lore of the resurrection of the body affects concepts of the individual life and subjectivity; and finally, the placement of ritual exchange in the context of race.

In the end, Barkan wryly admits that, although he has "sworn off the making of facile transhistorical parallels," he has chosen a story that "represents, after all, a late medieval organ transplant." He confesses that he has "rather coyly led the topic around to issues of demonstrable contemporary relevance, such as the relations between medicine and the miraculous and the various ways in which the presence of an alien organ serves to call into question profound and enduring beliefs concerning both flesh and spirit, both in individual experience and in the constituting of human beings as a society." He concludes with a cautionary affirmation: "In the space between the imaginative projection of . . . anxieties" about the "physical and metaphysical, human and divine" body in the early modern period "and the twentieth-century experience of recipient and donor lie all the nuanced particularities of history."

In the final chapter, "Afterthoughts: Continuing Reflections on Organ Transplantation," Renée Fox retrospectively explores the reasons that organ transplantation has engrossed her for so long, the kinds of personal and philosophical significance it has held for her, and, within a cross-cultural perspective, the aspects of American society and culture it has led her to contemplate. Numerous themes on which she reflects appear as leitmotifs in the chapters that precede hers.

Fox's chapter encompasses a wide range of phenomena and issues: the symbolic and anthropomorphic meanings of human organs and organ exchange; the sublimity and tyranny of the gift; the relationships between self, other, and "otherness"; the bases and boundaries of family and of kinship that extend beyond family; the nonscientific elements that are coded into the technical language of organ transplantation and into its underlying worldview; the human conditions, essences, and questions with which transplant medicine confronts the doctors and nurses engaged in it; and the bearing that organ transplantation has on issues of neoindividualism and market orientation in present-day American society.

Her chapter concludes with concrete examples of the ways in which organ transplantation and its ultimate meaning are being desacralized by excessive American ardor for prolonging life through this process (combined with the technical routinization of transplant surgery, its expansion, and the continuing shortage of donated organs). These developments have reinforced her previously announced decision to depart from the field of organ replacement after some forty years of intensive involvement in it as a participant observer, Fox says: and they have impelled her to bear witness, as she does in this chapter. She ends with a statement of gratitude for all that observing and reflecting upon organ transplantation has taught her, and of mounting concern about what she regards as the progressive medical, moral, and spiritual profanation that it now seems to be undergoing.

Notes

1.   Alfred Schütz, "Symbol, Reality, and Society," in *Collected Papers*, vol. 1 (The Hague: Martinus Nijhoff, 1941), 344.

2.   For a fuller account of this and other Japanese television presentations about organ transplantation, see Margaret Lock's chapter in this volume.

3.   R. E. Billingham, "Basic Genetic and Immunological Considerations," in *Symposium on Organ Transplantation in Man*, vol. 63 of *Proceedings of the National Academy of Sciences, U.S.A.* (Washington, D.C.: National Academy of Sciences, 1969), 1020.

4.   Andrew A. Skolnick, "Are There Too Many U.S. Transplantation Centers? Some Experts Suggest Fewer, Cheaper, and Better," *Journal of the American Medical Association* 271, no. 14 (13 April 1994): 1062.

5.   "Miscellaneous Medica," *Journal of the American Medical Association* 263, no. 20 (23–30 May 1990): 2721.

6.   Mark A. Hardy and Elliot R. Goodman, "Transplantation," *Journal of the American Medical Association* 271, no. 21 (1 June 1994): 1716.

7.   Manikkam Suthanthiran and Terry B. Strom, "Renal Transplantation" (Medical Progress review article, *New England Journal of Medicine* 331, no. 6 (11 August 1994): 368.

8.   Hardy and Goodman, "Transplantation," 1717.

9.   Skolnick, "Too Many Transplantation Centers?" 1062.

10.   Suthanthiran and Strom, "Renal Transplantation," 373.

11.   Jean Ladrière, *La science, le monde et la foi* (Tournai, Belgium: Casterman, 1972), passim.

12.   Victor Perera, "Behind the Kidnapping of Children for Their Organs," *Los Angeles Times* (Opinion section), 2 May 1994, M1.

2 *Laurence J. O'Connell*

The Realities of Organ Transplantation

Personal Statement

My interest in organ transplantation is quite personal. My aunt and three of her children have been afflicted with a rare genetic disease that leaves them a harsh choice: kidney transplantation or certain death. My aunt has already died. My cousins are struggling. The eldest has already undergone a transplant, and the others are waiting. Although I harbor deep reservations about the advisability of many organ transplants and I am concerned about our ability to do justice in the allocation of scarce organs, the plight of my own family seems to color my moral judgment. I remain ambivalent and morally conflicted in my feelings about transplantation.

The Park Ridge Center's research program is designed to break new the-oretical ground and to think critically about fundamental assumptions and foundational questions concerning health, faith, and ethics. Given my role as the center's president, as well as my personal experience, I am naturally enthu-siastic about this volume's emphasis on the human and cultural dimensions of organ transplantation and pleased that its purposes coincide with the center's interest in belief systems and their impact on health-related concerns.

Some argue that the debate about organ transplantation has run its course. I think not. We are presently moving toward an even deeper level of analysis and morally charged debate, as signaled by the chapters that follow.

Introduction

What does it mean to be *really* dead? Who has the last word? How do we know the opinion is right? Answers to these questions have changed in recent years, and we can expect them to undergo further revision in the not-too-distant future. The development and widespread use of life-support systems in clinical medicine, as well as advances in organ transplantation techniques and the need for organs, have been prompting a reconsideration of the traditional medical definition of death. Currently, we have three competing definitions of death, which hinge on cessation of function of the heart and respiratory functions, the whole brain, or the higher brain.[1] Everybody dies, but we are increasingly capable of extending our biological life beyond earlier limits. This has forced us to recognize that death's precise time of arrival is a socially constructed matter of interpretation.

Recent developments that have occurred in the field of organ transplantation are prompting us to revisit the debate about when a human being is dead.[2] Organs are now taken from non-heart-beating cadavers whose hearts could in some cases be started again.[3] And it is not always certain that sufficient time has elapsed for the complete cessation of all brain functions before the organs are harvested. Are we taking organs from people who are still technically alive?

Current medical technologies and techniques, coupled with a continuing shortage of human organs, have sparked renewed discussion of the definition of death and reignited interest in the web of complicated issues that surround organ transplantation. Organ transplantation has entered the mainstream of popular consciousness, but it has a disquieting presence. As level after level of meaning is laid bare and examined, basic human questions persist. Embracing so many deeply personal, socially complex, and culturally ambiguous aspects of our humanity, transplantation resists easy acceptance. A nagging sense of moral doubt and emotional discomfort fuels a relentless line of questioning: What does it really mean to donate body parts? Is it morally justified to repair and remake people with transplanted organs? What are the social, economic, and political ramifications of organ replacement?

This volume of essays represents a distinctive approach to such fundamental questions. Authors did not commit themselves to a particular method in advance; yet, as their conversations progressed and their insights matured over a period of two years, a common angle of vision emerged. And, in retrospect, a shared outlook is everywhere apparent. This unity-in-diversity undergirds the integrity of the whole and at the same time guarantees the free play of a plurality of voices and viewpoints.

The synoptic vision of these essays is rooted in an appreciation, usually implicit, of the organizing principles and basic thrust of the phenomenological method. The chosen path was not mapped out in any philosophically rigorous way but followed the course of the group's conversations. Each author captures the reality of organ transplantation and describes it from a different vantage point. As we shall see, the phenomenological method allows for widely divergent interpretations and, perhaps more important, explains how these variant interpretations can coexist without canceling one another. The phenomenological approach unveils the many layers of meaning that enfold a complex reality like organ transplantation and establishes a framework for common understanding.

A Phenomenological Point of Departure

In discussing phenomenology, Herbert Spiegelberg noted that "the difficulties of stating point-blank what phenomenology is are almost notorious."[4] The question, What is phenomenology? "is as irritating for the layman who hearing the word would like to know at least roughly what it means, as it is for the historian of philosophy or the philosophical specialist."[5] In the present context, a minimalist description suffices to confirm the relevance of a rich phenomenological approach for thoughtful reflections upon organ transplantation. As we shall see, it opens vistas of understanding that would otherwise remain closed.

Phenomenologists are not concerned with the ontological status of the objects of experience under investigation. Rather, phenomenologists are "interested in their *meaning*, as it is constituted by the activities of the mind."[6] For example, the fact that the unicorn in the garden might not really exist "out there" is not of particular concern to the phenomenologist *as* phenomenologist. Although the unicorn may not rollick in the garden behind our home, it does roam in the world of myth. What *is* important is that the unicorn, as object of mythology, is constituted in particular and appropriate acts of consciousness. It is the essential conditions of the unicorn as *meant* (intended) that constitute the subject matter of phenomenological inquiry. In short, phenomenology focuses on the meaning of an object rather than its place in the material world. The relevance of this approach to our topic comes immediately to the fore. The actual exchange of body parts simply establishes the biological point of departure for a much larger project, namely, the search for meaning. The donor, the recipient, the families of both, and society at large must constitute the meaning(s) of the transplant phenomenon. Transplant may be a medical marvel, but it is also a powerful generator of personal and social meaning. Phenomenology aims at locating and disclosing these multiple meanings.

A physician-scientist might say that a person is dead. And from a clinical point of view, this may be the case. Yet some would contend that the same person observed at the same moment from a particular religious point of view is not *really* dead and should not yet be treated as a corpse. In fact, the state of New Jersey has adopted a law that acknowledges the possibility of such divergent perspectives.[7] How can this be? Who is right? Under what circumstances would organ retrieval be appropriate in such a situation? Can such contradictory claims be explained or reconciled? Absent prior agreement regarding death, organ replacement presents an intractable medical and moral quandary.

The solution to such a dilemma hinges upon the *meaning* of death. What is understood when we say that a person is *really dead?* Here phenomenology can help by clarifying the meaning and applicability of the term *reality*. As we shall see, the reality of death means different things to different persons and peoples. Moreover, phenomenology will help us uncover the direct link between the particular historical and cultural contents for defining death and their expression in attitudes and practices that characterize transplantation in general. Our discussion of the reality of death is designed to illustrate and bring into clear view the common assumption that runs through this set of essays, namely, that the complex nature of transplantation demands kaleidoscopic rather than monochromatic treatment. While it may not be an organizing principle in the formal sense, the phenomenological perspective represents a unifying influence amidst the intentional diversity that marks the chapters that follow. In short, it provides the rhyme and reason for this unique series of reflections on the twentieth-century phenomenon of organ transplantation.

What Is "Real"?

Under what circumstances do we think things real? It was in response to this question that William James, the renowned Harvard physician-philosopher and early phenomenologist, developed his theory of the various orders of reality.[8] In considering the question, James concluded that our primitive impulse is to affirm the reality of any object given in the flow of experience: "Any object which remains uncontradicted is *ipso facto* believed and posited as absolute reality."[9] And a thing thought of cannot be contradicted by another, unless it initiates the quarrel by saying something inadmissible about the other. And if one object contradicts another, the experient must make a choice and bestow the accent of reality on one or the other, for no one can continue to think in two contradictory ways at once.

Suppose a two-year-old child who has never seen or heard about a horse is taken to an art museum by his grandfather. While meandering through the gallery, the child comes across a painting of Pegasus, the winged horse of Greek mythology. Standing before the depiction of Pegasus, the child asks, "What is it?" And the grandfather simply replies, "It is a horse." He doesn't explain that Pegasus is a mythological horse or that Pegasus, unlike the horses the child may encounter in the future, has wings. Now the child has no reason to doubt that Pegasus exists somewhere as a real horse and that real horses have wings. Since the child has no perception to annul his belief that horses have wings, he adheres to the *real* existence (as opposed to, for instance, the *imagined* existence) of winged horses. He has no reason to doubt that he will someday mount a winged horse.

"The sense that anything we think of is unreal can only come, then, when that thing is contradicted by some other thing which we think," observed James.[10] We are sure a burglar has entered the house at 3:00 A.M., *until* we hear the voice of our teenager, who supposedly was home at midnight. For a split second we find ourselves suspended, straddling the divide between belief and disbelief, until we can confirm what is really happening.

The belief that something is real can wax and wane, depending upon how one relates to it. For example, a former believer might say she has lost her faith in the existence of God. God is no longer real for her. In short, "the whole distinction of real and unreal, and the whole psychology of belief, disbelief, and doubt, are grounded on two mental facts—first, that we are liable to think differently of the same; and second, that when we have done so, we can choose which way of thinking to adhere to and which to disregard."[11] Thus the child in our example considered Pegasus real (that is, as existing in the outer world of material things) until he visited his grandfather's farm, where he learned that horses in the material world do not have wings. And, as a consequence of this inherent contradiction, he will be compelled in the future to regard this fabulous creature as a figment of the artist's imagination.[12] Similarly, the reality of God has evaporated for someone who has "lost the faith."

In James's opinion, "*the fons* [fountain] *and origo* [origin] *of all reality, whether from the absolute or the practical point of view, is thus subjective, is ourselves.*"[13] As a consequence, several or, more likely, an infinite number of "sub-universes" or various orders of reality exist, each characterized by its own special and separate style of existence.[14] Each sub-universe is a world unto itself; and "each world, while it is *attended to*, is real after its own fashion," and "*any* relation to our mind at all in the absence of a stronger relation with which it clashes, suffices to make an object real."[15] We are really terrified at the approach of a knife-wielding assailant, and we cry out, until we are awakened and reassured that it was just a dream. The reality of the dream world loses its hold on us when someone shakes us back into the world of ordinary perception. In James's view, then, reality is "an analogous term which we predicate in different ways depending upon the various 'sub-universes' to which we refer a given experience."[16]

Although William James drew attention to the various provinces, or sub-universes, of reality, he did not develop his originary insight. More thorough studies of multiple realities were conducted by several phenomenologists, including Edmund Husserl,[17] Aron Gurwitsch,[18] and Alfred Schütz.[19] With Schütz in particular we find a powerful philosophical mentor and methodological partner in our exploration of the meanings and realities of organ transplantation. His work provides a coherent yet multifaceted approach to the cluster of questions under consideration here.

Schütz's Finite Provinces of Meaning

Schütz follows James in emphasizing the primacy of perception: "William James rightly called the sub-universe of senses, of physical things, the paramount reality."[20] Schütz, however, refers to this paramount reality as "the world of daily life" or "everyday reality." He also prefers to speak of "finite provinces of meaning," upon which we bestow the accent of reality, instead of speaking of "sub-universes of reality." In changing the Jamesian terminology, Schütz intends to "emphasize that it is the meaning of our experiences, and not the ontological structure of the objects, which constitutes reality."[21]

Schütz's "Epochè of the Natural Attitude"

Our natural stance toward everyday reality is characterized by acceptance. We naturally narrow or abridge any form of radical skepticism that would challenge the reality of our day-to-day world. It is this "perspectival abridgement"[22] of consciousness that Schütz calls "the epochè of the natural attitude,"[23] or our very natural tendency to put in brackets any doubt that the world and its objects might be otherwise than they appear to us. We suspend any doubt in the existence of the outer world and its objects.[24] So everyday reality, "in which 'normal life' takes place and which persists in its massive facticity,"[25] is founded upon the epochè of the natural attitude. It is unreflectively assumed to be real. Its reality is taken for granted because it presents itself as self-evident.

Shifting the Accent of Reality

As long as our practical experience supports the unity and congruity of the world of daily life, we give this everyday world the accent of reality. Moreover, this reality seems to us to be the natural one, and consequently we are reluctant to relinquish our attitude toward it. The epochè of the natural attitude gives everyday reality "the appearance of an 'orderly, smooth roundness,' within which the life of an individual becomes plausible to himself as an orderly and seemingly necessary sequence of facts."[26] We are "at home" in the world of daily life or paramount reality, and we are usually content to remain within its confines. But, according to Schütz, certain experiences befall us that compel us to shift the accent of reality away from the world of daily life toward other finite provinces of meaning.

This transition from paramount reality to other finite provinces of meaning is experienced through "shock." We are shocked into the realization that everyday reality is not as monolithic as it might seem or as we might like it to be. Certain experiences do violence to the taken-for-granted consistency of everyday life, thereby giving rise to an intimation of novel and sometimes peculiar modes of reality.[27] We encounter various types of shock. For example, there is "the inner transformation we endure if the curtain in a theater rises as a transition to the world of the stage play; . . . or falling asleep as a leap into the world of dreams. But also religious experience in all its varieties—for example, Kierkegaard's experience of the 'instant' as the leap into the religious sphere—is a shock."[28] Disparate spheres or finite provinces of meaning exist as "alien enclaves"[29] within the paramount reality of everyday life. Thus, "while everyday reality is experienced as a totality, it is within itself variegated and stratified."[30] And these enclaves are entered by means of interruptions or shock experiences that undermine the unity and congruity of the taken-for-granted reality of everyday life. In other words, other finite provinces of meaning break in where the epochè of the natural attitude breaks down.

In explaining the dynamics of the shift from the world of ordinary daily life to some other finite province of meaning, Schütz drew upon the insights of Henri Bergson, who theorized that

our conscious life shows an indefinite number of planes, ranging from the plane of action on one extreme to the plane of dream at the other. Each of these planes is characterized by a specific tension of consciousness, the plane of action showing the highest, that of dream the lowest degree of tension. According to Bergson these different degrees of tension of our consciousness are functions of our varying interest in life, action representing our highest interest in meeting reality and its requirements, dream being complete lack of interest. *Attention à la vie*, attention to life, is, therefore, the basic regulative principle of our conscious life. It defines the realm of our world which is relevant to us; it articulates our continuously flowing stream of thought.[31]

Schütz was quick to grasp the relevance of Bergson's ideas to his own theory, immediately recognizing the "leap" or "shock" that precipitates the transition from the world of daily life to some finite province of meaning as "nothing else than a radical modification in the tension of consciousness, founded in a different *attention à la vie*."[32] When one's attention shifts, the specific tension of consciousness is altered, thereby effecting the withdrawal of the "accent of reality" from one province of meaning and shifting it to another realm.

Specific Epochè

"The transference of the accent of reality," according to Schütz, "consists in a specific 'epochè' peculiar to a given finite province of meaning."[33] Each finite province of meaning is founded upon a specific epochè that safeguards its "reality" against the same type of disintegration it originally visited upon the reality of everyday life. Indeed, "to the extent that the new reality is removed from the massive reality-confirmations of everyday life, it is *more* susceptible to disintegration than the latter, therefore *more* in need of a determined suspension of doubt."[34]

Because of the specific epochè that is operative in each finite province of meaning, each possesses a unique mode of consistency and compatibility that is definable in terms of those aspects of the everyday world from which the accent of reality is withdrawn in each case. "By no means will that which is compatible within province of meaning 'P' be also compatible within the province of meaning 'Q.'"[35] Winged horses and flying carpets might be compatible components within the world of myth, but neither fits into the world of daily life. Little boys who take their mother's Persian carpet to the roof are universally disappointed and sometimes seriously injured. They fail to realize that the world they inhabit is essentially different from the world of Aladdin, where flying carpets are common conveyances. And it is for this reason, says Schütz, that "we are entitled to talk of *finite* provinces of meaning. This finiteness implies that there is no possibility of referring one of these provinces to the other by introducing a formula of transformation. The passing from one to another can only be performed by a 'leap,' as Kierkegaard calls it, which manifests itself in the subjective experience of shock."[36]

An atheist, for example, is impervious to the presence or reality of God because the atheist has not elected to enter into a specifically religious province of meaning. So, when Catholics speak of the real presence of Jesus Christ, atheists predictably respond with disbelief. Their existential reach has a finite limit in this regard. They cannot make or choose not to make a leap of faith or directly enter into the enclave of religious consciousness.

In a more frightening illustration of the point, some people receive strange promptings, see bizarre visions, and embark on murdering sprees because they inhabit the world of sheer madness and caprice.[37] They are not treated as ordinary criminals, because society recognizes that sometimes they live in another world. Sadly, they are locked into a world of meaning that is absolutely real for them (and particularly dangerous for others). Thus each finite province of meaning operates on its own wavelength, so to speak. And unless the frequency is modulated and a leap is made, there can be no change from one channel (finite province of meaning) to another.

The Reality of Death: A Movable Moment

So what does it mean to be *really* dead? Who says so? How do we know? The phenomenological theory of multiple realities or finite provinces of meaning demonstrates that these questions have no clear-cut answer. The meaning, as well as the precise moment, of real death depends upon the particular province of meaning to which it is referred. What counts for dead in the world constructed by medical science (clinical death) may not be viewed as dead in other worlds or provinces of meaning. This explains why the moment of death is a social construct, that is, a shared convention among those who move within the same province of meaning. As Stuart Youngner reminds us in his chapter, in the world of clinical medicine, we have created a new class of dead persons by recognizing the irreversible loss of all brain function as a sufficient criterion for declaring a person legally dead.[38] Yet, he also notes, some members of both the Christian and the Jewish communities reject the notion of brain death in favor of the traditional cardiopulmonary definition, that is, the complete cessation of breathing and heart function. So what may be legally dead for clinicians may not be really dead for religious believers. This is not surprising to anyone who understands that both reality and death are analogous terms that we predicate in different ways, depending upon the specific province of meaning to which they are referred.

Zombies, the living dead, still roam the Haitian countryside; and Dracula defied death for centuries. The neurologically based brain-death criteria of clinical science are simply irrelevant to the circumstances surrounding the "deaths" of Count Dracula and the denizens of Haitian lore. Each inhabits its own sub-universe of reality or province of meaning. The lurid antics of zombies and the ultimate demise of Dracula by wooden stake are quite real, of course, when they are situated within the appropriate province of meaning. Mythical reality, religious reality, scientific reality, pathological reality, and the many other orders of reality must all be accommodated and seriously considered in our attempts to understand the human and cultural dimensions of organ transplantation. There is more to it than the comfortable world of "everyday reality in which 'normal life' takes place."[39]

Transplantation and the Phenomenological Approach

Issues surrounding organ transplantation cannot be reduced to monolithic interpretations. They are better resolved against the background of a phenomenological approach to the meaning and the concept of multiple realities. Several orders of reality exist, each characterized by its own special and separate style of existence. According to Schütz, "It is this particular style of a set of our experiences which constitutes them as a finite province of meaning,"[40] limited to their own area of operation. Each finite province of meaning—the paramount world of concrete objects and events, the dream world, the world of poetry, the world of religious experience, the world of imagination, the world of scientific theory, the world of the surgical suite, and so on—exhibits its own internal structures and incorporates its own set of requirements.

In keeping with a phenomenological understanding of reality, this volume on the human and cultural contexts of organ transplantation both celebrates and acknowledges the converging, and sometimes competing, provinces of meaning. Readers are invited to cross the threshold, that is, to join the authors in a move from everyday reality to a particular province of meaning. In stepping into another world, we are free to explore the inner and self-consistent logic, emotions, values, and beliefs that constitute that world, and learn how the dynamics of these sub-universes of meaning inevitably shape personal and cultural attitudes toward organ transplantation. Ranges of variegated and stratified meaning that inhabit the depths of our individual and communal consciousness are recognized and examined sympathetically on their own terms. Having followed our expert guides through various provinces of meaning, we return to the taken-for-granted reality of everyday life with a more sophisticated understanding of the issues that still shadow organ transplantation, and with the knowledge that these issues will undoubtedly persist. Organ transplantation taps into and energizes so many deep levels of meaning that superficial acceptance is simply impossible for the vast majority of those who seriously reflect upon it. It is our hope that these essays constitute a substantive point of departure for those who continue to struggle with the curious and essentially unsettling phenomenon of organ transplantation.

Notes

1.   See Robert M. Veatch, "The Impending Collapse of the Whole-Brain Definition of Death," *Hastings Center Report* 23, no. 4 (1993): 18–24.

2.   Renée C. Fox and Judith P. Swazey, *Spare Parts: Organ Replacement in American Society* (New York: Oxford University Press, 1992), 59–64.

3.   Stuart J. Youngner and Robert M. Arnold, "Ethical, Psychosocial, and Public Policy Implications of Procuring Organs from Non-Heart-Beating Cadaver Donors," *Journal of the American Medical Association* 269, no. 21 (1993): 2769–74.

4.   Herbert Spiegelberg, *The Phenomenological Movement*, vol. 1, 2d ed. (The Hague: Martinus Nijhoff, 1969), 1.

5.   Peter Thévanaz, *What Is Phenomenology?* (Chicago: Quadrangle Books, 1962), 37.

6.   Alfred Schütz, "Some Leading Concepts of Phenomenology," in Maurice Natanson, ed., *Collected Papers*, vol. 1 (The Hague: Martinus Nijhoff, 1941), 115.

7.   Veatch, "Collapse of the Whole-Brain Definition of Death," 23.

8.   See Abraham Gobar, "The Phenomenology of William James," in *Proceedings of the American Philosophical Society* 94 (1970): 294–309.

9.   William James, *The Principles of Psychology*, vol. 2 (New York: Dover Publications, 1950), 289.

10.   Ibid., 288–89.

11.   Ibid., 290.

12.   This, of course, does not mean that Pegasus is nonexistent. Pegasus is an existent; he is a mental object, and mental objects have existence as mental objects. As James says, "In the strict sense of the word *existence*, everything which can be thought of at all exists as *some* sort of object, whether mythical object, individual thinker's object, or object in outer space and for intelligence at large" (ibid., 294). In other words, "opposition between existence and non-existence does not coincide with that between reality and fiction or imagination" (Aron Gurwitsch, *The Field of Consciousness* [Pittsburgh: Duquesne University Press, 1964], 412).

13.   James, *Principles of Psychology* 2:296–97.

14.   Ibid., 292–93. For purposes of illustration, James concentrates upon eight sub-universes: "the world of sense or ordinary perception (the paramount reality); the world constructed by the scientist; the world of ideal relations and abstract truths held by all, and the logical, mathematical, and metaphysical

propositions expressing them; the world of 'idols of the tribe'—illusions, prejudices, superstitions; the various supernatural worlds of myth and religion; the various worlds of individual opinion; the world of dreams and imagination; and the worlds of sheer madness and caprice."

15. Ibid., 293, 299.

16. Richard Stephens, *James and Husserl: The Foundations of Meaning* (The Hague: Martinus Nijhoff, 1974), 111.

17. Edmund Husserl, *Experience and Judgment: Investigations in a Genealogy of Logic*, trans. James S. Churchill and Karl Ameriks (Evanston: Northwestern University Press, 1973), 171, 187, 344. Although Husserl considers the issue, he does not develop it thematically as Schütz does, for instance.

18. Gurwitsch, *Field of Consciousness*, 379ff.

19. The issue of multiple realities is taken up in several places in Schütz's works. For example, see Schütz, "Symbol, Reality, and Society," *Collected Papers* 1:207ff., and vol. 2, "The Stranger: An Essay in Social Psychology," and "Don Quixote and the Problem of Reality" (The Hague: Martinus Nijhoff, 1971), 91–105, 135–58.

20. Schütz, "Symbol, Reality, and Society," in *Collected Papers* 1:341.

21. Ibid.

22. P. L. Berger, "The Problem of Multiple Realities: Alfred Schütz and Robert Musil," in Maurice Natanson, ed., *Phenomenology and Social Reality: Essays in Memory of Alfred Schütz* (The Hague: Martinus Nijhoff, 1970), 216.

23. Schütz, "Symbol, Reality, and Society," 229.

24. Ibid.

25. Berger, "Problem of Multiple Realities," 215.

26. Ibid., 216.

27. My use of the term *modes* in this context is meant to reflect Schütz's contention that "the world of working daily life is the archetype of our experience of reality. All the other provinces of meaning may be considered as its modifications" (Schütz, "Symbol, Reality, and Society," 233).

28. Ibid., 344.

29. Berger, "Problem of Multiple Realities," 220. See also Schütz, "Don Quixote and the Problem of Reality," 2:136–37.

30. Berger, "Problem of Multiple Realities," 216.

31. Schütz, "Symbol, Reality, and Society," 212.

32. Ibid., 232.

33. Gurwitsch, *Field of Consciousness*, 398. It should be noted that in this context *epochè* is to be understood in the same sense as "the epochè of the natural attitude." It does not refer to the transcendental phenomenological reduction of Husserl.

34. Berger, "Problem of Multiple Realities," 224–25.

35. Schütz, "Symbol, Reality, and Society," 232.

36. Ibid.

37. This is not to imply that all otherworldly visions and voices can be dismissed as madness. In some places such visitations are culturally authenticated

and thus find legitimation and a claim to normalcy. Native American culture provides many examples. See Åke Hultkrantz, *Shamanic Healing and Ritual Drama: Health and Medicine in Native North American Religious Traditions* (New York: Crossroad, 1992). In an earlier essay, Hultkrantz draws upon the work of Henry Wegrocki, noting that "the 'abnormal' behavior of the hallucinating Indian is analogous to the behavior of the psychotic, but it is not homologous." See Åke Hultkrantz, "Health, Religion, and Medicine in Native North American Traditions," in Lawrence E. Sullivan, ed. *Healing and Restoring: Health and Medicine in the World's Religious Traditions* (New York: Macmillan, 1989), 332. This is an excellent illustration of James's main point, that is, that *reality* is an analogous term.

38.   In 1974, Willard Gaylin ignited a serious debate surrounding the shifting definition of death. Willard Gaylin, "Harvesting the Dead: The Potential for Recycling Human Bodies," *Harper's*, September 1974, 23–30.

39.   Schütz, "Symbol, Reality, and Society," 229.

40.   Ibid., 341.

3 *Stuart J. Youngner*

Some Must Die

Personal Statement

When I was a first-year medical student in 1967, I spent a summer talking with renal dialysis patients and their families at the Cleveland Clinic. I was fulfilling a requirement for a research project, but the experience turned out to be a formative one for me. It confirmed my interest in medicine as a humanistic profession.

The clinic had begun a program to teach patients and their families how to carry out the new and complicated technique of dialysis in the home setting. The patients and their families lived in a hotel near the hospital and came in every day for treatment or instruction. I spent my days "hanging out" with them, talking about their reactions to the dramatic change in their lives. There was excitement in the air; at that time dialysis was not only a new step for medical science but a controversial one as well, since there were more people who needed dialysis than machines to treat them. Hospital committees, using improvised criteria, selected who lived and who died. Some patients I worked with had been turned down by other programs.

Although home dialysis was supposed to be less expensive than hospital dialysis and could give patients a greater sense of independence, the emotional strain on both patients and their families was tremendous. The financial strain was great as well; before the federal End Stage Renal Disease Program (ESRDP) was enacted by Congress in 1972, dialysis patients had to pay out of pocket for this lifesaving, but expensive, therapy. The ESRDP is part of Medicare and pays most of the costs of dialysis and renal transplantation.

The patients I came to know felt very special and lucky. They wanted badly to live. But home dialysis was no picnic. Not only were the patients coping with end-stage renal disease and the rigors of dialysis, but also their relationship with the dialysis machine (to which they were attached and through which all their blood circulated for several hours three times a week) became a focus of fantasies, dreams, and jokes.

Those were exciting and frightening times. It was clear to health professionals and patients alike that we were moving into uncharted territory. Patients, families, and health professionals were perplexed by many boundary issues: the lines between life and death, between human and machine, between allowing to die and killing, and between medical progress and hubris. We spent long hours discussing these issues. But, over the next decade, when life-sustaining medical technology became commonplace, the wonder seemed to subside. Tens of thousands of Americans were now on chronic dialysis, waiting, often years, for transplantation.

I graduated from medical school and finished my training as a psychiatrist. When I began doing psychiatric evaluations of potential liver and heart transplant candidates in the early 1980s, many of the troubling questions that had so intrigued us in the early days were drowned out by an uncritical embrace of "medical progress" and the unidimensional, utilitarian ethic that accompanied it. When I listened carefully, however, the same questions, excitement, and fear were shared by patients, families, and many health professionals. Yet, these powerful sentiments were ignored or trivialized by the transplant community and public policy "experts" while they pressed to increase the organ supply.

I dreamed of bringing together a group of scholars who were firmly grounded in the humanities and the social sciences to enrich our society's conversation about transplantation, to reopen our eyes and ears to its complex meanings, and to reclaim some of the innocent wonder that home dialysis patients and their caregivers felt before "miraculous" technology became just another entitlement, market share, and standard treatment option. The Park Ridge Center valued my dream and brought it to fruition by sponsoring and hosting the project that resulted in this book. It was, without question, the most stimulating, enjoyable, and gratifying experience of my academic career.

Introduction

With the advent of organ transplantation, the myths, fantasies, and nightmares of past generations have become not only a reality but also a banality in the clinical and economic life of modern medical institutions. Today the standard of care for many life-ending diseases, organ transplantation has become a growth industry. Dying persons desperately want it, third parties pay for it, the news media promote it, and increasing numbers of medical centers clamor to join the no-longer-elite circle of transplant centers that provide it.

However, human body parts, the natural resources necessary for transplantation, are in short supply. The tensions created by this short-age remind us that transplantation retains its magical, irrational, and frightening aspects, which dog its progress like shadows—shadows that can darken when the bright lights of rationality and utilitarianism propel public discourse in an effort to obtain more and more organs. Thus, for example, while the public service announcements and human interest stories extolling transplantation multiply, so too do the grisly cartoons, jokes, and tabloid horror stories about the same subject.

Our society views organ transplantation simultaneously from two distinct and often contradictory perspectives. The first is the rational ethos of the Enlightenment, appropriated not only by medical science, academia, and public policy but also by mainstream religions. The sec-ond is the messier and less-well-articulated world of emotion, supersti-tion, and magic. In the context of human psychology, neither perspective is right or wrong. They simply exist and function together, an important and unavoidable quality of the human condition. With cool rationality alone, we would be computers or robots. Without it, we would be prey to our emotions and fantasies, unable to cope.

Our experience with human organ transplantation is an excellent illustration of the dynamic and often uneasy relationship between these two ways of seeing and understanding the world.

Primary- and Secondary-Process Thinking

Sigmund Freud's notions of primary- and secondary-process think-ing provide a helpful framework for understanding society's appar-ently contradictory attitudes toward organ transplantation. Secondary-process thinking is the most immediately familiar of the two. As Brenner notes, "It is ordinary conscious thinking as we know it from introspec-tion, that is, primarily verbal and following the usual laws of syntax and logic."[1]

The primary process, in contrast, characterizes unconscious or precon-scious thinking and dreaming. Compared with the secondary process, it is less objective and organized and "is ruled by emotions and hence full of wishful or fearful misconceptions . . . remote from any logic."[2] Primary-process thinking is carried out more through pictorial, concrete images; representation by allusion or analogy is frequent; and a part of an object may be used to stand for the whole. Similarities are not distinguished from identities, and mutually contradictory ideas can coexist peacefully. Primary-process thinking is a magical type of thinking. Not only may wish be equated with deed and fantasy with action, but the perpetrator of a crime or misdeed will be punished with the same injury he or she inflicted. In primary-process thinking, there is no sense of time; past, present, and future are all one.[3]

Primary-process thinking is easily recognizable in infants and small children, in seriously disturbed psychiatric patients, and in dreams, where fantasies and other internal stimuli are projected onto other persons or the environment as "delusions" or "hallucinations," indistinguishable from reality. Psychoanalysts from Freud to the present have observed that primary-process thinking is an integral, though subordinate, part of normal adult mental life, where it becomes visible in dreams, games, jokes, and slips of the tongue.

The primary and secondary process are in dynamic rather than static equilibrium. When the capacity of the secondary process is attenuated by sleep, metabolic disturbances, drugs, or severe anxiety, the primary process breaks through. Under these circumstances, the wishes and fears of the unconscious are perceived as real, and rational thought is replaced with magical thinking. Conversely, the irrational fears and delusions of the unconscious can be diminished by strengthening the secondary process, for example, by education or the reassurance of a trusted person or authority.

The inherent nature of transplantation provides both a stimulus and rich material for the primary process. In order for some to live and benefit from transplantation, others must die. When organs are transplanted, conventional boundaries between persons are violated. When organs are taken from newly dead bodies, bodies are mutilated. While the organ shortage grows, our increasingly desperate efforts to create new sources of organs inevitably provoke additional discomfort. For example, by recognizing brain death, we have created a new class of dead persons whose hearts continue to beat for days, weeks, and occasionally months. And by taking organs from baboons, chimpanzees, and pigs, we violate boundaries between species. I will argue that, at an even more subterranean level, organ transplantation represents a form of nonoral cannibalism.

Circumstantial evidence of the impact from these issues can be found in the very fact of the organ shortage, which persists despite: widespread medical and legal acceptance of organ transplantation; a radical expansion of criteria for determining death; laws that require health professionals to give families the donation option; and a federally funded, nationwide organ procurement and sharing system. This chapter will provide a more direct exploration by examining (1) the experience of patients who are waiting for or who have received organ transplants, (2) the treatment of organ transplantation in popular culture, (3) the link between our society's rapidly evolving but highly controversial acceptance of mercy killing and new methods of organ transplantation, (4) the experience and behavior of health professionals involved in procuring organs from brain-dead patients, and (5) the use of language in transplantation.

Case Studies

Mr. Anderson

I first met Mr. Anderson when I performed a routine psychiatric examination as part of his evaluation for heart transplantation. He was a large, well-built man in his late fifties who appeared surprisingly healthy considering he was nearing the end stages of a cardiomyopathy—a progressive weakening of his heart muscles, most likely due to a viral infection. Mr. Anderson lived in central Ohio, about a two-and-a-half-hour drive from Cleveland, where our transplant program was situated. He had been a career Marine Corps officer who retired at age fifty to become the manager of a small dry-cleaning business. He was married and had two children and four grandchildren.

Mr. Anderson's exam was unremarkable. He denied any psychiatric or social problems and had a positive attitude about transplantation. He expressed no concerns about taking an organ from another person into his body. I saw no evidence of depression or anxiety. I felt almost embarrassed when I asked him a routine question about whether he had ever had hallucinations. He was silent for a minute and then said, "Not exactly." He then recounted the following story.

One month before, when he had come up to Cleveland for his first evaluation visit, he had been informed that, if he were put on the waiting list, he would have to carry an electronic pager so that he could be reached instantly if a heart became available. He was also told that in order to save critical time, he would be flown by emergency helicopter to Cleveland.

This information made him quite anxious. He had been in two helicopter crashes before, once in Korea and once in Vietnam. The Vietnam crash had been the more serious. He was the gunner in a helicopter that was flying into a battle zone to pick up wounded soldiers. Coming in low over the trees, the helicopter had been shot out of the air and crashed in flames. Miraculously, Mr. Anderson had been thrown clear of the wreck with "hardly a scratch," but the pilot and copilot had burned to death.

Mr. Anderson denied any symptoms of posttraumatic stress disorder other than a fear of flying in helicopters. He had never been in one since the crash in Vietnam. While he drove back home, he had worried about flying again in a helicopter. When he arrived at home, his nine-year-old grandson greeted him, full of questions about the transplant. When the child asked Mr. Anderson where the heart would come from, the patient somewhat uncomfortably explained that it would come from a person who had died "in an accident or something." His grandson was surprised. He had assumed "they just have them on the shelf in the operating room." He then asked his grandfather if he would still love him once he had another person's heart in his body. "Of course I will," Mr. Anderson had replied. But that night he went to bed ruminating about the questions his grandson had raised. Later he awoke with a start when someone tapped him on the shoulder. The patient assured me he had not been dreaming. "I was awake," he said. "No doubt about it."

He recalled how he had sat up in bed to find the pilot and copilot of the helicopter that had crashed in Vietnam in his room. They stood silently in full battle gear, stared at him for a few minutes, and then beckoned with their hands for him to come. Mr. Anderson was terrified and began sweating profusely. The two men gradually faded away, leaving him trembling as he sat on the side of the bed.

Because of his Vietnam experience, Mr. Anderson was especially vulnerable to unconscious and primitive feelings of responsibility and guilt. As Renée Fox has remarked elsewhere, organ transplantation is both lifesaving and death ridden.[4] The vast majority of organs come from persons who have died from sudden, unexpected head injuries. Something must happen to one person for another to be saved. Of course, our rational minds tell us that these deaths are linked to organ procurement only after the fact. To Mr. Anderson the linkage became more problematic for several reasons. Like many survivors of catastrophic events, he harbored a tremendous sense of guilt and responsibility for the deaths of his helicopter pilot and copilot. The horror of this earlier episode both fueled and was fueled by the transplant situation, in which Mr. Anderson would have to take another fateful helicopter ride that would end with himself saved at the expense of another's death.

Mr. Anderson's defenses were further weakened when he saw transplantation through the eyes of his grandson, who hoped that hearts were to be found like equipment, on the shelf of the operating room, and innocently feared that his grandfather's love for him might disappear when the elder's original heart was discarded. Under the mantle of sleep, his primitive thinking gained ascendancy, awakening him to a terrifying hallucinatory morality play.

Ms. Jones

Ms. Jones, an uneducated woman in her sixties, began having a recurrent nightmare months after she had received a kidney transplant. In her dream, a dead man approached her calling her name, and like Mr. Anderson's fellow marines, beckoned her to join him in death. She would awaken terrified and remain anxious during the day. She was certain that the dead man in her dream was the person from whom she had received a kidney; she had been told he had died in a car accident.

In our discussions, she revealed that twenty-five years before, her six-year-old son had run out in traffic and was struck by an automobile. He had been taken to the hospital and placed on a mechanical ventilator, where it was determined that he had no brain function. This had occurred in the early 1960s, before brain death was widely accepted and before health professionals felt comfortable removing dying patients from ventilators (many are still uncomfortable doing this). Ms. Jones insisted she had been told that there was no hope but that, if she wanted the plug pulled, she would have to do it herself.

"I wanted to do it, but I was afraid," she told me. Her son died two days later, but she had always felt guilty—that she had not prevented the car accident and that she had wanted to turn off the ventilator but had not done so. After she verbalized her guilt about her son's tragic death, she was able to connect this guilt with her nightmares and the death of a donor. As a result, her nightmares subsided.

Ms. Smith

A twenty-five-year-old woman with a psychiatric diagnosis of border-line personality disorder was referred to me because of overwhelming anxiety. Ms. Smith had received a kidney transplant two years before and was now in the hospital because her body was rejecting it. When I spoke with her, she told me that she had become obsessed with the thought that her grandfather had been murdered and that she had received his kidney, which was now rejecting *her*. During out talk, Ms. Smith told me that when she was a child, she had been removed from her parents' home because they were sexually abusing her. She had been sent to live with her grandfather and uncles. Her grandfather was a "very nice man" but did nothing to protect her when her uncles sexually abused her.

She had loved her grandfather (who had died several years before), but she was also very angry at him for not protecting her. Her anger and guilt were reflected both in the fantasy that he had been killed to save her and the fear that his kidney was now rejecting her.

For most patients, concerns about the death of the donor surface in a less disturbing manner. Many of the people I interview volunteer that they are distressed that someone has to die. Several patients have assured me, without my asking, that they had signed organ donor cards since finding out that they would need a transplant. Naturally, many persons suppress their fears and fantasies or are reluctant to share them with psychiatrists or others who are "screening" them for transplantation suitability. Evidence indicates that complete suppression of these concerns may be a useful coping strategy in the perioperative period.[5] However, when patients are bothered by their fears, health professionals can be a source of education and reassurance. For example, a liver transplant candidate in her midthirties was worried that the donor of her organ would come back to "haunt" her. By talking with staff and with patients who had already received liver transplants, she was able to overcome her fears.

Examples of the ambivalence and guilt about donor deaths can be found in the medical literature as well. Levenson and Olbrisch report "gallows humor" among patients waiting for transplant: They not uncommonly "talk about fantasies of standing on the roof of the hospital with a rifle" or ask hospital staff "whether they have had any opportunities to run down pedestrians on their way to work."[6] In several instances, candidates for transplantation or their relatives "have coped by identifying 'healthy specimens' among the house staff and inquiring as to their body weights and blood types."[7] Frierson and Lippmann report that "patients often found themselves hoping for inclement weather because of a greater likelihood of fatal accidents to afford more organ donations. This so-called 'rainy day syndrome' was often accompanied by significant feelings of guilt."[8]

Popular Culture

The legacy of Burke and Hare and the modern myth of Frankenstein described so vividly by Ruth Richardson[9] and Leslie Fiedler[10] in this volume are very much alive in our collective consciousness. Stimulated by the steady diet of upbeat news stories, sermons, and public service announcements about transplantation and the need for more organs, fears that people will actually be killed for organs find free reign in popular culture. Horror books and movies tell tales of powerful and maniacal physicians (either functioning independently or as agents of even more powerful scoundrels) who take advantage of patients or other, weaker persons to obtain their organs. A recent series of the comic strip "Dick Tracy" concerned a nefarious conspiracy in which homeless people were shanghaied from a city shelter, killed, and used as organ sources.[11]

As noted earlier, the fears are often expressed as humor. In the movie *Monty Python's The Meaning of Life*, a group of medical people ring the doorbell of a family home. When the father answers the door, they ask him if he has signed a card donating his liver. When he replies in the affirmative, they barge into the house, tie him to the kitchen table, and proceed to remove his liver (without anesthetic and in front of his horrified family).

Fears about killing for organs are given impetus by proposals to allow criminals condemned to death to donate their organs as part of the execution process. Some prisoners serving life sentences have even asked to be executed so they could both end their miserable existence in prison and donate organs. In fact, allowing condemned inmates to donate their organs upon execution is a pet project of Dr. Jack Kevorkian, better known to the American public as the crusader for physician-assisted suicide.[12] Of course, such killings can be rationalized as different from the killings in *Coma*,[13] a novel and movie in which patients are killed and kept in suspended animation so their body parts and fluids can be used. After all, in the horror movies and books, the organ sources are unwilling victims of murder. In real life, the prisoners give consent or even initiate requests to have their organs taken.

These subtleties, however, are lost on the unconscious mind, where killing and organ procurement are linked concretely. Primitive but powerful associations are only reinforced by stories from China about executed criminals whose organs are taken whether or not they wanted to be donors.[14]

Even more disturbing are recurring stories in the press about innocent persons killed for organs. In 1992, newspapers reported that hundreds of patients at a mental hospital near Buenos Aires were allegedly killed by greedy staff members who sold their body parts and blood.[15] For several years, rumors have appeared that children from various South and Central American countries are being kidnapped and taken to the United States to be "fattened up" and then killed for their organs. More recently, foreigners have been attacked in Guatemala in a panic fed by rumors that Americans were coming to kidnap children, cut out their vital organs, and ship them to the United States for transplantation.[16]

An article in *Asiaweek* titled "Life for Sale" described the extensive and legal sale of kidneys (single kidneys from live donors) in India. It went on to describe a more disturbing story from Bangladesh:

Last year 400 children disappeared in Chittagong city, according to police. It's suspected that most of them were kidnapped for their organs. In October police in suburban Dhaka rescued 49 people and arrested two human traffickers. The men confessed that they were going to smuggle the group into India under the guise of finding them work. Once there they planned to sell some of them to human organ traders who operated through some hospitals in Bombay and Madras. The victims would be forced to donate their kidneys, eyes, hair and blood.[17]

None of these stories has ever been verified by reliable sources, and the transplant community in the United States has vehemently denied their veracity. Furthermore, no one has seriously proposed that any of these ghoulish practices actually occur in the United States. But the newspaper stories and rumors keep coming. Horror movies and novels continue to be produced and sold. To be sure, they exist at the margins. But they find their way to the collective unconscious, where they percolate, resonating with the popular myths that Leslie Fiedler describes,[18] breathing new life (or death) into the psychic legacy of body snatching for dissection, which Ruth Richardson so vividly portrays,[19] and playing on the fears, not merely of the paranoid and insecure, but of the poor and disadvantaged as well. Examining the historical relationship between organ transplantation, the determination of death, and treatment-limitation decisions helps to explain the darker side of our society's reaction to organ procurement.

Planned Death and Organ Procurement

Aside from living donors (who provide about 20 percent of donated kidneys in the United States), solid vascularized organs such as the kidneys, heart, and liver come from patients who are brain dead but whose hearts continue to beat. Brain death is a legal and clinical concept introduced in the 1960s that subsequently achieved widespread acceptance throughout the United States. The reasons for introducing it were quite rational: (1) to facilitate organ procurement and (2) to avoid legal concerns about turning off ventilators.[20]

A patient who suffers a massive head injury (for example, in a car accident or following a heart attack) can now be resuscitated and put on a mechanical ventilator. Moreover, physicians and nurses in the intensive care unit can now perform many of the integrative functions previously carried out automatically by the brain, such as regulating body temperature and blood pressure. Brain-dead patients are legally dead in every jurisdiction in the United States, yet they are a wonderful source of organs because their hearts beat spontaneously, pumping warm, richly oxygenated blood throughout their living bodies until their organs can be removed and quickly put on ice.

Brain death raises a profound problem that is relevant to our general discussion, but one I will not consider until later—namely, the cognitive dissonance engendered by the overwhelming signs of life in these dead patients. For the moment, however, I will turn to new methods organ transplanters have employed to increase the donor pool.

New Methods for Obtaining Organs

As organ transplantation has become more popular, the supply of brain-dead patients has not kept pace. In response to the organ shortage, transplanters have developed new techniques for retrieving organs from traditional corpses—so-called non-heart-beating cadavers (NHBCs). The University of Pittsburgh Medical Center has implemented a protocol in which the time of death (not brain death, but death by cardiopulmonary criteria) is controlled so that it occurs in the operating room, where organs can be quickly removed before they are damaged.[21] Patients who are potential candidates for organ donation under this protocol are ventilator dependent but not brain dead. They might be severely brain injured (but still have identifiable brain function) or might have completely intact cognitive function but are unable to breathe spontaneously (for example, patients who are quadriplegic from high spinal injuries). In either case, after the patient's family (or the patient when competent) asks that life support be removed, they can also request that organs be donated for transplantation. After an elaborate informed-consent process, the patient is taken to the operating room (if organ procurement were not in the picture, ventilator removal and death would occur in the intensive care unit), prepped for surgery, and the ventilator turned off. Two minutes after the heart stops beating, the surgeons come in and remove the organs as quickly as possible to reduce warm ischemia time.

Controlling the timing of death in this way would have been hardly imaginable a quarter century ago, when turning off machines that kept people alive was very controversial. To many persons, it seemed too close to killing. Health professionals and health care institutions were reluctant to turn off mechanical ventilators for fear they would be sued or prosecuted for murder. (In other countries that have had less experience with medical technology, the level of controversy remains high.)

Clinical practice and the law have undergone a dramatic evolution over the past two and a half decades. Competent patients or their surrogates may refuse any form of life-sustaining treatment, including mechanical ventilators and artificially provided fluids and nutrition. Today we turn off the ventilators not only of brain-dead patients but also of still-living patients with a spectrum of clinical conditions ranging from terminal illness to quadriplegia. However, this evolution in attitude and behavior has not likely run its course and has special relevance to organ procurement under protocols like the one in Pittsburgh.

At preconscious and unconscious levels, our society has accepted increasingly active forms of physician-assisted suicide and euthanasia, paving the way to open acceptance. Local newspapers and TV news regularly feature stories about Jack Kevorkian and his assisted suicides. National polls reflect a growing public acceptance of physician-assisted suicide and euthanasia, which have become widespread and socially sanctioned practices in one of our "civilized" European neighbors, the Netherlands. Prestigious medical journals such as the *New England Journal of Medicine* have published articles in which physicians have openly admitted helping patients end their lives and set forth comprehensive guidelines for this practice.[22] While voter initiatives to legalize physician-assisted suicide and euthanasia have been narrowly defeated in two states, one was recently approved by Oregon voters. In sum, then, it appears likely that physician-assisted suicide and euthanasia will be explicitly or implicitly tolerated in many jurisdictions in the United States within the next decade.

If this prediction proves accurate, one can easily extrapolate the likely scenario for organ procurement. If we ask patients, as the Pittsburgh protocol does, to become donors when they ask that their ventilators be turned off, why would we not allow them the same prerogative when we help them to commit suicide or put them to death at their own request?[23] Unless something unforeseen intervenes to disrupt it, the evolution from an ever-expanding array of treatment limitations to an equally expanding array of voluntary suicides and mercy killings is inevitable. The decision to allow euthanized patients to donate their organs would follow quite naturally, once the more controversial practices of suicide and mercy killing were to become sanctioned.

By controlling the time and place of death, the Pittsburgh protocol takes a critical symbolic step: It links the planned death of one human being to the procurement of organs for another (the transplantation of tissue from electively aborted fetuses is a second example). What makes the Pittsburgh protocol legally and morally acceptable is that both the death of the donor and the taking of his or her organs are voluntary. This same protection could exist if organ donation were linked to physician-assisted suicide or voluntary active euthanasia. An extensive informed-consent process and the total absence of coercion would be necessary to prevent the killing for organs, about which both Richardson and the modern myths of popular culture warn and for which they, perhaps, prepare us.

Public Policy Protections

From early on, the government and the transplant community have tried to dispel concerns that people will be killed or exploited for their organs. The National Organ Transplant Act of 1984 made clear that care of the potential donor and care of the potential recipient must not be provided by the same persons, and that transplant personnel should in no way be involved in treatment decisions before the donor's death.[24]

In contrast with the Organ Transplant Act, the dead-donor rule evolved as an informal policy; but like the Organ Transplant Act, it is intended to reassure the public that people will not be taken advantage of so that their organs can be used.[25] The dead-donor rule has two aspects: first, people must not be killed by or for organ retrieval; and, second, with the exception of completely healthy family members, people can have their organs taken only after they are dead, even if taking the organs will not kill them. So, for example, we are unwilling, even with a family's (or the patient's prior) permission, to take a single kidney from a patient in a permanently unconscious state.

Nonetheless, public opinion polls regularly reflect the fear of many persons that their care will be compromised so that they can become a source for organs.[26] Such fears are greatest among minority groups, who have good historical reasons for mistrusting organized medicine or for doubting that they will be protected by the law.[27] Already, demagogues in the African-American community have sought to play on these fears.[28] Appeals to informed consent and protection of the law are more likely to quell the irrational fears of those members of society who have the power, privilege, and experience to exploit those protections more successfully.

Brain Death: Another Layer of Confusion

When newspapers report on brain death, they regularly refer to the legally dead patients as being kept alive on life-support systems or in critical condition. Such ambiguous language is the rule rather than the exception when news media report about brain death. I recently witnessed a local TV anchorman describe a severely brain-damaged patient as "in critical condition but technically brain dead."

Such confusion is common even among health professionals, who stubbornly persist in describing patients who have lost all brain function as brain dead rather than simply dead. These patients, who are considered legally dead in all fifty states, are also characterized as being kept alive on "life" support, and as dying after that support is removed. Even though the legal time of death occurs when the patient is determined to have irreversibly lost all brain function, health professionals regularly fill in the death certificate with the time the heart stopped beating (after life support is stopped).

I alluded earlier to the cognitive dissonance stimulated by the phenomenon of brain death. Before the advent of medical technology, numerous indicators of death occurred more or less at once. So, for example, a person with a fatal heart attack would lose consciousness, stop breathing, become motionless and unresponsive, and have no detectable pulse all at approximately the same time. All the vital signs of life would vanish together. Now, however, medical technology has forced us to choose which signs of life are sufficiently important that their loss constitutes the death of the patient, while other signs of life persist.

The traditional view rejects the notion of brain death altogether, arguing that vital fluid flow, the movement of air and blood through the body, indicates life. Thus, the persistence of cardiac and pulmonary function sufficiently demonstrates that the patient is still alive. In the United States, this view receives considerable support in the fundamentalist Christian and Orthodox Jewish communities. In contrast, the more recent view holds that even with a spontaneously beating heart and air flow in and out of the lungs (by means of a ventilator), irreversible loss of all brain function (brain death) signals the death of the patient.

However, in the intensive care unit (ICU), where brain-dead patients are maintained, and in the operating rooms, where their organs are removed, nurses, house officers, and anesthesiologists are often confused and sometimes dismayed by these paradoxical patients. In the intensive care unit, nurses and physicians must "treat" these dead patients quite aggressively in order to maintain them for transplantation. They must attach them to breathing machines, monitor them for heart rhythm and blood pressure, give them fluids and nutrition, and when indicated, administer antibiotics and other medications. The medical staff must also closely monitor and adjust the patients' blood chemistry and oxygen levels. These dead patients are even candidates for full resuscitation should they suffer cardiac arrest. Yet, in the next bed may lie a completely conscious patient, who, at her own request, does not want to be resuscitated. ICU nurses often talk to brain-dead patients and are concerned when they are subjected to painful procedures.

Brain-dead patients pose an even greater emotional challenge for operating room personnel, who must maintain them through organ-retrieval surgery. Such a patient is prepped like any other surgical candidate and draped to reveal only the operative field. An anesthesiologist stands at the head of the patient to manage the mechanical ventilator and maintain homeostasis by giving fluids and drugs. The surgeons use sterile technique, tie off or cauterize bleeding blood vessels, and carefully cut and separate tissue planes. The patient's chest rises and falls with the rhythm of the ventilator. And it is not uncommon to give the dead patient a transfusion of fresh blood while his or her organs are being removed.

These similarities between brain-dead and regular surgical candidates add emotional force to the differences as the process unfolds. Instead of diseased tissue, healthy organs are removed, and then the meticulous attention to detail comes to an end. It becomes concretely clear that the purpose of the surgery is for another patient, not the one in the room. The mechanical ventilator is turned off, and the patient's newly emptied body is closed in one pass with coarse retention sutures. Some nurses and anesthesiologists describe the turning off of the ventilator as the most emotionally intense moment. Some say that not until then does the patient's spirit leave the room. Others frankly describe it as the second death of the patient. It is most upsetting for the unprepared and the uninitiated—young nurses or anesthesiologists or those who work at smaller community hospitals where organ procurement and transplantation are rare events.

The resulting confusion and cognitive dissonance were reflected in a study of ICU and operating-room physicians and nurses. Almost all participants intellectually accepted that brain-dead patients were indeed dead. However, when asked what makes brain-dead patients dead, fully one-third gave answers indicating that they really believed such patients to be alive, for example, "the patient will die soon, no matter what we do," or "the patient's quality of life is unacceptable."[29]

Cognitive dissonance was magnified in the case of an eighteen-year-old woman, whom I will call Janet, who was twenty-two weeks pregnant, suffered a spontaneous ruptured cerebral aneurysm, and was admitted to the intensive care unit, where an unequivocal diagnosis of brain death was made within twenty-four hours. Here, nurses and physicians cared for dead mother and living fetus. Eight weeks later a healthy baby was delivered by cesarean section, following which the young woman's heart, liver, pancreas, and kidneys were removed and transplanted into four waiting patients, three of whom were cared for in the same intensive care unit that had maintained the dead mother-donor.

Because the care of Janet was going to be both clinically and emotionally challenging (the first such case for the ICU), a small group of nurses volunteered to provide it. Heavily identified with the tragedy, they became very attached to both the dead mother and the living fetus, who had already been named. For many of the staff, taking care of the patient was a religious experience. Its mystical nature was enhanced by the fact that Janet had anticipated her death a week before it occurred, when she told her family that "if anything happens to me, I want them to do everything to save the baby." The ICU staff's mission was to bring a healthy baby out of the tragedy, and they constantly watched and worried over it. But they were also preoccupied with the baby's mother.

One nurse described what the day-to-day care of Janet was like. "We kept her immaculately clean and neat, even had her mother bring in a silk robe in which to dress her. I washed her hair every week," the nurse told me. "It was long, beautiful red hair, and it grew for eight weeks. I could sense the presence of her soul in her body." Another nurse sensed the presence of a soul hovering over the body, "watching us."

The nurses developed rituals, including putting a picture of the dead mother on the wall. They played music in the room, "for the baby," but were convinced that the mother's heart rate changed in response to it. The physicians, who spent much less time with the patient (the nurses worked one-to-one with the patient for ten-hour shifts), were less emotionally involved, although one of the obstetricians was clearly convinced that "the whole thing [had] a preordained purpose."

Not surprisingly, the medical staff constantly used speech indicating that the patient was alive. "Our job was to keep the mother alive until the baby was born," one physician told me. A nurse said, "We all *knew* she was dead, but we *felt* she was alive." The patient's mother told a physician, "Every time I leave, I think she is going to finally die, and each time I return to the ICU, she is still with us."

What is reality for family members who watched the living body of a dead girl nurture, grow, and issue forth a healthy baby? While Janet's hair grew longer and the nurses washed and combed it, was she *really* alive or dead to them? They could rationally say that she was dead and explain why; the signs of life told another story.

The Language of Organ Transplantation

Ruth Richardson argues that the language of organ transplantation is sometimes intended to disguise its darker side.[30] Language can also provide an unwitting representation of transplantation's more disturbing but subterranean aspects. The persistence of the term *brain-dead* to describe patients whose hearts continue to beat but who have lost all brain function, and the habit of referring to them as *alive* only to describe them as *dying* when their ventilators are turned off, does not reflect mere ignorance of the facts. The transplant community correctly perceives that, by using the term *brain death* instead of simply *death*, health professionals and journalists encourage the notion that a difference exists, that is, that brain-dead patients are not dead but constitute some other category of being. They are mistaken, however, in thinking that mere education will either eliminate the use of the term or solve the problem.

The fact that experienced transplant surgeons and nurses make the same slip on a regular basis is evidence that something more powerful than lack of knowledge is at work. The physicians and nurses who cared for Janet were intellectually aware that she was legally dead and that the fetus inside her was alive. They persisted in referring to both mother and fetus as alive because of the abundant signs of life emanating from both. As the mythologist Wendy Doniger insightfully commented when I described this phenomenon to her, "Why, it's just the way we persist in describing a sunset when we know full well on the intellectual level that the earth is moving around the sun, not vice versa."

Other words are viewed as politically incorrect by the transplant community because of their unpleasant connotations. *Procurement* of organs has an unsavory association with commodities and commerce, even prostitution. Some persons have suggested organ *retrieval* as preferable, but others have objected that retrieval implies that the organs belonged to someone other than the donor patient and that we are merely taking them back. Terms such as *heart-beating cadaver* or *neomort*[31] are offensive to many persons because they seem ghoulish or crude.

Another example supports the notion that transplant language can be sanitizing: most cadaver "donors" are, of course, no such thing. They have given no indication of what they want done with their organs when they die. The organs are most often donated by their families. It is more comforting, of course, to think of them as organ donors than as organ sources. Rather than view the language of transplantation as a product of ignorance or intentional disrespect, however, we should understand it as an inevitable expression of the complex and dynamic interaction between the rational-utilitarian and emotional-symbolic ways in which we understand or try to understand this wonderful and terrifying miracle of science.

Cannibalism

Ruth Richardson suggests that the word *harvesting* presents too benign an image of organ procurement. Some persons disagree, arguing that the word is disrespectful to the dead donors, implying that they are vegetables rather than human beings. An even more disturbing interpretation is possible—that harvesting imports the notion of cannibalism. Of course, in an entirely concrete sense, organ transplantation *is* a form of nonoral cannibalism, that is, the taking of the flesh and blood from one person into another. Historically, two general categories of cannibalism have existed—survival cannibalism and ritual cannibalism.

Survival cannibalism. Of the two categories, survival cannibalism is metaphorically closest to organ transplantation—taking in the flesh of another as the only means of preserving one's own life. Examples of survival cannibalism abound throughout history. Two that are part of our public consciousness concern the notorious Donner party, in which human cannibalism was widespread among a group of pioneers trapped by a winter snowstorm in the Sierra Nevada in the late nineteenth century,[32] and the more recent story of a group of Uruguayan rugby players and their families stranded in the Andes Mountains after an airplane crash. The latter story was published in a best-selling book[33] and has been made into two popular movies. The inherent drama and tragedy of these situations are not the only things that capture the public imagination; these situations also depict well-meaning people who overcome their own sense of repugnance and violate a strict social taboo in order to survive. In such cases, society seems to understand and forgive—as long as those consumed died naturally and were not unjustly killed.

Examples of survival cannibalism also offer insight into how rituals can be created or adapted to help overcome the extraordinary and terrifying nature of the act. For example, the Uruguayan rugby team (the Old Christian Club) used a cannibalistic ritual at the very heart of Christianity, communion, to make their own cannibalism more acceptable. "It's like Holy Communion," one of them said. "When Christ died, he gave his body to us so that we could have spiritual life. My friend has given us his body so we can have physical life."[34]

When death has to be planned and manipulated (this is, when people have to be killed for their flesh), the emotional and moral stakes are inevitably raised. Examples of cannibalism abound in British naval history and provide examples of how reasonable people in unreasonable circumstances (for example, starvation in a life boat) rationalized their choice of whom to kill.[35] The "fairest" way was the drawing of lots (for both the person to be killed and the killer). Less judicious were decisions to kill individuals because of their race or because they were children. One way to make such deaths more tolerable was to identify people who were "about to die anyway," thereby diminishing the harm to them. Sometimes these murders were rationalized as mercy killing.

One could argue that this same reasoning underlies our current acceptance of brain death. That is, in patients who have lost all brain function, we have identified a group of severely injured and dying persons who are so "beyond harm" that we feel justified in killing them in order to obtain their organs.[36] Since we would rather not think that we are killing them, we simply gerrymander the line between life and death to include them in the latter category.

Conceptual gerrymandering is even more apparent in proposals to label anencephalic infants (born with no cerebral hemispheres but entirely functioning brain stems) as dead, precisely so that their organs can be taken for transplantation.[37] Recently, the American Medical Association took a more candid approach: "It is normally required that the donor be legally dead before permitting the harvesting of organs. The use of the anencephalic infant as a live donor is a limited exception to the general standard because of the fact that the infant has never experienced, and will never experience, consciousness."[38]

The AMA did *not* suggest that anencephalic infants were dead, but rather that they were beyond harm and, therefore, could be killed for their organs. Of course, the AMA did not use the word *killed*.

Ritual cannibalism. Ritual cannibalism is often performed with the intent of incorporating desired qualities of the person who is eaten. While incorporation of the donor's personal characteristics (other than the health of his or her organs) is not the *intent* of organ transplantation, the early transplant literature is replete with examples of patients who either feared incorporating unwanted characteristics or were convinced it had actually happened. Renée Fox points out how little the current psychiatric and medical literature comments about this issue,[39] but it has not been ignored in lay literature, novels, or movies. Writing in the *New Yorker* in 1990, a general surgeon, Sherwin B. Nuland, describes his interview with a man named Cretella, who had received a heart transplant:

Toward the end of my visit, our conversation turned to a topic I had been hesitant to bring up. What does it feel like to live with another person's heart beating in your chest? It proved to be something Cretella was trying very hard not to think about.

"I don't know yet," he said. "I really don't know yet. When I catch myself thinking about it, I try to forget about it. You know—I think, What is it? A female? A male? Black? Orange? White?"

I asked him what he would want it to be.

"I don't know that yet, either. I can't answer any questions like that at all. I even get upset talking to you about it. When I talk about it, I get paranoid. I think mainly it's because I don't know what's going to happen tomorrow, and the reason for that is that I can be sitting here feeling fine and all of a sudden something clicks and I get nervous and everything just starts going. Something in my body changes, as if somebody pushed a button. I talked to another transplant patient—he's in his fifth year—and he says it still happens to him . . . you know, they tell you it doesn't make any difference what kind of heart you get. And I'm sitting there thinking, I don't believe that, I honestly don't believe it."[40]

In my own experience, transplant candidates and patients often express fantasies and worries about taking on characteristics of the donor. Mr. Anderson's young grandson, for example, was afraid that his grandfather would no longer love him after the man received a new heart. His "mistake" was an innocent and unrationalized representation of the emotional significance given to the heart throughout our society, even though we know that the brain is the real seat of our emotions. Mr. Anderson's grandson expressed concretely what usually remains in our subconscious or emerges in common metaphors when we speak of losing our hearts, breaking our hearts, and having good or evil hearts. These examples, to use Wendy Doniger's analogy, are like talking about the sun setting over a post-Galilean horizon.

Transplant candidates sometimes joke with me about adopting the sexual, ethnic, or other personal characteristics of donors. They rarely express their fears directly—either because they have successfully rationalized them or because the potential candidates are worried that candor would harm their chances for receiving an organ (in fact, it would not). Humor, of course, provides a window into the unconscious, deriving its energy from the partial exposure of what is usually hidden and forbidden. It is not surprising that cartoons and movies often present concerns about identity and transplantation in a comic as well as a horror mode.

I learned of a dramatic example of donor-personality incorporation when I was called by a producer of the "Phil Donahue Show," a somewhat sensational TV talk show. An upcoming broadcast would feature a group of heart transplant recipients in the New York City area who claimed that they not only had taken on personality characteristics of the donors, but also had come to know intimate details about the donors' lives—all without having received any information about them! Accompanying the heart recipients was a psychoanalyst who had them in a therapy group. I was asked to appear as "a voice of rationality and science," to provide "balance" for the show. (I declined.)

While thoughts and fears about incorporating personal qualities of the donor (or losing one's own identity) characterize transplantation, the converse distinguishes ritual cannibalism; that is, people are eaten with the express purpose of incorporating desirable characteristics. For the unconscious mind, the concrete or literal similarities are as important as the differences. The term *cannibalism* is itself used commonly to describe taking working parts from one machine (for example, an automobile) to fix another that is broken.

The association between organs and food becomes even more concrete when transplant surgeons are seen (by other health professionals, as well as by the public when viewing television) transporting organs in easily recognized brand-name coolers usually reserved for carrying picnic lunches. Transplanters also use Tupperware to transport tissues or wrap them in the same brand-name cellophane that sits on the shelves of our supermarkets. The Japanese film crew that taped a total body harvest in an American hospital for a Japanese national television program debating the merits of transplantation missed none of these culinary details.[41] One of my own patients made an inescapable connection when he expressed regret that someone had to die so that he could get a liver. "I wish I could go to the grocery store and buy one off the shelf," he lamented.

Conclusion

I have used the words and experiences of transplant patients, their families, and the health professionals who care for them to examine some of the powerful but often subterranean psychological forces that exist alongside the more rational, tidy, and "constructive" view of the official transplant and public-policy communities. Neither is right or wrong. Each must be understood on its own terms. To ignore the more rational side is to miss the wonderful opportunity transplantation offers to save, extend, and improve the lives of thousands of people. To ignore or dismiss the more subterranean side is to build transplant policy on an unrealistic view of the human psyche that is not only insensitive but also ineffective because of its naïveté.

The tragic and often violent death of others, the taking in of another's flesh to live, the confusion of boundaries, the mutilation of dead bodies, and the cognitive dissonance of brain death are all disturbing but inescapable aspects of transplantation and organ procurement. Society adjusts and accepts new practices, even when they stimulate powerful fears and taboos. Ruth Richardson chronicles how it took England four centuries of dissection to become comfortable enough for voluntary donation to triumph. Her observations about the Anatomy Act of 1832 and her view that it set back voluntary donation by a century should give us pause while we pursue public policies that ignore the deeply held fears and taboos of our society.

Notes

I would like to thank Robert Arnold, Rebecca Dresser, Renée Fox, Laurence O'Connell, Rina Youngner, and Julius Youngner for their thoughtful comments and suggestions.

1. Charles Brenner, *Elementary Textbook of Psychoanalysis* (New York: International Universities Press, 1973), 52.

2. Otto Fenichel, *Psychoanalytic Theory of Neurosis* (New York: W. W. Norton, 1972), 47.

3. Brenner, *Elementary Textbook of Psychoanalysis*, 52–54.

4. Renée C. Fox, *Essays in Medical Sociology* (New Brunswick, N.J.: Transaction Books, 1988), 170.

5. Francois M. Mai, "Graft and Donor Denial in Heart Transplant Recipients," *American Journal of Psychiatry* 143, no. 9 (September 1986): 1159–61.

6. James L. Levenson and Mary Ellen Olbrisch, "Shortage of Donor Organs and Long Waits," *Psychosomatics* 28, no. 8 (August 1987): 399–403, 400.

7. Ibid.

8. Robert L. Frierson and Steven B. Lippmann, "Heart Transplant Candidates Rejected on Psychiatric Indications," *Psychosomatics* 28, no. 7 (July 1987): 347–55, 350.

9. See Ruth Richardson's chapter in this volume.

10. See Leslie Fiedler's chapter in this volume.

11. Dick Locher and Max Collins, "Dick Tracy," *Pittsburgh Press*, 4 August–25 September 1991.

12. Jack Kevorkian, *Prescription Medicine* (Buffalo: Prometheus Books, 1991).

13. Robin Cook, *Coma* (Boston: Little, Brown, 1977).

14. "Grim Commerce in China," *New York Times*, 30 August 1994, A20.

15. "Patients Killed for Organs," *Guardian* (London), 14 April 1992, 10; "Journal: Patients at Argentine Hospital Were Killed for Organs," *American Medical News*, 18 May 1992, 92.

16. "Behind the Kidnapping of Children for Their Organs," *Los Angeles Times* (opinion section), 2 May 1994, M1; "Guatemala Gang Kidnaps US Girl, 7," *Boston Globe*, 12 April 1994, 6.

17. "Life for Sale," *Asiaweek*, 13 April 1994, 49.

18. See Leslie Fiedler's chapter in this volume.

19. See Ruth Richardson's chapter in this volume.

20.   Ad Hoc Committee of the Harvard Medical School to Examine the Definition of Brain Death, "A Definition of Irreversible Coma," *Journal of the American Medical Association* 205 (1968): 337–40; Stuart J. Youngner, "Brain Death: A Superficial and Fragile Consensus," *Archives of Neurology* 49 (May 1992): 570–72.

21.   Stuart J. Youngner and Robert M. Arnold, "Ethical, Psychosocial, and Public Policy Implications of Procuring Organs from Non-Heart-Beating Cadaver Donors," *Journal of the American Medical Association* 269, no. 21 (2 June 1993): 2769–74. For a more complete treatment of the University of Pittsburgh protocol, see Robert M. Arnold and Stuart J. Youngner, eds., "Ethical, Psychosocial, and Public Policy Implication of Procuring Organs from Non-Heart-Beating Cadavers," Special Issue, *Kennedy Institute of Ethics Journal* 3, no. 2 (June 1993): 103–277.

22.   Timothy E. Quill, "Death with Dignity—A Case of Individualized Decision Making," *New England Journal of Medicine* 324, no. 10 (1991): 691–94; Timothy E. Quill, Christine K. Cassel, and Diane E. Meier, "Care of the Hopelessly Ill: Proposed Clinical Criteria for Physician-Assisted Suicide," *New England Journal of Medicine* 327, no. 19 (1992): 1380–84.

23.   Robert M. Arnold and Stuart J. Youngner, "The Dead Donor Rule: Should We Stretch It, Bend It, or Abandon It?" *Kennedy Institute of Ethics Journal* 3, no. 2 (June 1993): 263–78.

24.   National Organ Transplant Act, Public Law 98–507, 98th Cong., 19 October 1984.

25.   Arnold and Youngner, "The Dead Donor Rule."

26.   J. M. Prottas and H. L. Batten, *Attitudes and Incentive in Organ Procurement*, Report to the Health Care Financing Administration, 1986; J. M. Prottas and H. L. Batten, "The Willingness to Give: The Public and the Supply of Transplantable Organs," *Journal of Health Politics, Policy, and Law* 16 (1991): 121–34.

27.   C. O. Collender, L. E. Hall, C. L. Yeager, et al., "Organ Donation and Blacks: A Critical Frontier," *New England Journal of Medicine* 325 (1991): 442–44.

28.   "Farrakhan Links Race to Transplants," *New York Times*, 2 May 1994, A18.

29.   Stuart J. Youngner, C. Seth Landefeld, Claudia J. Coulton, Barbara W. Juknialis, and Mark Leary, " 'Brain Death' and Organ Retrieval: A Cross-Sectional Survey of Knowledge and Concepts among Health Professionals," *Journal of the American Medical Association* 261, no. 15 (21 April 1989): 2205–10.

30.   See Ruth Richardson's chapter in this volume.

31.   Willard Gaylin, "Harvesting the Dead," *Harper's*, September 1974, 123–30.

32.   George R. Stewart, *Ordeal by Hunger: The Story of the Donner Party* (Lincoln: University of Nebraska Press, 1986).

33.   Piers Paul Read, *Alive* (New York: Avon Books, 1974).

34.   Ibid., 83.

35.   A. W. Simpson, *Cannabalism and the Common Law* (Chicago: University of Chicago Press, 1985).

36.   Arnold and Youngner, "The Dead Donor Rule."

37. John C. Fletcher and Robert D. Truog, "Anencephalic Newborns: Can Organs Be Transplanted before Brain Death?" *New England Journal of Medicine* 321, no. 6 (1989): 388–91.

38. "Anencephalic Infants as Organ Donors," *Opinion of the American Medical Association's Council on Ethical and Judicial Affairs*, CEJA Opinion 10-A-94; "Council: Use of Anencephalic Organ Donors Ethical," *American Medical News*, 27 June 1994, 9.

39. See Renée Fox's chapter in this volume.

40. Sherwin B. Nuland, "Annals of Surgery: Transplanting a Heart," *New Yorker*, 10 February 1990, 82–94, 93.

41. Margaret Lock discusses this Japanese TV program at greater length in her chapter in this volume.

4 *Leslie A. Fiedler*

Why Organ Transplant Programs Do Not Succeed

Personal Statement

My presence in a volume of essays on organ transplants may seem surprising to readers who know me only as a literary critic and long-time teacher in departments of English. As a matter of fact, I too was a little astonished when I found myself accepting an invitation to join a three-year project intended to end in the publication of a book addressed primarily (or so I surmised) to medical professionals, bioethicists, and government bureaucrats.

I had, to begin with, never thought very much about organ transplantation at all. Certainly, I had never contemplated donating any body part of my own, much less signing a pledge to do so, living or dead. I had, to be sure, lost a couple of my organs to the surgeon's knife during my long life; but they have wound up in the garbage disposal rather than the body of some stranger.

In any case, there seems something shamelessly chutzpahdik *in my addressing as an amateur an audience of specialists on a topic so clearly in their area of expertise and outside my own. Yet after all, I keep reminding myself, I have done so before, several times over indeed, beginning in 1978. In that year, I had published a thick, copiously illustrated book called* Freaks: Myths and Images of the Secret Self, *in which rather than analyzing—as I am accustomed to do—literary texts for their mythic content, I reflected on the ways in which our culture has mythicized people with congenital malformations, including dwarfs, giants, Siamese twins, and intersexes.*

56

In my book, I explored how and why such anomalous human beings were originally worshiped in awe or killed at birth in terror; then displayed as curiosities privately in courts and publicly at side shows; and finally came to be treated as patients by doctors, who attempted to cure them by chemistry, hormones, or radical surgery. And I concluded by pointing out that, when such medical intervention is counterindicated, "nonviable terata" are allowed to die.

My implicit disapproval of such therapeutic infanticide, in particular, seems to have annoyed many members of the medical profession; one of whom, indeed, at the end of a particularly heated argument with me on this topic, disrupted an otherwise friendly cocktail party by hurling a martini glass at me, barely missing my head. Nonetheless, ever since, I have been repeatedly invited to talk before groups of physicians, nurses, and bioethicists, presumably because I share their interests if not their points of view. Consequently, since I am reluctant to pass by any opportunity to talk about what moves me, whatever the motives of my sponsors, I have ended up speaking as an outsider to insiders, not just on teratology, but on gerontology, genomes, and child abuse, as well as broader topics like "What babies shall live?" or the images of doctors and nurses in literature and the arts, and finally, of course, "Why Organ Transplant Programs Do Not Succeed."

My original invitation to contribute to the colloquium on this subject suggested that more specifically I concentrate on the treatment of transplantation in popular fiction. And almost without thinking, I took down from my shelf the well-thumbed copies of two of the most popular of all popular books, Frankenstein *and* Dracula. *Rereading them, however, I was plunged deep into an iatrophobic nightmare from which I and (I began to suspect) many others have never fully awakened. But was this not, I thought, a clue to the answer for a riddle that has long vexed the medical profession: Why, despite our avowals to the contrary, do so many of us not give the much touted "gift of life"? That troubling question, at any rate, I have sought to pose as provocatively as I know how.*

From the start, there have been two major obstacles to the success of organ transplant programs, both of which can be called by the single name *rejection*. Most often that term is applied to a host body's stubborn refusal to accept the organs of another as its own; and since such reactions are purely somatic, physiological, chemical, their solutions are sought and sometimes successfully found in the laboratory. In ordinary usage, however, *rejection* implies volition, a psychological response not soluble by mechanical means. Less metaphorically, then, it can be used to describe the failure of the majority of our population to become organ donors, which has caused the ever-growing gap between supply and demand that so vexes the sponsors of transplant programs. Especially vexing to them, it seems to me, should be the refusal of young males (the optimum field for organ harvesting) to pledge parts of their bodies for posthumous donation, or of their surviving family members to permit their dismemberment after death.

To deal with this sort of rejection involves making changes not in the soma but in the psyche. This would be difficult enough in any case, but what makes it especially so is that the attitudes which underlie it are rooted in fears and fantasies below the level of full consciousness. Clear evidence of this is to be found in the fact that, when asked by pollsters, 90 percent of the same population that resists organ transplantation indicates a willingness, even an eagerness, to become a donor. There is, that is to say, a puzzling contradiction between what most potential donors say they are prepared to do and what most of them end up doing.

This is not mere hypocrisy. Rather it results from a profound, though quite unsuspected, contradiction between the conscious acceptance and the unconscious repulsion many of us—perhaps, to some degree, all of us—feel when confronted with a presumably benign surgical procedure that challenges our most deep-seated, primal notions about life and death, the self and the other, body and spirit: a procedure, moreover, conducted without any of the consoling rituals traditionally accorded the cadavers of our beloved ones.

In light of this, the naïve strategies of indoctrination currently used to persuade the young to become donors of their own body parts evidently will not work—certainly not the one I recently received through the mail, urging that required courses on the benefits of organ donation be given in all high schools as part of driver training. It is a persuasive technique equaled in its naïveté only by the Donor Award Patches currently being offered by the Boy Scouts of America to members who pledge to "give the gift of life." Both, moreover, use pious and humane metaphors presumably more effective in moving the general public than the horticultural ones, like *transplantation* itself and *harvesting*, employed by medical professionals talking to each other.

Yet though less dehumanizing, even these religioid figures of speech are likely to be greeted with skepticism by the streetwise disenchanted young men (many of them poor and/or black) who are the suicides or the victims of traffic accidents and urban violence, and who provide the eminently suitable *membra disjecta* for transplantation. Indeed, they are unlikely to persuade very many of any gender, race, or class at the deep psychic levels where instinctive rejection occurs and where what matters is not our conscious beliefs but the myths that possess the underminds of us all. It is, therefore, those myths—the unconscious grids of perception through which we see the world—that we must understand if we are to come to terms with the problem of psychological rejection. I say "come to terms with" rather than "overcome" because I am not sure that we can overcome this problem in the foreseeable future, if ever.

But where to find such myths is a question not easily answered. It is tempting to look for them in the creeds of the established churches, to which the majority of us at least nominally belong. This, however, turns out to be of little use, since, as the propaganda leaflet to which I earlier alluded proudly and truly asserts, "All the major religions support organ and tissue donation." Indeed, the many sects and denominations of America (including the Roman Catholic, as the latest revision of their official catechism makes clear) are less conflicted and divided on this issue than on such other ethically problematic medical procedures as euthanasia, abortion, and *in vitro* fertilization.

In any case, the myth systems to which we late-twentieth-century Americans pay lip service on whatever our sabbaths may happen to be are not those that determine our daily behavior. No more are the myths implicit in our politics, liberal or conservative, which—to make matters worse—tend finally to divide rather than unite an already heterogeneous, multiethnic society. The sole myth system that unites us all is found in popular culture, which constitutes in fact a kind of unsuspected secular scripture. Certainly we are exposed to the archetypal images that popular culture projects in print and postprint form for a much larger portion of our waking lives than we spend listening to sermons or political speeches. Moreover, precisely because we are not aware that we are being indoctrinated as we watch, listen, or read in quest of entertainment and escape, we are less apt to resist the implicit messages.

One subgenre of popular literature deals centrally with technology, including medical technology, and with the bioethical problems posed by its impact on our lives. This is, of course, science fiction, to which it is, therefore, tempting to turn first, especially since it is at the moment a favorite form of the mass audience. But science fiction did not come into its own until the late 1920s, by which time the basic myths that trigger psychological rejection had already received their classic expression. Moreover, only quite recently have writers in that genre felt able to confront head-on the new procedures that have made organ and tissue transplantation available to a large number of patients, and consequently a topic of general interest.

The stories, in any case, when they do not project juvenile fantasies about transplanted members taking control of their host bodies, tend to be more ideological than mythological. In fictions, that is to say, by highly esteemed writers in the genre (like Robert Silverberg's "Caught in the Organ Draft," or Larry Niven's "The Patchwork Girl" and "The

Jigsaw Man"), transplantation is represented as a form of exploitation. Sometimes it is portrayed as being imposed on the powerless young by a dictatorial gerontocracy, eager to add to its other privileges that of indefinitely prolonged life. Sometimes it is described as a stratagem of the very rich, who seduce the desperately impoverished into selling their own flesh, or, where such sales are forbidden by law, hire criminals to rob the graves of anonymous paupers and kidnap, drug, even murder the living poor.

Both of these scenarios seem updated versions of familiar nineteenth-century tales about "resurrection men," the bodysnatchers who provided corpses for dissection in anatomy classes of medical schools and hospitals. This time around, however, doctors, though villains still, are portrayed not as the instigators of such atrocities but merely as accomplices after the fact. In any case, these latter-day tales of "organ-legging" serve to foster similar fears and resentment of the medical profession, feeding a preexistent iatrophobia, which ever since the 1960s has been endemic in our society. To make matters worse, these tales have passed into the lore of the streets, in which they are reported as having actually happened. Occasionally, indeed, they do—chiefly in Third World countries like India—but even when the reports are apocryphal, they make it into supermarket scandal sheets, where, though in due course denied and disproved, they are still believed by the credulous.

Nonetheless, no late-twentieth-century grave robber has as yet been mythicized like those of the last century—the notorious Burke and Hare, for instance. Nor, for that matter, have any of the characters in more recent science fiction entered the communal nightmares that trouble our sleep. Such mythological status has, however, been achieved by the protagonists of four popular novels, which still in reprints and new postprint versions attract the mass audience and continue to haunt the nightmares we all share.

The first of these, Mary Shelley's *Frankenstein*, was written when the nineteenth century had barely begun; and the other three, Bram Stoker's *Dracula*, Robert Louis Stevenson's *Dr. Jekyll and Mr. Hyde*, and H. G. Wells's *Island of Dr. Moreau*, appeared in the last decades of that century. All of them, that is to say, were published not only before transplantation had become viable but also before science fiction, that literary genre that anticipates the technology of the future, had found a proper name and a distinctive identity. All four, though not quite science fiction, seem forerunners of that form at its most bleakly dystopian, but they more closely resemble a related though finally different genre, the horror story.

Beginning in the late eighteenth century with the Gothic romance or tale of terror, and imported into this country by Edgar Allan Poe, such fictions have remained favorites of American readers down to the present day, most notoriously perhaps in the super best-sellers of Stephen King. Earlier examples of the form, however, typically seek to make us shudder by evoking the occult and supernatural; whereas three of the mythic books we are examining deal solely with what is, though terrifying, naturally explicable, the fourth, *Dracula*, treats both the natural and the supernatural.

What all four try to frighten us with are primarily the new horrors that have come to haunt us after the Age of Reason had presumably laid to rest forever all traditional demons and bugaboos. These are, of course, the horrors created by modern science and technology, particularly in the field of medicine, whose procedures most of us sooner or later become all too familiar with at first hand. Driven by pain and fear we entrust ourselves to such healers, even though their methods for averting death and prolonging life challenge our most dearly held beliefs about mortality and immortality. Small wonder then that, in our most archetypal fictions, doctors tend to be portrayed as villains, who, having hubristically usurped the divine power to create and destroy, end by bringing disaster on themselves and those they hold most dear.

More specifically, Wells's Dr. Moreau is portrayed as attempting, with an utter disregard for the pain inflicted, to take the process of evolution into his own hands: turning beasts into men by vivisections, plastic surgery, and hypnosis. Stevenson's Dr. Jekyll, on the other hand, experiments only on himself, releasing by psychochemistry all the dark impulses we normally repress for the sake of civility—and simultaneously altering the fleshy envelope of his body, which his potion makes younger even as it turns it repulsive. In the end he is trapped in that body, becoming a serial murderer, whose last victim is himself.

Bram Stoker's *Dracula* seems at first glance anomalous in this regard: although there are two doctors in the major *dramatis personae*, neither is identified as a villain. The first, Dr. Seward, a psychiatrist, however ineffectual, is clearly on the side of good, while the second, Dr. Bram Van Helsing, is portrayed as the enemy of the villainous vampire. On closer examination, however, Van Helsing turns out to be a disconcertingly ambiguous figure, as much an alter ego as an antagonist of that villain.

To begin with, Van Helsing, too, is a stranger in a strange land, speaking English with a foreign accent. Moreover, though he is introduced as "one of the most advanced scientists of the day," having (as we learn eventually) "revolutionized therapeutics by the discovery of the continuous evolution of brain matter," the only scientific means he uses to thwart the vampire is blood transfusion. For the rest he depends on Old World charms and amulets like wreaths of garlic, crucifixes, holy water, and stakes driven through the heart. As a matter of fact, although one of Dracula's cognomens is Vlad Teppish (Vlad the Impaler), it is the good doctor we actually see impaling the vampire, as well as presiding over a similar ritual mutilation of Lucy Westenra, Vlad's first female victim. In any case, Van Helsing, for the most part, quite like the foe he seeks to destroy, operates in the realm not of modern science but of ancient magic, black and white.

Even transfusion seems finally to belong to that realm, being like vampirism an attempt to prolong life (the vampire, after all, aims not to kill but to make "undead") by transferring vital fluids from one body to another. Additionally, the transfusions from multiple donors, including Van Helsing himself—which he sets up in his earlier vain attempts to save Lucy—end by making her in a sense polyandrous. As when Dracula later forces Mina (Lucy's friend and his second intended female victim) to drink from his veins, Van Helsing's therapeutic mingling of blood calls into question the sanctity of Christian marriage. He perpetrates, that is to say, a travesty of sexual union, which undercuts the orthodox belief that only a man and his wife can and should be made one flesh.

It seems to me quite evident, in any case, that Stoker's fantasy about the irruption of vampirism into the modern world was initially triggered by the invention of blood transfusion, which is, of course, the precursor of organ and tissue transplantation, along with the bioethical problems it poses. Stoker, however, does not deal with those problems as explicitly as Mary Shelley does in *Frankenstein*, which—prophetically, as it were—confronts head-on the dark side of harvesting the body parts of the dead to prolong life. Her hyperbolic "fairy tale" was suggested, she informs us in her introduction, by an overheard conversation about recent experiments in which inert matter was revivified by the passage of an electric current. But in her actual text she never describes the process by which a patchwork of cadaveric parts is transformed into a living being.

What she does depict is the horror of digging up graves and dissecting corpses. Indeed, she does this twice over: once when she relates the creation of the original male monster; and again when she tells how, in response to that monster's demand, Frankenstein begins to fabricate a mate for him. Though he rejects the first creation and never completes the second, Frankenstein pays dearly for both impious attempts to manufacture more-than-human creatures by what amounts to a total body transplant.

Nor does it mitigate his guilt that, as Shelley makes clear from the very start, his motives are benign and his methods scientific. Old-fashioned necromancy, we learn early on, he has long since abandoned as delusory as well as evil. It is therefore in the university laboratory rather than the lairs of magicians that he seeks to discover "the cause and generation of life." And in this sense he is the prototype of the modern white-jacketed surgeon transplanting hearts and livers rather than the heir of alchemists searching for the *elixir vitae.*

To be sure, Shelley never refers to Frankenstein as a doctor, calling him only Victor or Baron. But in the popular mind, he rapidly came to be thought of, and has remained forever, Dr. Frankenstein; his name without that honorific title has been attached instead to his monstrous creation, whom Shelley left nameless. It seems a little surprising all the same that *Frankenstein* so deeply moved its readers long before the hospital had become a major institution, the practice of medicine a prestigious and rewarding (though ambivalently regarded) profession, health care a large part of every national budget, and bioethics a subject of obsessive concern. But surely this is no more surprising than the fact that it has continued to move readers (as have the three other books with which I have linked it); none of them, in fact, has gone out of print to this very day, despite the changes of fashion in literature and lifestyle. After all, they are essentially mythic works, which is to say, they exist out of time, in the eternal now of the collective unconscious.

For the same reason, these books have been felt from the very start as being in the public domain: the property not of their nominal authors but of the mass audience worldwide. Shortly after publication, they were translated into other media: first stage plays, then horror films, TV shows, and eventually comic strips and comic books. Finally, they have escaped from all media and are transmitted by word of mouth—the cognomens of their sinister protagonists turned into common nouns, familiar even to those who have never encountered their stories on the page or on the screen. This is less true of *The Island of Dr. Moreau* than of the others, but *Frankenstein* and *Dr. Jekyll and Mr. Hyde* have been thus transmogrified scores of times, while the versions of *Dracula* have reached the hundreds. At the moment I am writing this, indeed, a movie is being released called (a little misleadingly, I gather) *Bram Stoker's Dracula.*

More typically, however, in the course of such metamorphoses the names inscribed on their original title pages have been forgotten by most readers and viewers. Moreover, as only the few like me are aware, much else has been lost, added, or radically changed in the process— not just style and structure, which is inevitable, but theme, plot, and character. Finally, however, even we happy few have to grant that these tales (once again like all true myths) should be stripped by the popular mind of all that it instinctively senses is extraneous, even as it fills in what it feels to be blanks. First of all, subthemes of the original texts that are ideological or personal rather than archetypal and universal tend to disappear in the later recensions. Such subthemes include Bram Stoker's many allusions to new technologies of information storage and retrieval, as well as his references to the impact on traditional morality of the feminist movement of late Victorian times, Mary Shelley's repeated allusions to birthing and mothering, and R. L. Stevenson's reflections on the oedipal encounter of fathers and sons.

Meanwhile, characters absent from the original *dramatis personae* have come to play important roles in the ever-developing myth. Especially notable among these are the sinister cripple, Igor, who serves as Frankenstein's lab assistant; the even more monstrous bride, who rejects his monster; and the various female characters who have been added to the initially all-male cast of *Dr. Jekyll and Mr. Hyde* to provide occasions for romance or titillating sexual assaults. In addition, certain characters included from the start have been drastically altered; the monster himself, for instance, whom Shelley imagined as fully literate and superarticulate in at least two languages, has become a stuttering analphabetic with bolts in his head.

What has remained untouched, however, or rather what has become ever more clearly defined thanks to such changes, is the mythological core of these tales. At the core, the archetypal doctor is portrayed as an enemy (all the more dangerous because of his good intention) of those traditional beliefs that long enabled us to live at peace with our fragile bodies and our sense of their inescapable mortality. Typically in a lonely setting, which symbolizes his alienation from the rest of humanity, that doctor creates out of himself or the scraps of his dead fellows a creature intended to be better than his imperfect self, perhaps even immortal. Inevitably, though, that creature turns out to be a monster, and his creator even more of one for having dared to usurp the prerogatives of a superhuman creator. That archetypal scenario will, of course, continue to be imagined and reimagined for as long as humanity continues to fear death, calls on science to forestall it, and resents it for doing so.

Moreover, just as the telling of that mythic tale has no foreseeable end, it has no discernible beginning. Indeed, one reason for the instant success of books like *Frankenstein* and *Dracula* is their readers' feeling that the tale they tell is one they have always known without quite being able to formulate it. Even in medieval and early modern times, when society still put its trust in magic rather than technology to conquer the ultimate horror of death, mythic stories embodying that horror and that trust were already being formulated. The best known of these is *Dr. Faustus*, which has come down to us in a play by Christopher Marlowe and a long epic poem by Goethe, along with later plays and operas based largely on them.

Faustus, an ill-fated experimenter, not only succeeded in rejuvenating himself but also created the homunculus, a living human being of miniature size. His methods, to be sure, were not medical (despite his title, he was a magus rather than an M.D.) but thaumaturgic, beginning with evoking malign spirits and culminating in a pact with the devil. Closer to the techniques of present-day science were those of the alchemists, whose search for the elixir of life also became the subject of many-times-told tales. But though their art was the forerunner of modern chemistry, in their own time they, too, were also portrayed as black magicians risking damnation in a quest for forbidden knowledge.

In our time, however, when many of us have ceased to believe in damnation or indeed in any form of otherworldly life after death, the pursuit of immortality in this life has come to be regarded, on the conscious level, as a benign activity. On the one hand, research in cryonics and cloning is generously supported, and the moribund are provided, at great expense, with prosthetic devices, artificial life-support systems, and of course, transplanted organs, including the mythological heart itself. On the other hand, we are being constantly urged to avoid suspected carcinogens and foods high in cholesterol, including such long-time staples as tobacco and whiskey, coffee, sugar, eggs, and milk, even as we pop vitamin pills and rack our decaying bodies with dieting, jogging, and aerobics. It is as if we were secretly convinced (though we do not confess it openly) that with one more food forbidden, one more exercise regime required, one more miracle drug or surgical procedure perfected, we will all live forever.

Nonetheless, at a deeper level of the psyche, the dark side of our old ambivalence about the quest for immortality keeps suggesting that perhaps this whole strategy is wrong, misguided—finally monstrous; that forestalling death indefinitely is as impious as hastening it was traditionally thought to be; that, in the eloquent words of Shakespeare, "We must endure our going hence even as our coming hither. . . . the readiness is all." Surely, such a conviction underlies the covert rejection of transplantation—not despite but precisely because of its success in prolonging life. Or so, at least, the mythic tales I have been examining would seem to indicate.

5 *Ruth Richardson*

Fearful Symmetry: Corpses for Anatomy, Organs for Transplantation?

Personal Statement

I am a historian. I was invited to join the Park Ridge Center's group as a result of my work on the history of whole-body procurement. My interest in attitudes toward death and the human body, I think, derives in part from finding Johannes Nohl's book The Black Death *on a lower shelf in my parents' bookshelves when I was about three years old. Its medieval woodcuts of the Dance of Death fascinated me. As an adolescent, I later experienced at first hand the ways in which our London working-class family traditionally dealt with death.*

Historical interest in the subject came later still, when as an adult student at university, a reading of Frankenstein *moved me to ponder whether Mary Shelley had any personal knowledge of bodysnatching. Researching the subject for an essay developed into a major research project concerning the popular culture of death and the history of anatomical training and experiment in Britain since the Renaissance. My book* Death, Dissection and the Destitute *was the result of a decade's research.*

I am currently Wellcome Research Fellow in the History of Medicine in the Department of Anatomy and Developmental Biology, University College, London. I live near Mary Shelley's birthplace, with a doctor of medicine interested in medical ethics and law who has among his patients several long-term survivors of transplant surgery.

66

Introduction

The twentieth century has become accustomed to perceiving itself unique. Scientific and medical progress, many believe, confront us with moral and ethical problems which are entirely novel, quite unlike those of previous ages. This belief in the newness of our own preoccupations pervades consideration of ethical problems generated by the transplantation of human organs. While there may be some basis for this perception—the surgical transfer of living parts from one human body to another is indeed a relatively new phenomenon—the human imagination had certainly conceived of such a possibility centuries before it existed in reality.[1]

Transplantation is a recent development in a much longer historical process. The history of modern surgery in the Western world springs from centuries of exploration of the human body, fundamental to which were dissection and experimentation upon the bodies of the dead. This chapter considers current problems in obtaining organs for transplantation in the light of this long historical perspective. Difficulties encountered by past practitioners in procuring whole bodies for dissection, and the ways in which contemporary legislators dealt with the antecedents of present-day difficulties, offer empirical answers to some of the most serious public policy questions in organ procurement today.

Although I glance briefly at the United States, my main focus here is the British Isles. My chapter's title derives from the famous poem "The Tyger," by William Blake:

> Tyger, Tyger, burning bright,
> In the forests of the night:
> What immortal hand or eye,
> Could frame thy fearful symmetry?
>
> In what distant deeps or skies,
> Burnt the fire of thine eyes?
> On what wings dare he aspire?
> What the hand dare seize the fire?
>
> And what shoulder, and what art,
> Could twist the sinews of thy heart?
> And when thy heart began to beat,
> What dread hand? & what dread feet?
>
> What the hammer? what the chain,
> In what furnace was thy brain?
> What the anvil? what dread grasp,
> Dare its deadly terrors clasp?

When the stars threw down their spears
And water'd heaven with their tears:
Did he smile his work to see?
Did he who made the Lamb make thee?

Tyger, Tyger, burning bright,
In the forests of the night:
What immortal hand or eye,
Dare frame thy fearful symmetry?

The poet questions whether the Tyger's fiery rapacity could conceivably have been created by the same God that made the meekness of the Lamb. This chapter seeks to ask a similar question of modern surgery.

Dissection for Anatomy and for Transplantation

The activities involved in the dissection of the dead for anatomical study and for transplantation bear close affinities. Both depend upon an accessible supply of dead bodies. Each damages the dead body for the sake of what is generally seen as a greater good. Both processes break cultural taboos.

Since at least as early as the Renaissance the dissection of the dead has been of profound importance to the treatment of the living. Its role has been crucial but often indirect: by way of its contribution to the professional and individual knowledge base and to individual training. In dissection for anatomy the dead body is systematically excavated and dismantled, often over a long period of time, for the purposes of learning. In medical education, dissection has permitted individuals the opportunity to understand, learn, and experience at first hand the architecture of the body; to acquire clinical detachment toward the body—what the famous anatomist William Hunter described as a "Necessary Inhumanity"; and to develop manual technique in the use of scalpel, saw, and other tools. Each of these learning processes is basic to the practice and development of the skill and discipline of surgery.

Dissection of the dead has provided the basis for professional knowledge and understanding of anatomical structures and pathological processes. Exploration and experimentation on the dead body have permitted improvements in the understanding of disease and have assisted in improvements in diagnosis and operative procedures. In past and present, tools and techniques developed upon the dead have been crucial to attempts upon the living.

The removal of body parts from the dead for the use of the living also has a long history. Parts were often extracted from corpses undergoing dissection so that surgeons could comprehend reasons for the success or failure of their procedures. Human parts were preserved by drying, bottling, salting, or pickling, and were stored as anatomical preparations in museums for use in teaching and research. Bones, too, were extracted for use in skeletal preparations.

Transplantation is a modern development of dissection and surgery. As a discipline, it has evolved from and built upon knowledge gained from centuries of exploration and experiment upon the dead and the living. The so-called retrieval process in transplantation is much more swiftly accomplished than is generally the case in dissection. The dead body is systematically excavated, but not always completely dismantled, in order that organs and tissues may be reused in the living bodies of others. Transplantation is of direct value to the treatment, and often to the survival, of others. Transplantation and its allied disciplines have increased knowledge of the body's immune system, of tissue typing, and of the preservation and storage of organs and tissues removed from the dead for later use.

Obtaining Corpses and Their Parts

The great majority of bodies used for dissection, and most organs used for transplantation, in the United Kingdom today have something in common: they are gifts. This is, however, a comparatively recent phenomenon. Teaching and research in human anatomy were historically rendered difficult and sometimes impossible by a scarcity of corpses upon which to work. Because the mutilation of the dead breaks deep-seated taboos in Western culture, historically anatomists met with noncooperation and sometimes outright hostility from the public in obtaining the basic material for their work.

The current public policy debate on ways to increase the supply of transplantable organs seems to favor two possibilities: *financial inducement*, and what has become known as *presumed consent*. Many readers may be surprised to learn that very similar suggestions were being raised in Britain 150 years ago as means by which to obtain corpses sufficient to meet the needs of anatomists, and that each scheme has undergone effective trial in the past. Both policies had serious adverse consequences. Financial inducements to secure corpses led to theft and eventually to serial murder. Presumed-consent legislation, which appropriated the corpses of the poor *without* their consent, provoked enormous opposition and yielded only a meager supply, and that of poor quality. Moreover, the bad feeling generated by the legislation served to delay for more than a hundred years the development of a satisfactory level of public donation.

The history of whole-body procurement prefigures in a number of interesting ways the current situation in obtaining organs for transplantation. I have written this chapter in hope of facilitating discussion of how best to obtain an ethical source of transplantable tissue while respecting the fears and anxieties of the public concerning organ donation, requisition, and purchase. The historical affinities revealed here may assist in a more critical awareness of some of the ethical difficulties we face today.

Historical Summary

From the inception of surgery in the early Renaissance, those who sought dead human material for dissection have suffered shortage. Put simply, a perception of shortage is not a new problem. Public hostility to the dissection of the dead ensured that demand for corpses always outstripped the legal supply. Except, perhaps, in war—when surgeons hardly require dead bodies because they learn their skills upon the living—there has never been an era of glut.

In the United Kingdom, prior to the Tudor period there was no legal supply whatsoever. Statutory provision dates from the early sixteenth century, when the patronage of King Henry VIII permitted an act of Parliament in 1540 (Anno 32 Henrici Octavi c.42), bestowing upon the Companies of Barbers and Surgeons the annual gift of four executed criminals' corpses. Dissection was recognized in law—and by the public—as a mutilation, a postmortem punishment, a terrible aggravation of the death penalty. Hence derives the medical profession's association with the gallows and with the infliction of punishment, an association which persisted without intermission until the nineteenth century.

Demand increased over time, as scientific interest in human anatomy grew during the seventeenth and eighteenth centuries. Paying patients added to the pressure by seeking better treatments and better-qualified doctors. Despite extensions of the original grant by statute in 1565, 1663, and 1752, the number of gallows corpses consistently fell short of the profession's requirements. The great anatomist William Harvey, who published his work demonstrating the circulation of the blood in 1628, had reached his findings by access to an alternative source: Harvey dissected the corpses of both his father and his sister. His case, though probably atypical, offers a lucid illustration of one of my key themes: *once the need for human dissection material was recognized, a supply was obtained; and once the supply was obtained, it was found to fall short of demand.* Shortage both intensified demand and prompted illicit supply. A similar pattern repeated itself throughout the period between Henry VIII's enactment and the early nineteenth century.

It was probably in the period 1675–1725 that the human corpse began to be bought and sold like any other commodity. Corpses, skeletons, and preserved body parts were sold behind closed doors. The inadequacy of the legal supply led students and professional surgeons to seek elsewhere, and grave-robbing probably served well in a quiet way for a considerable period of time. Opposition made the work hazardous, however, and a class of entrepreneurs—bodysnatchers, or "resurrectionists"—soon arose to procure merchandise for a lucrative black market. Anatomy schools, being established in this period, sold the dismembered parts to students at a profit.

The public viewed dissection just as the law envisaged: as a fate worse than death, to be avoided at all costs. Loathing of dissection may have derived from fears that the process somehow damaged the soul, caused haunting, or denied the possibility of resurrection.[2] Popular opposition to dissection was vocal, and often violent. Friends of executed criminals fought with dedication at gallows to save their dead from the surgeons, and the resulting riots were often violent and dangerous. Here concern may have been less with eschatology than with the fact that public hangings were often bungled affairs, and attempts to revive the hanged occasionally met with success, in which case the criminal could be freed. To such people, dissection was regarded not only as worse than death, but as likely murder.

Gallows riots prompted anatomists and their suppliers to focus increasingly on the buried dead. Churchyards were vulnerable to predation, particularly in and around London and in the vicinity of towns and cities with schools of anatomy. Ports and other places on coastal and canal routes of navigation, and even unexpectedly distant villages, could find their burial grounds rifled of the freshly dead. Poorer folk suffered the greatest risk; the wealthy could always purchase additional protection in the form of extra-thick and cast-iron coffins, private vaults, and other security devices.

Wherever their handiwork was discovered, bodysnatchers were subject to violent physical attacks, forcible recovery of stolen bodies, vociferous pursuit, and prosecution. Cases are known in which they were seriously injured and even killed by protesters. Bodysnatchers perceived these as the risks of the job: when secrecy was maintained, theirs was an extremely lucrative profession.

In times of shortage and difficulty, prices rose, and other methods had to be tried—bribery, importation from abroad, theft prior to burial— which could be hazardous and costly. Anatomists attached to teaching hospitals were cushioned from the worst shortages, since they had access to the dead in institutional mortuaries.

The mid-1820s seem to have been a crisis point, when, in an attempt to peg prices, a group of London anatomists formed a cartel to deal directly with the resurrectionists. But competition between the private schools was so fierce that professional unity fractured. Those willing to offer higher fees immediately received the best supplies.

For over a century bodysnatchers bore the brunt of popular execration and legal penalties alike, but in March 1828, a prosecution at Lancaster Assizes entirely changed the situation. An anatomist was convicted of possessing a dead body, knowing it to have been obtained unlawfully. The judge announced that however necessary exhumation for dissection might be, the only corpses legally available to the profession were those granted by statute from the gallows. Surgeons and anatomists were suddenly vulnerable to the taint of criminality they had managed to avoid for so long.

The case provided a cue for parliamentary activity. Within forty days a House of Commons Select Committee was established to investigate the problem of corpse shortage and to look into the possibility of augmenting the legal supply. The committee was formed by a group of politicians who had already decided what its recommendations would be: that requisition was the preferred mode of procurement, and that the bodies of the dead poor should be obtained from institutions. Several alternative means by which the profession might obtain dead bodies *by consent* were discussed by contemporaries, but such ideas were not given a hearing. Instead, the Select Committee's work was hastily completed, so that its *Report* could be submitted to the House of Commons before the parliamentary recess, in June 1828.

Although they had received warnings from well-informed witnesses, none of the members of Parliament on the Select Committee knew that, while they were taking evidence and composing their report, two enterprising Edinburgh men had found a simpler method of procuring fresh corpses: murder. Ten people had already met their deaths, and six more would follow. Burke and Hare's murdering career ended not by forensic discovery or detective policing, but after a Halloween party, when curious guests discovered the body of the final victim concealed in bedstraw.

All the victims had been very poor vagrants, mainly women, the men being elderly or handicapped in some way. They had been plied with whisky and smothered. Their bodies were sold to the nearby anatomy school of Dr. Knox, who approved of their freshness and asked no questions. The murderers had been well paid, and whenever they delivered a body they were always told to get more. Here was the first known case in which the fees offered by anatomy schools had served as a premium for murder. The public and the profession were aghast. It had suddenly dawned on society that poor people had become worth more dead than alive. One practitioner perceived the enormity of the situation: "Shall it be said that we owe it to that science which professes to alleviate human suffering [that] her votaries be encouraged to encourage . . . Murder?"[3]

For political reasons, the passage of the Anatomy Act requisitioning the bodies of the poor was delayed until a further case of murder for anatomy—or *burking* as it became known—was discovered in London in 1831. Here, the murderers were reputed to have confessed to the deaths of sixty victims. Almost immediately, a new bill was submitted to Parliament and passed with little opposition. It remains the basis of modern law in this field in much of the English-speaking world. By defining *institutions* such as workhouses and hospitals which housed the poor as "lawfully in possession" of the dead, it permitted the confiscation of the bodies of those dying without relatives to "claim" them, or without sufficient money to pay for their own funerals.

Requisition promoted resentment, and resistance. Dissection, which for centuries had been used to punish and stigmatize the worst of crimes, now did the same for poverty. To die without provision for burial became the key indicator of social failure. The Victorian poor became famous for doing everything possible to avoid this fate. A variety of expedients was used: purchases of burial insurance soared, bodies were kept at home for long periods, postmortems were requested when family or friends died in institutions, house-to-house and public-house collections were made, to save even the poorest from falling into the hands of the doctors. Suspicion of medical men and infirmary staff was widespread in poor communities. The fear of dying without adequate burial provision survived well into living memory, and persists among the elderly poor in the United Kingdom even today.

Resistance to requisition had a significant impact on the number of corpses the legislation had been expected to yield. Shortages persisted, and the quality of supplies deteriorated as the nineteenth century progressed. The old supply from grave-robbing and the gallows, for all its disadvantages, had at least provided a proportion of good specimens. Bodies made available under the new law were generally poor physical specimens, as they tended to be those of very elderly, injured, diseased, or vagrant people without family or friends to save them.

Moreover, voluntary bequests of corpses for dissection, which prior to the Anatomy Act had been increasing, now declined. Potential donors, believing an adequate supply was provided by law, saw no need to bequeath their bodies. The secrecy with which the act was implemented—intended to foster ignorance among those liable for requisition—served also to keep potential donors in the dark concerning the medical need for their donations. More than a century was to pass before voluntary bequest was again contemplated as a feasible source of corpses for dissection.

Toward the end of the nineteenth century, the issue of the confiscation of the institutionalized dead once again became a matter of political contention. Democratically elected councils, which now controlled supplying institutions in all parts of the country, were changing their political complexion, and an understanding of the class nature of the legislation manifested itself in contemporary debates, which were reported widely in the press. An increasing number of districts voted to refuse to consign their dead to medical schools for dissection. It was a widely held view that the poor had enough grief in their lives without this addition, and that instead of confiscating the bodies of the poor, doctors ought to bequeath their own bodies for dissection. Failure to do so was taken as a sign of professional hypocrisy.

What had been a chronic shortage soon became acute. By the early twentieth century, welfare provision for the elderly resulted in fewer deaths in institutions, and mental institutions were virtually the only source of corpses. When even these corpses were denied, the profession was driven to appeal for public generosity, and it did not take long to become evident that they were pushing at an open door. Bequests for dissection rose from 3 percent of all bodies dissected in 1934 to 6 percent in 1940. By the 1960s, between 70 and 100 percent of bodies were freely donated. The sense of national cohesion created by the situation in Britain during World War II perhaps contributed to this historically unprecedented public generosity. Doubtless, too, the establishment of the National Health Service in 1949 promoted greater public trust toward the medical profession, and a more benign view of scientific medicine. Change did not occur overnight, but historically speaking, the postwar era has seen a very significant and remarkable change in public attitude. Today, more bodies are offered than are required.[4]

The situation in the United States has followed a course broadly similar to that in Britain, but with differences of detail, particularly in chronology. The principle of requisition as recommended by the House of Commons Select Committee in 1828 was swiftly adopted in the state of Massachusetts, even *before* it was enacted in Britain, but it took a considerable time before a majority of other states followed. Criminals were still being dissected, and medical schools remained dependent upon bodysnatchers, in several U.S. states into at least the second decade of the *twentieth* century. As David Humphrey has observed, "The passage of anatomy acts . . . did not signify that Americans had come to regard dissection as a legitimate use of the body after death. In practice, if not always in conception, the anatomy laws confined dissections to a voiceless, widely-scorned segment of society. The procurement, dissection, and disposal of cadavers became for most citizens an invisible process and a distant issue." The social origins of the corpses obtained for medical schools under the various U.S. anatomy acts were similar to those in Britain, but it should be noted that in the United States the very poorest classes contained disproportionate numbers of Native and African Americans.[5]

This summary of the last half-millennium of medical difficulty in obtaining human bodies for dissection situates the more recent problem of the shortage of human organs for transplantation in its proper historical context (see table 5.1). The sustained sense of shortage to which the summary bears witness highlights an important affinity between obtaining and dissecting human bodies in the past, and obtaining and transplanting human body parts in the present day. Modern problems of organ shortage may seem less remarkable when viewed in its light.

Affinities between Past and Present

Before looking at the matter of shortage and how it might be resolved, I should like to glance at a number of other parallels between past and present, such as those between the predicament of anatomists then and that of transplanters now. Nor can we forget the predicament of the dying, whose corpses were so coveted then, as they are for different reasons now.

Disquiet about Donation

In the past, many people regarded dissection as beneficial in the abstract but undesirable for themselves in particular. Today, many people recognize and appreciate the value of organ transplantation yet do not themselves wish to contribute to the supply of human organs. As was also the case in the past, these feelings span barriers of class and education, and even medical personnel may be found among those harboring such reservations.

Table 5.1. Corpses for Dissection in Britain: Summary

• Inception of demand for corpses to dissect prior to legal supply (medieval period)
• Growth of profession and increase of demand
• Limited legal provision for dissection: gallows corpses (1540 Act of Parliament)
• Legal supply insufficient
• Alternative supply of corpses obtained (Harvey, early seventeenth century)
• Profession develops; demand for corpses increases
• Sustained pressure for increased supply
• Legal supply augmented, but insufficient (1565, 1663, 1752)
• Supply of corpses augmented by other means (grave-robbery)
• Brokerage established, price mechanism in place (sales, body-snatchers, c. 1700s)
• Demand for corpses outstrips supply; costs rise
• Supply of corpses augmented by other means (transport from afar, bribery, and so on)
• Demand for corpses outstrips supply; costs rise
• Professional cartel regulates corpse costs and supplies (London, 1820s)
• Competition fierce: professional ethics fracture
• Corpse prices higher still
• Corpse supply augmented by murder (Burke and Hare, 1828; Bishop and Williams, 1831)
• Means of promoting voluntary corpse donation ignored (Select Committee, 1828)
• Law requisitions institutionalized dead; public fears remain (Anatomy Act, 1832)
• Voluntary donation of corpses declines
• Requisition prompts resistance and avoidance strategies (burial insurance, and so on)
• Legal corpse supply shrinks and is of poor quality (elderly, sick, neglected)
• Chronic corpse shortage, then acute shortage (early 1900s)
• Profession appeals for public generosity (between World War I and II)
• Voluntary donation of corpses increases (after World War II)
• Adequate supply of corpses obtained by voluntary donation (1960s to the present)

Source: Ruth Richardson, *Death, Dissection and the Destitute* (Penguin, 1989).

Animal and Mechanical Substitutes

Substitutes for corpses—such as animals, casts, wax and mechanical models, bottled preparations, preserved specimens, printed plates, even artificial corpses—were used in the past to obviate shortage. All proved less than adequate, but anatomy schools were obliged to depend upon them to a degree their proprietors, and their students, disliked.

In the last thirty years, a number of substitutes for live human organs have been tried or planned. Some, such as mechanical heart valves, have been a great success, but others have proved disastrous. Most recently, the use of animal organs has been tried, and we expect shortly to hear of the results of experiments with organs and other parts from genetically engineered pigs.[6] Both past history and present experience reveal a low level of success for most of these substitutes. No adequate substitute for the human source has yet been found.

Futures Markets and Rewarded Gifting

In the early nineteenth century, a significant number of doctors appear to have been comparatively satisfied with the existing system of "authorized stealth"; after all, financial incentives to bodysnatchers had served to produce an adequate supply of corpses for over a century. Corpse deals with bodysnatchers worked, cemented by a bond of mutual secrecy and interdependence—a sort of honor among thieves. Some doctors, however, found shortage intolerable and supported ideas for alternative sources by which the law could accommodate increasing demand. Such ideas focused mainly upon offering incentives to donate, such as sale during life, the offer of money to the relatives of the dead, or the abrogation of death taxes on the estates of those bequeathing their own corpses for dissection.

The idea of purchasing corpses directly from the relatives of the dead surely offered a cheaper alternative to purchasing from resurrectionists. The fact that anatomy schools remained dependent upon bodysnatchers suggests that custom, tradition, notions of decency, and attachment to the bodies of the dead prevented such approaches being made, even in cases of terrible poverty.[7]

In the 1820s and 1830s, the founder-editor of the *Lancet*, Thomas Wakley, campaigned passionately against the idea of *any* offer of payment whatsoever. He believed any association between financial benefit and the bodies of the dead would perpetuate the material motive for burking. A similar objection prevailed among other critics: "Will not an unprincipled executor or relative be as likely to kill a helpless and forlorn wretch, dying perhaps in an obscure garret, and attended only by his heir, as a resurrection man will be to 'burk a lost traveller, or stray apprentice in the dark'?"[8]

Sale during life had other problems altogether. A caller's suggestion that a weekly sum might be paid to a poor woman said to be interested in selling her body at death prompted such an overreaction by the anatomist Sir Astley Cooper that it appears likely he may have had his fingers burnt before: "The truth is that you deserve to be hanged for making such an unfeeling offer," he scribbled in reply. A contemporary humorous poem suggests the difficulties inherent in this sort of transaction.[9] On his deathbed, a bodysnatcher, Jack Hall (a London cockney pun on *jackal*), is attended by a "swarm" of twelve doctors, whose interest in his demise is evidently much greater than in his survival. It emerges at last that more than one bargain had been made:

> Ten guineas did not quite suffice,
>   And so I sold my body twice;
> Twice would not do—I sold it thrice,
>   Forgive my crimes!
> In short I have received its price
>   A dozen times!

Such cases may indeed have occurred among the numbers of interesting human specimens anatomists were keen to obtain for their museums. It would not have been difficult for a fraudster to extort fees from a series of interested anatomists by similar means, and to leave nothing but contention behind.

Nowadays, cloaked in new titles such as *rewarded gifting* and *futures markets*, the very same mechanisms are being mooted as means to promote organ donation.[10] Those raising such ideas seem to be unaware that their arguments are neither new nor original. They should know that these ideas were disposed of as practical alternatives by doctors and lawmakers 150 years ago.

"Presumed Consent"

In the present day, from time to time, suggestions are raised, particularly in the medical press, that we should extend the law covering organ transplantation in line with a policy referred to as *presumed consent*. This is one of the many misnomers with which the language of transplantation is peppered. Here, lip service is paid to the *need* for consent, but in practice its existence is irrelevant, because it is *assumed* to exist. *Presumed consent* is public-relations-speak for the denial of a need even to *seek* consent.

Advocates of this policy appear oblivious to the fact that it has ancient and rather ugly antecedents: its descent can be traced back in law by way of the Anatomy Act directly to the Tudor law which sequestered for public dismemberment the corpses of hanged murderers. Those raising these suggestions today should acquaint themselves with the fact that it took hundreds of years for the medical profession to shake off its associations with coercion, punishment, and the executioner.

The British government in 1832 legislated to sequester the corpses of the socially disenfranchised. The existing legal precedent was the dissection of murderers who had so transgressed all moral norms that the old Tudor law justified inflicting the ultimate mutilation in the name of a just punishment. However, in the case of the nineteenth-century poor, no such transgression had taken place: most inmates of Georgian and Victorian hospitals and workhouses had reached that situation through sickness, injury, or old age, having been decent members of society all their lives. Under the new law, their wishes were neither sought nor observed. No statutory provision was made for the registration of such wishes, and indeed, it is known that the Anatomy Inspectorate actively suppressed the recording of such wishes where this occurred spontaneously.[11] The principle became established in British law, and thus in the law of other nations, that because the condemned might be denied the right to prevent the mutilation of their bodies after death, the hospitalized living could suffer the same denial.

These historical precedents, I believe, help clarify current dilemmas. If public policy were to be changed in the direction of "presumed consent," a great deal would be at stake. Historically, legislation of a similar complexion, intended to obtain an increased supply of whole bodies for anatomy, had a number of unforeseen effects:

- The number of voluntary donations plummeted.
- Those liable to requisition devised ways to avoid that fate.
- The new supply was smaller than that already existing.
- The new supply was less useful than that already existing.
- The profession found itself the object of profound mistrust and violence.
- The profession was sullied by its coercive role in denying autonomy.

In our current situation, the profession also risks alienating hitherto supportive public opinion and, moreover, risks the introduction of dangerous possibilities into the hospital.

What Is a Corpse?

In the bodysnatchers' day, the human corpse was viewed with a mixture of fear and solicitude. Its latent power was enhanced by uncertainties concerning its physical and spiritual attributes: both the spiritual status of the dead body and the definition of death were foci of doubt. Theologians declared the corpse carrion while yet debating whether the spirit left the body or retained some association with it until the final trumpet. Tales of revival after hanging and drowning, of premature burial, and of people sitting up on the dissecting table had wide currency, as did ghostlore.

In a sense, all these matters are still with us today. The precise definition of life, and of death, and the mystery of the spirit or soul, remains open to discussion, debate, doubt, hope, and faith. The adoption of cremation as a means of disposal and the wide reporting of out-of-body experiences suggest a public willingness to believe in some sort of disassociation between body and soul/spirit at death. Nevertheless, the timing or organ removal is currently based upon physical definitions of death rather than spiritual ones.

In some Victorian hospitals, dissection was done with "indecent if not dangerous haste,"[12] so tales in contemporary folklore of dissections on living individuals may have had some basis in reality. Matters are pressed with even greater urgency today than they were in the days of the bodysnatchers. After all, the process of dissection upon a fresh body can take place over a period of several days, whereas organs—in order to be usable—must be removed as soon after death as possible. Although one hopes that an objective requirement for speed does not degenerate into overalacritous haste, the fact that it did so in the past when the pressure on doctors was not so great should alert us to this possibility today.

The definition of death is, if anything, even more problematic today than it was in the past. Even the medical profession seems undecided whether heart or brain death is the correct criterion, and seems to want it both ways. Redefinitions of death, which seem always to revise it nearer to life, serve only to confuse the situation. The current medical pressure toward the use of the heart-dead rather than the brain-dead is a particularly worrying development in this respect.[13]

The public is confused, only half persuaded, often doubtful, which is hardly surprising when one considers that the bodies from which organs are removed must be classified as dead, while their organs must yet be alive enough to be useful. In popular terms, this might mean that the human donor is still half alive. The physical and spiritual status of the bodies from which organs are removed is a simmering problem and seems likely to remain so.

Freshness, Preservation, and Grief

The ability to preserve human bodily material for any length of time remains another problem. Just as was the case for whole bodies in the past, today we have only limited means of keeping human organs for more than a short period of time after disembodiment. Deterioration seriously affects their therapeutic and financial value. Freshness is therefore at a premium today, just as it was in the time of the resurrectionists.

But the freshness of bodies has an analogue in the freshness of survivors' grief, and the modern need to obtain living tissues can involve intrusion upon very fresh grief. Organs are generally taken from individuals kept physically alive on life-support machines, which can allow relatives time to come to terms with the death and to make a positive decision. The ethics of taking organs from *non-heart-beating cadavers* are much more questionable. I share the alarm expressed by Renée Fox in the concluding chapter of this volume concerning the ethical and moral safety of this process.[14]

The potential for difficulties and conflicts between medical professionals and patients' families, between caring professions, and within the consciences of individuals is considerable. The medical profession has had to work hard to gain the trust of relatives, especially because there is a high level of public awareness—resulting from books and films such as *Coma*—that, in an intensive-care setting, medical power over life and death is great, relatives are dependent upon the information they are given, and the patient's capability for self-determination is nil.

In the past, incursions upon mourners' grief caused enormous distress. Hasty, ill-advised, and unethical behavior by some doctors— especially toward the dying or the dead—resulted in public mistrust of the entire medical profession. Cases are known in which popular distrust was sometimes expressed in violence against doctors, occasionally to the extent of riot. Several British and U.S. medical schools and hospitals were attacked by rioters protesting against dissection without consent, and on both sides of the Atlantic, medical schools were actually destroyed as a result.

We have recently witnessed opposition of a related kind against abortion clinics on both sides of the Atlantic. Happily, no similar events have yet occurred to stigmatize transplantation. Nevertheless, it is worth observing that the activities precipitating both nineteenth-century anatomy riots and twentieth-century anti-abortion campaigns concerned medical professionals who had involved themselves too closely on the wrong side of the life-death divide. Without serious circumspection, there is a danger that a similar tainting process may spread to transplantation.

Aspects of the Market

Like the teaching of anatomy and the historical activity of surgery, most transplantation today is undertaken in a medical marketplace of sorts. As with corpses in the past, organs now have internationally ascertainable value. Market conditions, and the characteristics of individual organs (freshness, age, tissue type), can affect therapeutic desirability and therefore value. As was the case with suppliers of dissection material in the past, organ brokers now tend to be a different professional group from the surgeons actually doing the transplanting or organs. Professionals benefit from the business, but as was the case with bodysnatching and requisition, the victim/donor receives nothing in return. Reciprocity is not a feature of the system.[15]

In the past, medical benefit accrued to those further up the social scale, who could purchase expertise gained on the living and the dead in public institutions. In many parts of the world today, the direction of benefit remains recognizably similar.

Sale of Body Parts

In the grave-robbing era, the value of whole bodies was enhanced by the facility with which the corpse could be quarried for teeth, hair, skeletons, and so on. Parts extracted were sold to those who could use them, such as dentists and wigmakers, and to those who assisted medical research and study, such as articulators of bones for medical skeletons, and medical-specimen makers. Profits were to be made at every stage.

Today a similar process is under way, involving the quarrying of as many live organs and tissues as possible from any one body—organs, eyes, skin, bone, membranes, glands—all of which have therapeutic, research, and potential money value. A recent report concerned a U.S. case of a man shot in the head, whose body was quarried for parts. It was later discovered that he had been HIV positive. Efforts to trace those who had received tissues from his body revealed that fifty-four parts had been removed from his body, but that only forty-eight of them could be traced.[16] Apart from the spread of HIV to a large number of people, this case illustrates two fundamental points: first, the enormous potential value of a single human body as a result of the transplantation process, and second, the fact that the administrative tracking of live tissue is so inadequate that fatally infected tissue can apparently become lost in the system.

Bodysnatchers who dealt in dead human tissue in the past were free of government surveillance and control. Even under the Anatomy Act, anatomists' breaches of law and of decency were overlooked for the sake of keeping matters quiet and the public in the dark. Today, those who obtain and deal in live human tissues may believe themselves similarly placed, as society's control of this field remains seriously inadequate.[17]

Dangers of a Market in Human Flesh

It is a truism of market economics that goods much sought after, but in short supply, fetch high prices. The scientific and therapeutic importance of the human corpse in the past was reflected in its commercial valuation. The attachment of money value to the human body provided the incentive to crime. High prices, severe shortages, and fierce competition between "consumers" all served to weight events in that direction. Doctors obtained human bodies in ways beyond the law of the day—such as grave-robbery and theft from gallows or institutions—by offering money for their procurement.

The historical summary (see table 5.1) identifies several key factors which, in the 1820s, permitted corpse "procurement" to develop into something far more sinister and dangerous:

- increasing demand for human tissue
- shortage of donors and public resistance
- competition among users/consumers
- money values attached to human tissue

In Burke and Hare's day, these were reinforced by two closely related factors: the ease of concealing the identity of the human source, and the ease of destroying evidence of crime.

Perhaps one of the most remarkable and chilling of the many affinities between the two eras under consideration is that *all* these factors are to some extent active today in the new field of transplantation. The benefits accruing from the quarrying of a single human body are comparatively as great, or indeed greater, today than they were at the time of the Burke and Hare murders. The theft, or surreptitious removal, of body parts is already known to have occurred.[18] The incentive to procure premature death in order to procure human organs already exists.

Identity and Anonymity

In nineteenth-century anatomy rooms, identifying characteristics were routinely obliterated from the dead to prevent the reclamation of corpses by relatives. It is worth remembering that this practice of anonymization was observed in Edinburgh in 1828 by those who purchased bodies from Burke and Hare. The murderers were protected rather than exposed by their customers. Signs of violence upon a body were easily overlooked or removed, either because the manner of death itself meant such signs were few or equivocal, or because forensic evidence could be destroyed by medical collusion. The "London Burkers" had devised— some thought they had been advised of—a way of dispatching their victims which left no marks. The ease and the rapidity with which both victims' identity and evidence of crime could be disposed of in the dissecting room materially assisted successful homicidal activity over long periods of time.

Similar problems and possibilities exist today. High values attached to organs, severe shortages, and fierce competition between "consumers" are all factors currently operating to various degrees in the international organ market. As corpses did in the past, organs now have value. Attempts to establish and sustain cost equilibrium within countries, such as organ exchange, have helped stabilize the situation and have kept transplantation a nonprofit endeavor in many parts of the world. Professional self-regulation has attempted to ensure ethical practice. However, despite the endeavors of the profession, government agencies, and lawmakers, a global medical marketplace exists, and its imperatives may operate within countries, even within institutions.[19]

Reputable agencies, of course, do all they can to obtain organs responsibly and to distribute them fairly and usefully. Routine anonymization is a component in this process. The most obviously worrying modern scenario, along lines suggested by past experience, might be in the contamination of networks served by such reputable and well-regulated organ brokerages by the infiltration of illicitly obtained material.

A recent discovery at a Colombian medical school of thirty murdered corpses was reported to have been the work of a gang murdering down-and-outs for dissection.[20] Here we can witness a Burke and Hare situation replicated in the present day in a Third World country which does a great deal of other illicit trade with the United States and other Western nations. It may be only a matter of time before such goods enter Western routes of supply. The poor bookkeeping revealed in the HIV case mentioned above could serve to assist such activity.[21]

That such activities are possible can be expected after documented cases of organ theft. A London surgeon was exposed in 1988 as having removed a kidney from a Turkish man who insisted he had traveled to London in ignorance of what was to happen to him. The case revealed the existence of an international trade in organs, carried by (witting or unwitting) live donors.[22]

A more recent report concerned a mental institution in Buenos Aires from which fourteen hundred people "disappeared" between 1976 and 1991. Bodies exhumed during the investigation were said to have had eyes and other organs missing, and blood drained. Several living inmates of the institution had apparently been recorded as already dead, probably in preparation for their demise. The institution's doctors were reported to have used the purloined tissue in an off-site private hospital for wealthy patients.[23]

Back in the 1830s, the cartoonist who went by the pseudonym Paul Pry registered a protest against the Anatomy Bill, then going through Parliament. His cartoon featured a scene of dismembered human parts hanging on hooks outside a shop, just as butchers' meat was then customarily displayed for sale. A doctor's servant was shown with a shopping list of the parts required for his master. At first I thought it only a bitter visual comment on the prospective legislation, until I read the diary of an apprentice surgeon who described just such a display of body parts at an anatomy school, each with a price tag attached.

The profits potentially available today from organ retrieval and transplantation are such as to ensure that—just as was the case for corpses in the past—every freshly dead human body has a high therapeutic and financial value. In the 1990s, Taiwan is reported to be removing organs from executed criminals. A professor of surgery at Taiwan University is reported to have said this in justification: "The only difference from usual organ donation is that the brain death is caused by execution."[24] A modern Paul Pry could just as well be sketching his comment today.

Urban Legends

Prior to the discovery of the Burke and Hare murders, stories had been circulating which suggested that murders were occurring, and that children were being stolen, for dissection. Such tales were dismissed as popular fantasy by contemporary doctors and journalists. Some well-informed individuals, however, did recognize that they might have some basis. The Select Committee received warnings in 1828 that the high prices then being offered for corpses constituted a danger to human life.

Tales of this sort are circulating once again. Now described as "urban legends," these stories are generally passed by word of mouth, and emerge occasionally in the press. They have worldwide circulation, spreading notions that the market in human body parts has promoted the theft of organs from living individuals, the murder of defenseless people (particularly of children) for their organs, and even the kidnapping and farming of babies in the Third World to accommodate transplantation projects. These rumors are so plausible, and so serious in their import and effects, that the U.S. Information Agency has been driven to counteract their potency with a campaign to deny their veracity. Governments, organ-obtaining agencies, and folklorists appear equally eager to deny the credibility of such tales.[25]

It seems to be unknown, or at least unrecognized, that tales with a similar theme circulating in the 1820s turned out to have more truth in them than did contemporary denials, and that their accuracy was

proved beyond doubt by the discovery of burking. It may be worth
remembering that the doctor implicated in that case, Dr. Knox, believed
that murdered bodies could have been discovered at any anatomy school
in the country—that it happened to be at his school was simply bad luck.
Whether his belief had any objective basis will probably never be known.

Semantic Massage

During the anatomy debate of the 1820s and 1830s in the United Kingdom, apologists for requisition consciously replaced words which had
known and familiar meanings with less emotive or more positive or
scientific-sounding terms. *Dissection* became *anatomical examination*. The
unasked became the *unclaimed*.

Dishonest language bespeaks dishonest intentions. Such substitutions
denied the reality of the activity contemplated; they served to cast problematic matters in a favorable light and to dehumanize the people whose
bodies were the real topic of debate. Even the murderer Burke used the
medical-scientific term *the subject* in referring to one of his victims.

Euphemism was utilized to promote requisition in the past, and is
being used so again today. We have already glanced at *presumed consent*.
I propose now to look briefly at four other terms: *HBPs, harvesting,
procurement*, and *donor*.

HBP is an acronym for *human body part*, an abbreviation which neatly
truncates both humanity and emotive meaning. To refer to a human
heart as an HBP is to edit out its physical and emotional resonance, to
annul the cultural import of the enterprise involved in its removal. The
acronym conveys scientificity, abstraction, and impassivity, whereas the
reality is human, physical, and of passionate importance. *HBP* makes
human organs sound as if they are car parts or industrial components.
The dehumanizing process could not be more clearly demonstrated than
in the reduction of the word *human* to the letter *H*.

A favored euphemism in the United Kingdom for the extraction of
HBPs from a human body is currently *explantation*—at once less emotive
and more technical in tone than the simpler and more straightforward
extraction or *removal*. The word features the noun *plantation* and centers
on the organic image of a *plant:* both words perhaps bear a relationship
to the much-preferred term to describe the process—*harvesting*—a term
which exudes pastorality: a fantasy of fertility. The term suggests season-
ality and natural ripeness, engendering a sense of physical well-being.

Harvest is a time of fullness and plenitude. Thoughts of death, and of
the plundered body, are banished.[26] Harvesting implies that the person
from whom organs are taken is a mere thing, a botanical entity—a

pumpkin, a squash, passive in the way a quiet country field is passive, or passive as a vine or a tree—one whose organs are merely a crop to be taken at will, or even by right. In normal speech, *harvesting* presupposes anterior intention in the planting of seed, its growth, natural development, and ripening for later harvest, storage, and use. Such an image in the context of organ transplantation is both fallacious and disingenuous. Human organs are grown and develop in the embryo, the child, and the adult to support the organism in which they grow. Human organs do *not* grow in order to be cropped by third parties, however laudable the ends in view may be. That human organs can be so treated is an extraordinary fact, but the activity involved should not be dressed up in terms which misleadingly suggest that *that* is all they are for. Only on animal farms could this be so.

Such evocative imagery prompts three further thoughts: First, harvesting is traditionally done in the broad light of day, whereas the removal of organs invariably occurs in windowless rooms under the glare of artificial light. Second, the harvesting of field crops was traditionally done with a sickle or scythe, the same implements used by the Grim Reaper, Death, to sever the thread of life. Last, something deeply important at harvest time is entirely missing here: there is no *Thanksgiving*.

Procurement is another of these unhappy words. Procurement is done by lawyers, to obtain objects animate or inanimate required by clients: land, goods, livestock, and so on. The term has undertones of weapons procurement for the destruction of unknown individuals at a distance. Historically, *procuring* has been associated with prostitution: procurers tote young women or boys for the gratification of lecherous old men. The procurer, or procuress, has been an intermediary between self-interested exploiter and victim. All usages focus upon the recipient's, not the provider's, wants and needs.

The word *donor* means giver, benefactor. In transplantation, however, it is invariably used glibly or fallaciously, to imply a gift where no gift is recognized. No reciprocation is envisaged toward the giver of organs. Discussion of the donor often undergoes swift slippage to the *cadaver*,[27] a less emotive and more clinical word than *corpse* or *body*, as if some embarrassment or guilt impels flight from the notion of the giver and the gift.

Those who employ these terms reveal unspoken attitudes. Seeking to romanticize the endeavor and conceal unpalatable truths, each term serves to cast the enterprise in a more positive light. Each usage in its own way serves also to devalue, even deny, the humanity of the donor—denying in the process the humanity we all possess.

In this discourse, the enormous value of the donor's gift has been denied, lost sight of.[28] The donor has become a thing, a nothing: a means rather than an end.

Demand, Shortage, and Resistance to Donation

Let us return again to the most conspicuous parallel between past and present in the historical summary: the constant refrain of shortage. We know that over the course of several centuries, anatomical discovery and teaching by dissection were hampered by a chronic shortage of corpses on which to work. Shortage was itself the result of a dual process, constituted on the one hand by the growing demand for human bodies for dissection, and on the other by very low rates of donation occasioned by public resistance to mutilation of the dead. The parallel with modern circumstances is manifest: we believe we have witnessed something similar.

Demand

Since the inception of transplantation a generation ago, demand for body parts has grown prodigiously. Not only has the number of medical professionals involved in the area burgeoned, so too has the variety of organs and tissues which can usefully be transplanted. New discoveries have been made whereby old medical conditions have been found to benefit from transplantation. Experimental surgery extends the field. Some of this effort is certain to be wasted, just as it was in the nineteenth century, when doctors dissected the corpses of cholera victims to seek the cause of death. No one will know which new ideas work, however, until they are tried. New treatments, experimental work, specialist training, and professional zeal require human organs and tissues for their continued sustenance. Publicity has promoted public hope of benefit from transplantation, increasing patients' expectations and their demand for transplantation as a treatment.

Factors Influencing Shortage

Despite the growth in demand, the number of organs potentially available is limited. Resistance certainly exists, but other factors also serve to limit the number of likely donors. So, although the old relationship between shortage, demand, and resistance still applies, it has become less simple.

Only a limited number of organs for transplant can appropriately be taken from "live" donors. There are neither sufficient "dead" donors, nor facilities in which to sustain them. Although organs are generally obtained from individuals defined as "dead," their organs must be sufficiently alive to be useful. Individuals in this intermediate state must also be in a location conducive to the removal of organs, that is, in an intensive-care unit. These requirements severely limit the pool of potential donors, who are usually individuals who have received swift treatment for near-fatal head injuries.

Whatever the potential level of public willingness to donate—and we shall consider this in a moment—it has effectively been limited by life-protecting legislation. Road-safety measures such as speed limits and the compulsory use of seat belts have significantly reduced the number of suitable donors in the United Kingdom. At a recent colloquium in London, one speaker suggested that the simplest way to produce more organs for transplant would be to repeal legislation requiring the use of seat belts in cars, crash helmets for motorcyclists, and speed limits on roads.[29]

Many more organs would be available for transplantation in Britain were it not also for a shortage of intensive-care facilities. At the same colloquium, a doctor stated that in his own local hospital in 1991–92, six suitable donated bodies had been lost to transplanters because of a shortage of such facilities. Had even half this number been available in every local hospital nationwide, the United Kingdom would have had a surplus of transplantable tissues.[30]

For all these reasons, waiting lists for transplants are growing faster than supply, and unmet demand seems likely to increase. The medical ethicist Alan Weisbard has expressed the view that there may *never* be enough organs to meet demand, since even if increasing numbers are donated, more medical conditions benefiting from transplant treatment will emerge, and technical improvements in surgical operations and better medications will be discovered. Unless the genetically engineered pigs come up trumps, for the moment it seems we must contemplate a situation in which shortages persist.[31]

Resistance to Donation

The argument is often made that public resistance to donation is the root cause of organ shortage. This argument seems to have considerable influence upon legislators and medical journalists.[32] However, the small pool of potential donors, the impact of life-protecting legislation, and the shortage of intensive-care facilities reveal that organ shortage cannot be attributed solely to a failure to give.

Resistance to the donation of organs does exist, and it does contribute to the chronic shortage of transplantable human material. Those whose job it is to try to obtain consent from potential donor families know all about it. In public opinion polls, people express positive attitudes toward transplantation and donation, but agencies express disappointment at real levels of organ availability. Resistance is thus evidenced in the disjunction between what people say and what they do.

With few exceptions, in almost every known culture in the world, ancient and modern, postmortem mutilation has been regarded as something inflicted only upon the corpses of enemies or malefactors. Western religious teachings embody and have often fostered the ancient notion that the care of the dead body influences the fate of the spirit/soul, that bodily coherence is somehow analogous to spiritual coherence. In addition, special meanings are associated with specific organs, particularly the heart and the eyes.

As with dissection, the removal of parts from the bodies of individuals breaks deep-seated cultural interdicts against mutilation. Indeed, the argument has even been made that, if individuals can be divided up in such a way, the entire concept of individuality is at stake.[33] The transfer of parts from one human body to another compounds this breakage with the pervasive fear of the physical survival of the dead, which itself taps into and is evidenced in the vast lore, literature, and movie culture of ghosts and revenants.

Medicine has always been involved in matters of life and death, but the production of novel medical artifacts—dead body with living parts, living body with parts from the dead—is, historically speaking, a new departure which impinges upon fundamentals of human life. As Leslie Fiedler shows in this volume, fear of such artifacts has spawned a swarm of monsters, from Frankenstein on.

At the heart of resistance to organ donation lies fear. Some derives from the currency of very old human attitudes toward the body and toward the dead—fear of bodily mutilation, fear of inflicting pain upon the dead, belief in the sentient corpse, fear of retribution from beyond the grave. But much of the fear may not, in fact, be irrational. It may be based upon informed deductions from knowledge—both public and private—of the powerlessness of the "brain-dead" and of the attitudes, behavior, powers, and priorities of doctors and of the institutions in which they work. Possible donors often express the fear that were they to carry a donor card, in an emergency their own life might be considered less important than someone else's—that doctors might be more interested in their death than in their survival; that their body parts might be perceived by others as more valuable than their life; that they would be worth more dead than alive.[34]

The definition of death is itself the locus of a cluster of cultural difficulties, one component of which is a concern that medical definitions of death may not accord with reality.[35] It is not difficult to dismiss such fears as manifestations of irrationality. But such a glib dismissal itself deserves examination: the label of irrationality has a long history of being applied to unpalatable truths. These fears do have a rational basis. Medical professionals are under increasing institutional pressure to obtain organs for transplantation. Pressure is exerted by knowledge of the need for organs, patient organizations, television programs, newspaper stories in a largely uncritical medical press, by presumed-consent legislation in some countries, financial considerations, new techniques of "organ retrieval," and by periodic tinkerings with definitions of death. Knowledge of these pressures seeds popular doubt, and the public is not without justification in fearing their end result. Deaths have been precipitated before to serve the best of medical motives.

Like public opposition to bodysnatching, public resistance to donating organs does exist. It is even measurable to some degree. In the United Kingdom in 1992, of those who were asked to donate the organs of brain-dead relatives for transplantation, 30 percent declined.[36] Although this level of noncooperation is disappointing, it compares extremely well with the equivalent refusal rate for dissection less than a century ago, which was 100 percent.

Discussion

It seems to me that rather too much emphasis is often placed upon public resistance to donation, and rather too little upon the public's generosity. Do we look at the 30 percent who refuse to donate or the 70 percent who agree? Whether the pitcher is half full or half empty depends on one's focus.[37]

Anatomists and surgeons have worked on the bodies of the dead since at least the Renaissance. Transplantation was barely heard of before the 1950s, at which time the number of donations made for transplantation was zero. In the 1980s, more than 400,000 transplants were performed in the United States.[38] In 1992, the last full year for which I have been able to obtain official United Kingdom figures, 5,200 transplants took place.[39] Seen in its proper historical context, such a rate of growth—from zero to a 70 percent donation rate in forty years—should be recognized, understood, and appreciated for what it is: remarkable, astonishing, extraordinary.

It is here that the most crucial *difference* between the 1830s and the 1990s is to be found. In Britain, our current source of whole bodies for dissection *and* of organs for transplantation derives not from executed criminals, not from theft or from murder, or from purchase or from presuming upon the consent of the powerless. It derives from the gifts of individuals who personally, or by way of their families, have decided to give their own bodies freely and for the benefit of others. This remarkable change—unique in the history of medicine—is the fruit of *a process of evolution* which has taken over four hundred years to reach its present stage. We have seen that, during that time, many other means of obtaining bodies were tried and found wanting. Balance was finally achieved in whole-body procurement only by dealing honestly with the public and by appealing to people's best motives.[40]

During the historical period in which *transplantation* was successfully developed there was no pressing necessity to contemplate purchase, inducement, or coercion, because at that time the needs of *anatomy* were increasingly being met by public gift. To have proposed inducements or threats at that stage would have been absurd. Public appeals were made for organ donors, and the public responded. Had the response been like that of the Tudor, the Stuart, or the Georgian eras, only the organs of executed criminals would have been available; and the post-capital-punishment supply would have been zero. Few indeed would prefer such a scenario, in which doctors might once again have to resort to stealth and theft. Indeed, the public's generosity can even be said to have helped *cause* the present shortage. Without such generosity, the rapid growth in demand could not have occurred at all.[41]

Donated supplies of human corpses for anatomy have become adequate to the needs of British anatomists as a result of a developing self-reflectiveness within the profession of anatomy itself, a reflectiveness which has engendered a deeper understanding of the *limits to the benefits* of anatomical endeavor. The traditional primacy of dissection in the curriculum has been questioned and downgraded, and many medical schools now have a more realistic estimate of its importance in the making of caring doctors. In anatomy, the profession has, as it were, come of age. Transplantation is still a long way from this stage, being only just out of its first flush of youthful enthusiasm.

The great utilitarian philosopher Jeremy Bentham bequeathed his body for anatomy when he died in 1832. The dissection was to be done by his friend the anatomist Thomas Southwood Smith, before an

invited audience at an anatomy school in London: an entirely unprecedented event quite as singular as the "subject" himself.[42] The audience
which filled the tiered seating around the slab was packed with the old
man's admirers, including key parliamentary figures who had assisted
Bentham's Anatomy Act through its parliamentary stages, as well as
intellectuals such as Bentham's philosophical disciple, Mill.

A decade earlier, Southwood Smith had published a highly influential
article, "The Use of the Dead to the Living," which argued for the
requisition of the bodies of the poor. In the intervening period, however,
he had grown to appreciate the ethical implications of his own arguments, and had realized their error. Southwood Smith rightly foresaw
that the coercive nature of the new Anatomy Act would do nothing to
diminish popular fear of dissection; nor would it provide an ethical, or
an adequate, source of corpses for anatomy. He now understood that
the only way to achieve this ethically in the long term was to encourage
individuals to give their bodies by voluntary consent.

Southwood Smith, a physician and a Christian preacher, began his
oration by speaking of Bentham as foremost among the benefactors of
the human race, the very Newton of social philosophy. He paid respect
to the dead man's courage in bequeathing his body, and to his abhor-
rence of the prejudice against dissection. He spoke sympathetically of
bereavement, and of the natural emotional attachment toward the dead
body. Such feelings had their foundation in the human heart. In his view,
however, they belonged to that class of feelings "which require control,
and sometimes, even sacrifice."[43]

While he was speaking, a thunderstorm broke, shaking the building.
Between flashes of lightning, which illuminated both the speaker and
his subject through the great glass roof light above the slab, Southwood
Smith continued in a clear unfaltering voice. He spoke of Bentham's
desire to set an example to others to rise above their prejudice, and
asked how the public could be expected to sacrifice their own feelings
for the public good when the best-educated shrank from the obligation?
Requisition, because done without consent, ultimately fostered fear and
loathing against the enterprise. In enforcing requisition without consent,
he observed, its supporters actually revealed their *own* prejudice and
fear of becoming subjects themselves. Turning full on his audience, he
delivered a powerful broadside at the invited guests, the public supporters of requisition without consent, and at those he knew would later
read his oration in print: "It is our duty, not by legislative enactments to
force others to submit to that which we are unwilling should be done
to ourselves, but to set the example by making a voluntary sacrifice for
the sake of a good which we profess to understand and appreciate."[44]

No more apt or eloquent analysis could have been made upon an entire generation of politicians, philosophers, and medical professionals. His words, I believe, have stood the test of time, and they serve as a text for those who fulfill these roles today.

Conclusions

Our historical situation is one in which, through ignorance or haste, the terrible results of earlier methods of obtaining bodies risk being repeated again, in order to obtain organs. Shrill voices are currently being raised which seek to evoke a sense of crisis, so as to urge a revival of legalized coercion by

- resurrecting the notion of "lawful possession" by institutions;
- promoting "presumed-consent" legislation;
- proposing the offer of money for the purchase of organs or to induce donation; or
- redefining death closer, and still closer, to life itself.[45]

The history of whole-body procurement reveals that the long-term outcome of financial inducements was murder, and that coercive requisition, besides being unethical, was publicly reviled and resisted. Each policy had very long-term adverse effects on popular culture and memory, and served to perpetuate profound public mistrust of the medical profession. As for the *re*-redefinition of death, it is self-evident that that way danger lies. Those who promote such options, it appears, are either ignorant or negligent of the implications of their suggestions.

Failure to appreciate the social and historical importance of the gift of human organs and the proper limits of medical enthusiasm serves to allow such shrill voices the ascendancy. Our civilization has achieved a remarkable level of public generosity toward the public good in this field, a fact which seems hardly to be appreciated by the very profession which has benefited most from it. The poet-philosopher George Santayana warned that ignorance of the past condemns us to repeat its errors.

Conventional histories of medicine seek to convey a linear development of progressive improvement right up to the enlightened present; surgeons' stories about heroic surgery in the past serve to justify it in the present.[46] But history is *not* necessarily progressive. One view of the past, which we prefer not to examine, leads from the slingshot to the megaton bomb.[47] In the recorded history of surgery there have been a great many false turnings, mistaken theories, and also a great many casualties along the way. Human beings can choose paths which lead toward catastrophe. The purpose of this chapter is to help us look down the path before we take it. We have been by this way before.

The poet-philosopher Blake asked whether the Tyger and the Lamb could have been made by the same creator. The past history of anatomy serves to remind us that the surgical profession has both lamblike and tigerish potential: that in the past, the study of the dead for the benefit of humankind graduated to theft, secrecy, dishonesty, and burking. Enthusiasm for what they perceived as medical progress led individual doctors to ignore or disregard the derivation of the bodies on which they worked. The end result was murder.

There is a very real possibility that a kindred form of enthusiasm in our own time may have kindred results. Indeed, Renée Fox and Judith Swazey have observed precisely this in the present day, when they describe among transplanters an "almost predatory obliviousness" to the source of organs.[48] Ignorance in this field is as dangerous as complicity.

On the day I completed this chapter, a broadcast on BBC radio reported a controversy erupting in Germany concerning the number of specimens still being used in anatomical teaching which originally derived from individual human beings who perished in the concentration camps. Later the same day, I was invited to attend an ecumenical service organized by the chaplains of all the London medical schools, in thanksgiving for those men and women who had donated their bodies for teaching and experimentation in the previous year. No reader can fail to grasp the ethical implications of each of these modes of obtaining dead bodies for teaching medicine.

A society whose ordinary members recognize the value of the medical enterprise, and are willing personally to assist it without requiring bribery or coercion, is a mature and a decent society. Those who choose to *reject* the value of such generosity and such gifts are mistaken if they believe that a return to the old ways of coercion, secrecy, and stealth will yield an increased supply. Those others who cite "lawful possession" to justify removing parts from what are referred to as "non-heart-beating cadavers"[49] or who believe that presuming upon consent is the way forward should think again about what they are actually proposing. None of these other directions offers an ethical way for a humanitarian society knowingly to go. As in the past, overenthusiasm for what is currently regarded as medical "progress" may serve to threaten social progress.[50]

Historically, the only *adequate* source of entire bodies for dissection—reached only in the final line in the historical summary above (see table 5.1)—proved also to be the only *ethical* one: donation for which consent was freely given. This is the lesson we should accept from the past. Donated organs, like donated blood supplies and donated whole bodies, minimize public danger, ethically and medically.[51]

An ethical source of human organs concerns us all, not just the transplant community. This should not be a private dialogue within the profession, or even only between ethicists and the transplant profession. There is a strong *public* interest here. Life and death decisions should not be made for the rest of us in cozy committees behind closed doors.[52] The history of anatomy shows that honesty and openness with the public is not only ethically preferable, but is also safer for society, and in the long term greatly preferable for the profession.

The public good is best served by a historical understanding of the course, *and the pace*, of cultural change in this most tender area of human consciousness. Such an understanding allows both an appreciation of how far we have already come, and the resolution to keep our nerve. It is imperative for the health of Western society that the human rights of the sick without a future be balanced against those of the sick with a possible future. Each is equally human, and their lives are equally sacred.[53] We deny or disregard the humanity of the first at the peril of our own.

Notes

I should like to thank my colleagues at the Park Ridge Center for the many fruitful discussions which have contributed to this chapter; also Stuart Young-ner and Brian Hurwitz, who have commented on successive drafts; and Renée Fox, who has inspired and encouraged me. I would also like to acknowledge the support of the Institute of Historical Research, University of London, the Leverhulme Trust, and the Wellcome Trust.

    1.   See the chapters by Wendy Doniger and Leonard Barkan in this volume.

    2.   Margaret Lock's chapter in this volume refers to the currency of a similar view in present-day Japan.

    3.   Hare turned King's evidence (confessed and served for the prosecution) and was freed. Burke's public execution was celebrated with carnival by the Edinburgh populace. His corpse, appropriately perhaps, was delivered up for public dissection. The full story may be found in Ruth Richardson, *Death, Dissection and the Destitute* (London: Penguin, 1989), chap. 6 passim.

    4.   Other cultural influences were also moving in a similar direction. For example, the incidence of cremation rose from 1 percent to over 50 percent between 1930 and 1970. See ibid., 258–60.

    5.   David Humphrey, "Dissection and Discrimination: The Social Origin of Cadavers in America, 1760–1915," *Bulletin of the New York Academy of Medicine* 49 (September 1973): 819–27.

    6.   Artificial organ disaster is exemplified in the Jarvik-7 Heart fiasco studied

by Renée Fox and Judith Swazey, *Spare Parts: Organ Replacement in American Society* (New York: Oxford University Press, 1992), chaps. 5–7 passim. For pigs, see C. Meek, "Organ Crisis," *British Medical Association News Review* (November 1992): 16–17; "World's First Pig with a Human Heart," *London Evening Standard*, 11 March 1993; D. Fletcher, " 'Human' Hearts Bred in Pigs for Transplants," *Daily Telegraph* (U.K.), 12 March 1993.

7.   Even today, to accuse someone of being willing to sell their granny is a shaming aspersion in British idiom.

8.   Cited in Richardson, *Death, Dissection and the Destitute*, 175.

9.   Thomas Hood, *The Works of Thomas Hood*, edited by his children (London: Moxon, 1869–73), 4:211–27. Hood was author of "The Song of the Shirt" and a friend of Charles Dickens.

10.   See the chapters by Thomas Murray and Renée Fox in this volume.

11.   Richardson, *Death, Dissection and the Destitute*, 241.

12.   Writing many years later of his period at St. Bartholomew's Hospital, London, in the 1820s, Sir Robert Christison stated, "There was . . . usually a race between the relatives and the students—the former to carry off the body intact, the latter to dissect it. Thus dissection was apt to be performed with indecent and sometimes dangerous haste. It was no uncommon occurrence that, when the operator proceeded with his work, the body was sensibly warm, the limbs not yet rigid, the blood in the great vessels fluid and coagulable." Robert Christison, *The Life of Sir Robert Christison*, edited by his sons (Edinburgh: Blackwood, 1885–86): 192–93.

13.   For a fine discussion of this point, see Renée Fox, " 'An Ignoble Form of Cannibalism': Reflections on the Pittsburgh Protocol for Procuring Organs from Non-Heart-Beating Cadavers," *Kennedy Institute of Ethics Journal* 3, no. 2 (June 1993): 231–39. See also Robert M. Arnold and Stuart J. Youngner, "The Dead Donor Rule: Should We Stretch It, Bend It, or Abandon It?" *Kennedy Institute of Ethics Journal* 3, no. 2 (June 1993): 263–78. See also the chapters by Stuart Youngner and Laurence O'Connell in this volume.

14.   Renée Fox's courageous article " 'An Ignoble Form of Cannibalism' " attacks a protocol agreed upon by ethics committees at Pittsburgh, translating obfuscating language so that *planned terminal management* means the subjection of "patient/donors to inhumane and irreverent deaths, increases the suffering of their families, and exposes the nursing and medical personnel involved to new forms of emotional and existential strain" (p. 234).

15.   D. S. Kittur et al., "Incentives for Organ Donation?" *Lancet* 338 (7 December 1991): 1441–43.

16.   E. Hunt, "Fifty Transplants from HIV Donor," *Independent* (U.K.), 29 March 1992.

17.   T. Patel, "France's Troubled Transplant Trade," *New Scientist*, 3 July 1993.

18.   Arthur L. Caplan, *If I Were a Rich Man Could I Buy a Pancreas? and Other Essays on the Ethics of Health Care* (Bloomington: Indiana University Press, 1992), 150.

19.   Christian Wolmar, "World Kidney Trade Generates Huge Profits for

Doctors," *Independent* (U.K.), 6 December 1989.

20. "Remains Found of 30 Colombians Killed for Sale to Medical School," *Manchester Guardian* (U.K.), 3 March 1992.

21. A well-policed system of genetic tagging for all tissues used in civilized countries could help prevent this.

22. The case involved Dr. Raymond Crockett, a leading U.K. transplant surgeon, charged with serious professional misconduct by the United Kingdom General Medical Council after kidneys from four Turks were transplanted into private patients at the Wellington Humana Hospital in North London in 1988. In evidence, a former president of the British Transplantation Society said that, in Japan and Haiti, organs were taken in redemption of loans. See Wolmar, "World Kidney Trade."

23. V. Chaudhary, "Patients Killed for Organs," *Manchester Guardian*, 11 April 1992; M. N. Castex, "Argentina: Alleged Murders at Psychiatric Institute," *Lancet* 339 (2 May 1992): 1103.

24. Amnesty International Secretariat, "Executions and Organ Transplantation: Taiwan," facsimile letter from Shu-Hsun Chu, M.D., professor of surgery, National Taiwan University Hospital, 17 July 1992. The same kind of idea has recently been raised as a serious suggestion in the United States. See R. D. Guttmann, "On the Use of Organs from Executed Prisoners," *Transplantation Reviews* 6, no. 3 (July 1993): 189–93.

25. United States Information Agency, "The Baby Parts Rumor Erupts in Honduras," April 1993; United States Information Agency, "The Baby Parts Myth: The Anatomy of a Rumor," May 1993; V. Campion-Vincent, "The Baby-Parts Story: A New Latin American Legend," *Western Folklore* 49 (1990): 9–25. My thanks to Paul Smith, professor of folklore at Memorial University Newfoundland, who drew my attention to Campion-Vincent's paper.

26. The notion that the dead are being plundered is from Renée Fox and Judith Swazey, *Spare Parts*, 207. See also notes 13 and 14 above.

27. This observation was made by Renée Fox at one of our Park Ridge Center meetings.

28. Thomas H. Murray, "Gifts of the Body and the Needs of Strangers," *Hastings Center Report*, April 1987: 30–38. See also the chapter by Thomas Murray in this volume.

29. In March 1993, the King's Fund Institute held a conference on improving the supply of organ donors at the Cavendish Conference Centre, London. The event seemed to be intended to produce a consensus in favor of *presumed consent*. The audience, however, took the opposite view. The opinion cited came from a speaker on the floor of the conference.

30. Ibid.

31. This observation was made by Alan Weisbard at one of our Park Ridge Center meetings.

32. This argument has been the means by which requisitioning legislation using the device of so-called presumed consent has achieved passage in such European countries as Belgium and Austria. See C. Meek, "Organ Crisis."

33. The English philosopher Derek Parfit, professor of philosophy at Oxford University, made this argument in a public lecture at Senate House, University of London, December 1992.

34. R. A. Robbins, "Signing an Organ Donor Card: Psychological Factors," *Death Studies* 14 (1990): 219–29.

35. For a fuller discussion of reality and the determination of death, see Laurence O'Connell's chapter in this volume.

36. United Kingdom Transplant Support Service Authority (the distribution network for organs in the U.K.), personal telephone communication.

37. Arthur Caplan asks, for example, "Why has encouraged voluntarism failed?" and recommends a policy of *required request*. See Caplan, "Why Has Encouraged Voluntarism Failed?" in *If I Were a Rich Man*, 148. Elizabeth Ward, founder and president of the British Kidney Patient Association, demands presumed-consent legislation on the grounds that the donor card has failed to yield enough organs. Ward, "Waiting for the Call That Never Comes," *Daily Telegraph* (U.K.), 20 July 1993.

38. Caplan, *If I Were a Rich Man*, 146.

39. United Kingdom Transplant Support Service Authority, personal telephone communication.

40. Murray, "Gifts of the Body"; J. M. Prottas and H. L. Batten, "The Willingness to Give: The Public and the Supply of Transplantable Organs," *Journal of Health Politics, Policy and Law* 16, no. 1 (Spring 1991): 121–33.

41. The dependence of transplantation programs upon cultural factors, and particularly upon public generosity, is well illustrated in Japan, where levels of both donation and transplantation are low. See Margaret Lock's chapter in this volume.

42. Ruth Richardson and Brian Hurwitz, "Jeremy Bentham's Self-Image: An Exemplary Bequest for Dissection," *British Medical Journal*, July 1987, 195–98.

43. Ibid.

44. Ibid.

45. Arnold and Youngner, "The Dead Donor Rule."

46. Barry D. Kahan, "Cosmas and Damian in the 20th century?" (editorial), *New England Journal of Medicine* 305 (30 July 1981): 280–81.

47. D. Gross, "Rescuing the Past," *Telos* 86 (Winter 1990–91): 23–32, discussing the views of Theodor Adorno.

48. Renée Fox and Judith Swazey, *Spare Parts*, 206.

49. C. Ferguson et al., "Non-Heart-Beating Organ Donors," *British Medical Journal* 308 (23 April 1994): 1103.

50. For a dissentient view on whether transplantation actually represents medical progress in a U.S. context, see Renée Fox and Judith Swazey, *Spare Parts*, 208–9.

51. Murray, "Gifts of the Body."

52. The Pittsburgh protocol seems to offer a fine model of what to avoid. See Renée Fox, " 'An Ignoble Form of Cannibalism.' "

53. Enthusiasts for organ removal currently aim to redefine the moment of death in potential donors to suit their own views, and to cite "lawful possession"

as a pretext to remove parts *without consent* (Ferguson et al., "Non-Heart-Beating Organ Donors"). Remarkably, Elizabeth Ward ends her appeal for presumed-consent legislation in a U.K. national newspaper (see note 37 above) with the following passage: "Sooner or later we all have to come to terms with the loss of someone close, but it is far easier when we know that death was inevitable, and that all that could be done to save his or her life had been done." Ward's concern and sentiments apparently apply exclusively to the *recipients* of organs, not to the unwitting "donors."

6 *Thomas H. Murray*

Organ Vendors, Families, and the Gift of Life

Personal Statement

The realm of gifts was mysterious to me. I liked receiving them, and was quite happy to give them, to be sure. But some things about gifts were puzzling. What is so bad if you forget to acknowledge a gift? How can it be that sometimes we are obliged to make a gift? Why do I feel more constrained in how I treat a gift than in my treatment of something I obtain for myself? I may never have cleared these mysteries up had it not been for a bizarre case that inexorably drew me in. The case involved a man whose cells were used by a researcher to develop a patentable, and potentially lucrative, cell line. The man, John Moore, protested that a wrong had been done and, as people do these days, sued.

The Moore case prompted me to think about the relationship between medical researchers and the people who donate the tissues that make research possible. I concluded that the best way to understand the relationship was to think of it as involving a gift—a gift of the body. That conclusion turned out to be the beginning, not the end, of my process of understanding. To understand the ethical implications of such gifts, I plunged into the (relatively meager) philosophical and theological literature on gifts, and, more important, into the eye-opening anthropological and sociological literature. I found much there about the role of gifts in society in general, along with compelling insights into organ and tissue donation—the sometimes life-preserving gifts of the body.

No other research I have ever done has caused such a transformation in my personal life. Reflecting on the moral significance of gifts and their role in human relationships has provided new, and I firmly believe, more insightful ways of thinking about those relationships. It has helped me to understand better the limitations of the economic model of human affairs, an understanding reflected in my chapter in this volume. And it has sharpened my appreciation for the intimate and enduring relationships that give meaning and structure to our lives. I now know much better what gifts are about. But I'm still bad about writing thank-you notes.

If we were to have a widget shortage, economists would tell us how it could be resolved. What gets people to produce more widgets is an increase in the price of widgets. The ordinary workings of supply and demand in a market would increase the price and, hence, the supply.

We do have an organ shortage. Many people die for lack of an appropriate transplant. Economically minded scholars have a diagnosis and a prescription, but our public policies forbid markets in transplantable human organs. The effective price paid to a prospective organ supplier—typically the close relative of a young person who has died suddenly from a catastrophic accident—is zero. This is an insufficient incentive to supply organs, the economist argues. Surely, a price greater than zero would increase the supply, just as raising the price of widgets would lead to a greater supply of widgets. The solution? Permit financial incentives in organ recovery that would effectively raise the price paid to organ suppliers.[1]

In this chapter, I consider three proposals to introduce financial incentives into organ recovery: a "futures market" in which individuals contract to sell their organs after death, with a price of several thousand dollars per recovered organ paid to their estate; discounts on health insurance to people who sign over their organs to their insurers, which would be taken upon their death; and the oxymoronically named "rewarded gifting," under which families of organ providers would be given a modest amount toward funeral expenses.

The proposals to use financial inducements to spur more organ donations raise questions of two kinds. First, as a practical matter, would financial incentives increase the number of organs for transplantation? Second, are financial incentives in organ recovery a good idea? Or would permitting markets for organs so compromise important values that we would be justified in forgoing the lives that might be saved by organ transplants?

The first question is empirical. We do not know the answer, although market enthusiasts are confident that people will respond to money here as they respond to it in most circumstances. Organs are like widgets and cars and turnips and daffodils. They belong in the market, and they are affected by the same incentives that affect other commodities in the market—or so the argument goes.

But proponents of financial incentives for organs make an important, and dubious, assumption here: Do people really think that organs are like cars and so on, such that they will respond to money for organs in the same manner as for those other objects? One way to approach this is to ask how many widgets would be supplied at a price of zero. The answer, I presume, is few, if any. Yet thousands of organs are supplied each year, not as many as might be made available or could be used, to be sure, but a significant proportion of the theoretically available supply. People, that is, are willing to donate organs, and in that way organs differ from widgets.

In addition to examining critically the empirical presuppositions of market approaches to organ recovery, we should look at where the logic of the market takes us. In my case (and in the spirit of Jonathan Swift), it led to a modest proposal inspired by the arguments of the market proponents.

A Modest Proposal

One problem with the proposals to obtain more transplantable organs by offering financial incentives is that, even if these proposals were successful, the organs might still come up short of the number that would be useful. Dazzled by the arguments offered in those other proposals, I was inspired to think up a new one that has the capacity to supply all the transplantable organs that might be needed, in pristine condition, when they are needed.

The idea is simplicity itself: Have a lottery! It could take either of two forms. In the first (modeled after Henry Hansmann's proposal, to be discussed later), instead of your paying for a ticket, we would pay you. Furthermore, the fewer people participating in the lottery, the more money you and the other players would receive. In that way, the financial incentive is directly tied to the supply, and medical needs for transplants would determine the demand. In the second (modeled after Lloyd R. Cohen's proposal, also to be discussed later), you can get your ticket free of charge, but you don't actually receive a payoff until your number comes up. To be completely accurate, you would not receive the money yourself; it would go to your estate. In both lotteries, the people whose names are picked would become multiple organ donors—every

usable part of their bodies would be removed, painlessly and under
ideal conditions for preserving the organs and tissues. The winner, of
course, would never wake up.

The advantages of this proposal are legion. As long as enough players
are in the lottery, we would obtain all the organs we need, with the added
bonus that they would be in pristine condition. Many lives would be
saved; in fact, for each lottery winner, we would be trading the loss of one
life for the saving of several. All the testing, tissue matching, and such
could be done well in advance so that matches are optimized and waiting
is minimized. The participants would all be volunteers, so there could be
no question about whether the source of organs had consented to having
them removed and placed in other people; we would only be enforcing
a contract. Nurses and doctors would not have to confront families with
messy choices about whether to release the organs of their newly dead
relatives; everything would be signed and sealed in advance, and the
family would have nothing to say about it.

The reader might be wondering by now whether I am serious about
this proposal, whether I think such an organ-taking lottery would be a
good thing. To put any such doubt to rest, let me say that I think this
would be a terrible idea. It is an idea, however, entirely in the spirit of
other proposals to increase the organ supply with financial inducements.
It follows the logic of the marketplace into its darkest corners, certainly,
but I do not believe that it distorts that logic. This "modest proposal"
builds upon three key commitments in market ideology: a firm belief in
the power of money to motivate people, a strong tilt toward a morality in
which the highest goal is to increase overall wealth, and a commitment
to the ultimate importance of individual choice as both a fundamental
moral warrant and the best way to achieve Pareto's optimal outcomes,
that is, a distribution of goods and services in which it would be possible
to make someone better off without making anyone else worse off. I offer
this with tongue firmly in cheek, though not as a parody or humorous
exaggeration, because I do not believe that it is much of an exaggeration.
I offer it, rather, to suggest in a provocative way where the economic
analysis of organ recovery goes wrong. It goes wrong, in the first place,
because of the way in which it frames the problem.

Framing the Problem of an Organ Shortage
from the Economic Point of View

Taking organs from one human body and placing them in another is
anything but a simple and straightforward business transaction. The
acts of recovering and transplanting human organs have profound

psychological, social, religious, and even mythological dimensions. I may ponder whether to get strawberries or raspberries at the grocers. The choice of what car to buy could have important financial and safety implications for me, as well as provoking questions of self-identity (a snappy, youthful Miata? a sleek and elegant Cadillac? or a safe and practical Taurus or Accord?). But none of these economic decisions seems to have much in common with the decision of whether to pass on my own or a deceased family member's organs and tissues to someone else, quite possibly an anonymous stranger.

Or do they? The three proposals I examine here all take the market as an appropriate framework for thinking about organ recovery. The intuitive appeal of a market solution is strong. Markets celebrate individual preference and choice. In ideal markets, people make their own decisions and live with the consequences of those decisions, so the theory goes. Consent and choice are powerful moral warrants, reasons for judging that a particular action, such as holding people accountable for the consequences of their choices, is morally justified. In theory, markets also effectively maximize wealth—the sum total of goods in a society. If a particular transaction would make both of us better off, then in a free market we are inclined and able to make it. People with organs to spare—their own or their dead relatives'—might well consider themselves better off if they trade those organs for cash, while on the other side, a person dying for lack of those same organs might well consider himself much better off with less money but with a healthy heart or liver or lung or pancreas. Making the trade—cash for flesh— would be, in the economist's lingo, a Pareto-optimizing move.

Their close allegiances with some popular moral ideas, coupled with their ideological resonances and enormous flexibility, have made economic analyses of social issues pervasive and important, but they are not necessarily insightful or useful guides to understanding and action. Economic analysis is not merely a set of neutral analytic tools but rather a prism through which to view the world. Whether that prism allows us to see more clearly or obscures our vision of organ recovery is an open question. I will try to illuminate the matter with a close and careful reading of the three proposals, especially the first two, by Cohen and Hansmann, which are clearer, bolder, and more radical than the third, by Thomas G. Peters.

My concern is that framing the problem of an organ shortage in economic terms distorts our vision. It picks out a few features and disguises or obscures other, vital ones. In the culture of the contemporary United States, where the market plays such a dominant role, thinking of any shortage in economic terms—including a shortage of transplantable organs—seems intuitively plausible. The presumptions are largely hidden behind a facade of what appears to be neutral, technical analyses—a facade that can best be penetrated by closely examining the analyses themselves to reveal what lies behind. It is important to see first whether organ recovery and the human beliefs and practices important to it are described adequately. Then we will be better prepared to ask whether the economists' solutions are morally defensible.

The first issue, then, is whether an economic analysis provides us with a full and faithful description of the problem. Does it capture the features that strike us as important? Does it distort our understanding of the situation? Does it leave anything of importance out? When the proposal moves from description to prescription, do the inadequacies of the description infect the prescription? In what ways? The best, indeed the only, way to answer these questions is in the context of the specific proposals. I believe that framing organ recovery in market terms misses much that is humanly important. If the description/diagnosis is badly flawed, then we can have no confidence in the proffered cure.

Three Proposals to Increase Organ Recovery by Financial Incentives

Lloyd R. Cohen, a lawyer and economist, proposes a futures market in transplantable organs.[2] Henry Hansmann, a professor of law, proposes that people willing to have their organs taken be given a reduction in their health insurance premiums.[3] Thomas G. Peters, a transplant and general surgeon, proposes that families of deceased persons whose organs are taken be given a "death benefit."[4] What the three proposals have in common is the conviction that financial inducements are appropriate and likely to be effective means of increasing the supply of transplantable organs. Before examining their assumptions, consider the bare bones of their proposals.

Cohen is not bashful in proclaiming the virtues of a market: "A cash market in transplantable organs would prevent much needless death and suffering."[5] He suggests a futures market in which individuals would contract to make their organs available after death—in his words, make a "prospective contingent sale"—with various sums to be paid to their estate for each organ and tissue successfully recovered. Hospitals would become "bailees" of the newly dead body, "required to take as much care with it as with his wallet and watch."[6] Hospitals that fail in their legal duties would be sued for negligence. The family's role? "Should some doctors still feel inclined to ask the relatives of the deceased for permission, and acquiesce in a negative response, they will receive a sharp blow to their wallet when they are successfully sued by another relative who is the named beneficiary under the organ sales contract; such requests for permission will quickly become extinct."[7]

Cohen's "ballpark estimates" for the value of major organs is five thousand dollars apiece; for other tissues, such as corneas, skin, and bone marrow, lesser amounts should suffice. He considers briefly other barriers to organ recovery but concludes unsurprisingly that the "problem . . . is not at bottom psychological and religious: it is economic."[8] His solution is to give people unambiguous property rights in their own bodies and to establish a cash market in futures rights for human organs.

Hansmann appears to share Cohen's faith in markets, although he structures his plan quite differently. Hansmann proposes that health insurers purchase the right to claim organs and tissues from the newly dead by offering in exchange a small reduction on insurance premiums. When people fill out their insurance forms, they could check off a box that promises them a slightly lower annual premium in return for surrendering ownership of their organs after death to whatever organization holds the rights to them. Hansmann estimates the amount of the reduction at roughly ten dollars per year.[9] He would permit a secondary market in organ rights, so that insurers could sell them to some sort of broker. A national registry of those who have sold their rights would be established and, presumably, before a physician could disconnect a brain-dead individual from respirators, IVs, and the like, he or she would have to get clearance from the manager of the registry. If a broker owned the rights to the decedent's organs, then organ-preserving measures would have to be continued until the organs could be removed from the body.

Hansmann is more modest about the virtues of a market in transplantable organs than Cohen is. Assessing the likely success of such a market, he writes: "It is at least possible, however (though by no means certain), that overall donation rates would be significantly higher under such an approach than they are, or could easily be brought to be, under the current regime."[10] He admits that it "would be foolish to suggest that the market offers a magic solution," but he asserts that "the present blanket prohibition on any form of payment seems extreme." He concludes that "there is a good case for reforming federal and state law to permit judicious experimentation with suitably regulated markets both to procure and to distribute human organs."[11]

Peters, a physician, has a much simpler plan. Rather than instituting a market or reorganizing the current system of organ-procurement organizations, Peters would have organ-procurement organizations offer each potential donor family one thousand dollars, described as a death benefit, and contingent upon successful recovery of at least some organs. He claims that his plan, far from commercializing transplantable organs, could actually discourage markets in organs, by increasing the supply of inexpensive ones. Like Hansmann, he would like to see his idea put to the test: "Unless proven otherwise by soundly designed pilot programs, I submit that a death benefit payment would save lives that are now lost, lives that should be more important to us all than adherence to concepts and rules that we have promulgated ourselves."[12]

A Note on the Misuse of Language

Confusion in language reflects and encourages conceptual confusion. Each proponent of paying for organs refers to the sources of those organs as donors.[13] Whether they do this out of habit, for that is how we now refer to the humans whose organs we recover for transplantation, out of misplaced delicacy in not wanting to use such terms as *vendor* or *supplier*, or because they do not grasp the distinction between a gift and a sale does not matter. (These authors at least avoid using that execrable oxymoron *rewarded gifting*, a euphemism employed by others in defending plans such as Peters's.)

A donor is "one that gives, donates, or presents," and a donation is "the action of making a gratuitous gift or free contribution esp. to a charity, humanitarian cause, or public institution," according to representative definitions of the terms.[14] To promise someone payment for a donation makes it something other than a donation; it makes it a sale. Gifts and sales are two very different means of transferring goods, with drastically different implications for the relationship between the parties involved. At this juncture, I want only to point out this misuse of language, which stems mostly I suspect from an underlying confusion about the social and moral significance of gift relationships as opposed to commercial relationships. I will discuss the significance of the distinction in terms below.

The same ideological worldviews that give rise to the confusion between donations and sales lead to other problems for proponents of paying for organs. In particular, proponents encounter difficulties in explaining what motivates people to give organs and tissues. Thus, in addition to their shallow understanding of motivation in organ donation, market proponents may have fundamentally misdiagnosed the underlying problem of the shortage.

Accounting for Donor Motivation

The discussions of donor motivation touch on three major questions. First, what motivates people to allow their own or their relatives' organs to be taken? Second, why don't more people provide organs under the current system? Third, why do people oppose financial incentives for providing organs?

What motivates approval for organ recovery? Cohen, in his long article, actually has very little to say about why anyone would consent to provide organs under the current system. Look at his general description of why people do what they do:

> I would rather not serve on committees, grade exams, or clean public toilets. While extensive discussion with a psychiatrist might reveal the psychological or ontological root of my aversions and even eliminate them, that is hardly the most efficient way of overcoming them. I perform the first two noxious activities despite my antipathy because I am compensated for doing so, and if sufficiently compensated I would even overcome my deep-rooted neurotic aversion to human excrement and perform the third task as well. . . . [In a poll, prospective donors] were unwilling to donate because they were being asked to assume costs without being offered a sufficient compensating benefit.[15]

According to Cohen, consenting to donate my own or my relative's organs is a "noxious activity" just like serving on committees, grading exams, or cleaning public toilets. And just as with those other noxious activities, the way to motivate people to provide organs is to supply sufficient quantities of the Great Motivator—money. Pay enough, and people will overcome their "neurotic aversions." Cohen has difficulty explaining why anyone would provide organs under the current system of donation. In the absence of money, what could move people to do such a difficult thing as donate organs? Given his assumptions, Cohen can have little useful to say. His basic strategy is to downplay the successes of a gift-based system and to bewail the failure to provide more organs.

Hansmann likewise has very little to say about what motivates people to donate organs. He sees costs, largely psychological ones, to individuals, but mentions no benefits to the donors. Money, again, is seen as the most important motivator. He refers scornfully to descriptions of the current system as voluntary, saying, "It might be more accurate simply to call it 'uncompensated.' "[16]

Hansmann does make a peculiar inference from the phenomenon of living-related kidney donations. He equates the risk of donating a kidney to driving a modest distance to work. Observing that people do accept such risks, for the right price, he concludes that the phenomenon "suggests that such transactions are efficient in the economic sense— that is, that the organ is worth more to the recipient than it is to the donor—and thus that there will commonly be a price that will make both donor and recipient better off even in the absence of altruism."[17] There may well be a price at which sellers will be willing to participate in the unconscionable "organ lottery" I described earlier, or to play Russian roulette for the entertainment of a perverse audience. Our capacity to find a price does not guarantee that both parties are "better off," nor does it prove that the community is served by permitting a market of that sort. Hansmann's argument is tautological given his premises, but it proves nothing once one questions those premises.

Peters has had direct experience with the current organ procurement system. He chides the reader for presuming that people are or should be altruistic when deciding whether to donate a relative's organs. He offers a cautionary tale about a prospective source of organs whose older brother responded to the request by saying, "I hated that s.o.b.! Go ahead and cut him . . . take his organs! Where do I sign?"[18] He allows that some decisions may be motivated by something vaguely describable as altruism, but reminds us that the motivation behind actual decisions may be more complex. Though he lacks the ideological fervor of Cohen and Hansmann, Peters agrees with them that money motivates, though in his case the decision is made by and the money is directed to the relatives rather than the would-be source.

Why do some refuse to donate? Cohen acknowledges three sorts of barriers to organ donation. Some people fear that physicians will hurry death along if they know the patient's organs will be used in transplantation. About what he dubs "religious and aesthetic concerns," Cohen notes correctly that theological barriers to organ donation are inconsequential for most Americans because their religions support the practice. He does not make clear what he means by "aesthetic" objections.[19] Finally, he cites as a barrier people's unwillingness to think about their own death.[20] To no one's astonishment, he diagnoses the failure as "fundamentally economic." The people involved in donating "all lacked sufficient incentive to carry out their assigned tasks in shifting these vital organs from those who no longer required them to those who had a vital need for them."[21] Given his conception of human motivation, Cohen could not have concluded otherwise. Weighing against the decision to donate organs—a "noxious activity"—are aversions, at least some of them neurotic or otherwise irrational. With enough money, the balance will shift. The aversions may be quite strong, and it could take substantial sums to overcome them.

Hansmann sees it differently. He offers a similar account of human motivation and the role of financial inducements, but he is offering people only an estimated reduction of ten dollars a year on their health insurance premiums; not surprisingly, he does not find that resistance to parting with organs is powerful. He argues that most people are not opposed in principle to donating their organs: "presumably they fail to donate only because of inertia, mild doubts about their preferences, a slight distaste for considering the subject, or the inconvenience involved in completing or carrying a donor card."[22] Choosing whether to donate an organ, in Hansmann's portrayal, seems about as significant as choosing whether to carry out the garbage or go to a movie. Inertia, mild doubts, slight distastes, inconvenience: this list does not appear to exhaust the factors influencing decisions whether to donate your own or your relative's organs. Instead, the list trivializes such decisions.

Peters suspects that the decisions of potential donors' families are affected by superstition, anger against "the establishment," and beliefs that the "disadvantaged in society are again being exploited." His proposed death benefit might tip the balance in some cases, he argues.[23] He is particularly concerned with "populations now giving the fewest organs, needing them the most, and being underserved by the present donation system."[24] Judging from the references he cites, these unspecified populations are African Americans, who are less likely to donate organs and more likely to need them, especially kidneys, than other ethnic groups in the United States. Because African Americans presumably are among the same people he describes as disgruntled and disadvantaged, it seems fair to infer that he has special hopes for inducing them to supply organs in exchange for the thousand-dollar death benefit he proposes.

Why do people oppose financial incentives for organ suppliers? Cohen offers the most original explanation for opposition to a market in organs. He cites the policies of three physicians' associations that threaten to expel members who participate in organ commerce. His explanation? "To the extent that [current transplant surgeons] have an adequate supply of organs to keep them well employed, restricting supply not only provides them with a necessary input at a lower price, but also, by indirectly limiting the potential supply of transplant services, gives them a measure of monopoly power."[25] Cohen professes he had to overcome a "naive faith in the beneficence of physicians" in order to suspect the monopolistic "knavish motives" behind their opposition to organ sales. One does not have to believe that surgeons are saints to find Cohen's account implausible on this point. I have yet to meet a transplant surgeon who did not complain loudly and at length about the shortage of organs and the crying need to do something about it. Transplant surgeons suspicious of organ markets seem to have the same roots for their opposition as most people who oppose these markets: concerns about the inappropriateness of commerce in vital human organs, concerns about justice, a feel for the awesome nature of such gifts, and some uneasiness about shutting families out of the process.

Having disposed of surgeons who dislike organ markets, Cohen takes on the rest of us. He accuses us of holding "widely shared beliefs and values hostile to trafficking in human body parts" that rest on "misleading and outdated ethical metaphors and analogies."[26] He describes four kinds of transactions for which a market might be considered morally objectionable: sales that degrade the seller, such as selling oneself into slavery; sales in which only the wealthy can purchase what we believe should be available equally to all; sales of what a person does not own, with children as a possible example (though Cohen appears to be sympathetic to the idea of a market in children); and sales of what cannot be sold without being transformed into something inferior, such as transforming friendship into paid companionship.[27] He judges all these possible objections to organ sales as either wrongheaded or irrelevant.

Hansmann is less interested in general opposition to the sort of market he proposes than in whether it would work in practice. He grants the possibility that true donations might dry up if people saw a market for their organs, and that fewer organs might actually be supplied. Despite citing evidence that payment may depress blood donations, his faith in the market triumphs, although cautiously. He worries also that some people whose organs might have become available under the current system would not check the appropriate box and hence be unavailable in his market, or that people would be afraid that doctors and hospitals, now having a financial incentive to acquire organs, would be "less than zealous in sustaining life."[28] Hansmann also acknowledges the opposition to commodifying organs but complains that he cannot "find a clear statement of precisely what is meant by commodification or why it is undesirable."[29]

Peters worries that our emphasis on altruism and our opposition to financial incentives may mean "imposing our own values on persons who may not appreciate those values at all. We may be coercing some families to accept concepts foreign to them at a time of great personal loss."[30] In response to the complaint that paying for organs would benefit the rich disproportionately, he once again emphasizes what he perceives to be the advantage to minority patients in need of organs. He cites evidence that transplanted kidneys survive best in patients of the same race, and that certain categories of patients, such as "immunologically sensitized black women," have great difficulty finding compatible donor organs. He argues that "black cadaveric donors, who might match with such recipients, are being lost with the current organ donation process."[31]

The three pleas for financial incentives give very flimsy and unconvincing accounts of why people donate organs and why they object to markets for them. Cohen and Hansmann give the standard economist's account of humans as individualistic, more-or-less rational pursuers of their own satisfaction. (Unlike more modest economists, who regard their theories as reasonable accounts of how markets operate in the world, Cohen and Hansmann appear to take the more radical stance of wanting to turn the entire world into a market.) This understanding of human nature must attempt to explain away nonmarket transactions. Hansmann does this most clearly.

Hansmann tries to explain why people object to selling children. He argues that such sales incur "substantial external costs or benefits that cannot be internalized without excessive transaction costs."[32] This market defect, he claims, prompts societies to make parents "internalize a set of norms that induce them to provide care for their children whether or not they feel that what they get in return yields them adequate compensation."[33] Ethics, in this case the moral obligations of parents to their children, constitutes nothing more than a second-best response to market failure.

Hansmann continues this theme, asserting that another "reason for using norms of right and obligation rather than market exchange to govern a set of transactions is that the cost of employing market mechanisms would be high relative to the value of the transactions involved."[34] What sort of transactions does he have in mind? Those within families and among friends and co-workers. We use ethics rather than cash in these relationships because "establishing prices for all such transactions would be unduly complex and time-consuming."[35] In other words, the reason I didn't charge my children every time I fed and burped them or, when they grew older, helped them with their homework, hugged and kissed them, or comforted them when they cried was either that the transaction costs were too high or that the "value of the transactions" was too low to justify the costs of establishing a market.

I feel that I have just paid a brief visit to Wonderland. I do not doubt for a moment that a creative scholar can give an account in economic terms of the entirety of human affairs. The concepts economists use are sufficiently powerful and flexible that they can wrap themselves around just about anything. But we must be careful not to confuse the ability to tell a Kiplingesque "just-so story"—how the camel got its hump; why we don't let parents sell their babies—with an authentic, persuasive, and insightful explanation.

The economic story of my relationship with my child has got it absolutely backward. The value of the transactions between my children and myself is not only high but incommensurable with the market transactions I conduct outside the family. Further, in a very important sense, the point of participating in market transactions is to provide the material necessities that permit humanly valuable relationships to survive and flourish.

Hansmann offers his economic theory of morality: "It is advantageous to assign as many transactions as possible to the category of market transactions since this 'economizes' on morality. Where the 'invisible hand' of the market works well in advancing social welfare, there is no reason to expend the substantial social effort necessary to develop and inculcate a (possibly very elaborate and perhaps rather rigid) set of norms to guide transactions."[36] Make no mistake about it: this is a bizarre account of morality, however internally consistent it may be with the economic view of the world. Perhaps its greatest intellectual flaw is that it presumes exactly what must be shown. It presumes that the economist's model of human nature is not merely plausible or useful in understanding certain phenomena but also fundamentally and exclusively correct. It presumes that the only valid measure of human flourishing is the maximization of wealth measurable by the economist's own instruments. And it presumes that the only source of value is money.

An Alternative Perspective on Markets, Justice, and Organs

In their most recent book on organ transplantation, Renée C. Fox and Judith P. Swazey place the current enthusiasm for market approaches in context.[37] The 1980s witnessed the first explicitly commercial endeavor in the United States to buy and sell organs. The International Kidney Exchange, Inc., established by Dr. H. Barry Jacobs, planned to import kidneys from poor countries and sell them to Americans.[38] Jacobs's plan quickly evoked resounding condemnation both from professional groups and from the U.S. Congress. Nonetheless, by the end of the 1980s and into the early 1990s, the idea of market incentives for organ procurement had reemerged. Fox and Swazey argue that "it is more than coincidental that a market approach to organ donation gained momentum during the 1980s, a decade when a certain view of the market has not only become more prominent and 'attractive' in the economic sector of American society" but has become more prominent in other spheres as well.[39]

The market analysis of organ recovery is seductive because it seems like such a realistic and sensible approach, especially in light of our recent political history. It evokes many of our culture's values and assumptions: autonomy, liberty, and private property; a belief in the power of money as a motivator; and a view of markets as fair and efficient institutions for producing and distributing goods. Market advocates like Cohen and Hansmann take the moral and practical superiority of markets for granted, and they assume that all other schemes for producing and distributing goods are second-best, if that (recall Hansmann's ideas about morality as a regulator of human behavior).

Money may well be the dominant good in American culture at this time, and markets may be widely used to distribute goods,[40] but there are many goods that money should not be able to buy, and for which the market is not the appropriate system of distribution. To name only a few, we should not be able to purchase a desired legal verdict, a Pulitzer Prize, or a child. These and many other goods have a meaning and value that places them outside the market. What we need is an alternative interpretation of goods and the principles by which goods are distributed among people; an interpretation that captures more faithfully the complexity of our most deeply held ideas about the meanings of those goods and about distributive justice. One promising interpretation is found in the work of Michael Walzer.

Walzer's theory of justice as complex equality is particularly helpful in understanding what is troublesome when all things are measured by one standard of value and when one good, such as money, dominates the distribution of virtually all other goods.[41] Complex equality is a response to tyrannies of the sort described by Blaise Pascal in this pensée cited by Walzer:

The nature of tyranny is to desire power over the whole world and outside its own sphere.

There are different companies—the strong, the handsome, the intelligent, the devout—and each man reigns in his own, not elsewhere. But sometimes they meet, and the strong and the handsome fight for mastery—foolishly, for their mastery is of different kinds. They misunderstand one another, and make the mistake of each aiming at universal dominion. Nothing can win this, not even strength, for it is powerless in the kingdom of the wise.[42]

Injustice in the form of tyranny consists in the domination of one social good over others. At different times in human history and in different places, the dominant good has varied, from sacred office to wealth and status by birth to political power. In the contemporary United States, the dominant good is money.

Also crucial to Walzer's theory is an account of social goods, ranging from membership in a community to security, love, office, and material things. Each of these sets of goods has a socially constructed and shared meaning, and each carries with it notions about how it should be distributed within its particular sphere. Recall Pascal: physical strength does not determine who is most wise and, therefore, whom we should respect as our teacher; the wisest may not be the best athlete, and so has no claim to prevail in the sphere of athletic competition solely by virtue of his or her wisdom. Each sphere is autonomous, and the goods within each sphere ought to be distributed according to the meaning of justice within that particular sphere.

Tyranny reigns when one sort of good is too readily converted into another—when money, for example, buys office. A market approach to organ recovery is not, strictly speaking, tyrannical in Walzer's or Pascal's sense. Tyranny would rule if the distribution as well as the recovery of organs were determined by money. (Market proponents seem to be sympathetic to a market approach to distributing organs, but they steer clear of emphasizing it, perhaps because they recognize that most people would regard it as a moral outrage.) The danger in an organ-procurement market is more subtle.

Financial incentives for organ recovery try to convert one sort of good—the organs and tissues that constitute the human body—into another sphere. Our culture has a long history of treating the human body as something distinct from commercial property. Though we make exceptions for certain replenishable products such as hair and plasma, we frown upon schemes to buy and sell organs or body parts. Imagine the public response to a wealthy bidder who offers fifty thousand dollars apiece for freshly severed human arms: we would, I think, block any such transactions immediately. We made a similar response to the entrepreneur who obtained a license to import transplantable human organs, passing no less than a federal law banning interstate transport of human organs for profit.

The dead human body likewise has been an object of great moral concern and social meaning.[43] Different cultures have had different ideas about what counts as respectful treatment of the dead, but few if any regard the newly dead human body as an object of moral indifference.[44] The Anglo-American legal tradition treats the body as "quasi property," a category that confers many of the responsibilities of possession with none of the privileges, certainly not the right to profit by sale. The leading book on tort law has this to say about cases dealing with the disposition of dead bodies:

In most of these cases the courts have talked of a somewhat dubious "property right" to the body, usually in the next of kin, which did not exist while the decedent was living, cannot be conveyed, can be used only for the one purpose of burial, and not only has no pecuniary value but is a source of liability for funeral expenses. It seems reasonably obvious that such "property" is something evolved out of thin air to meet the occasion, and that in reality the personal feelings of the survivors are being protected, under a fiction likely to deceive no one but a lawyer.[45]

I have some sympathy for the judges who ruled on such cases. They faced a difficult task. They had to adjudicate disputes over where bodies should be interred, whether burial or cremation would be done, the alleged stealing of bodies, and other such matters. And they had to rule with the legal tools at hand, tools better adapted for regulating commercial relationships. Yet their judgments suggest the understanding that the newly dead human body possesses a greater moral significance than mere commercial property.[46] So they were forced to come up with a legal category that captured, however imperfectly, the meaning and moral importance of the newly dead body.

I also want to reflect for a moment on the tort scholar's theory about the real source of the judges' concern: protecting "the personal feelings of the survivors." I think he is on the right track, as long as we take the relationship of the survivors to the newly dead person as something weighty and worthy of both our moral respect and sympathetic public policies. In this light, financial incentives for organ recovery can be seen as an attempt to transform the relationship that a family has to the remains of its newly deceased relative. The relationship is transmuted from one of intimate social and moral connectedness to something more like the relationship the owners of old cars have with their vehicles, which are now being stripped of still-useful parts in a salvage yard: impersonal, with the hope that a little utility and a little money can be extracted from the now lifeless hulk.

It is important to stress again the profound difference in meaning and moral significance between, on the one hand, such commercial acts and what they connote about the relationships between the custodians of the body and, on the other, acts of donation, in which families choose to make gifts from the body of their newly deceased relative.[47] Such gifts convey something beyond and other that what we think the now-dead person would have wanted, although respect for that person's memory and wishes is what one would expect from those who loved that person. These gifts may convey a sense that our loss intensifies our sympathy for other families who are imminently facing similar losses for want of a healthy heart or liver or kidney. They may offer some consolation in our grief, or a sense that our relative in some way lives on in another. They may permit us to affirm our belief that our relative's characteristic generosity (if he or she was generous) continues to enrich others' lives even after his or her death. I can imagine more meanings of the gift here. The point is that financial incentives intrude violently on these manifestations of the gift and on the meaning of the relationship between the family and the newly dead person.

Financial incentives for organs pose dangers of two kinds. First, they threaten to transform some deeply held conceptions about the moral significance of the body of a newly dead person. Those conceptions are relevant to whether we regard the body as a form of property that belongs in the sphere of the marketplace, to our sense about the meaning of death within a family, and to the relationship of surviving family members to the newly dead individual. A very practical reason also provokes worry about allowing money to intrude into such matters: to the extent that financial incentives misrepresent the moral meaning of the newly dead body, they may diminish people's willingness to part with organs—their own or those of their family members. Paying families for organs may inspire a reaction against the entire enterprise of transplantation, as well as increase the grief of surviving family members.[48]

The narrowly economic view of people and their morality is deformed, shrunken, and defective. It fails to understand why people value human relationships, how relationships based on and succored by gifts are significant, and what genuine human flourishing consists in. The economic view cannot grasp why people would donate their own or their relative's organs, or why people object to markets for organs. The solutions it offers are based on these defective explanations and are as likely to diminish the number of transplantable organs as to increase them. Even if they were to result in a modest increase, the social cost in values damaged and meanings distorted might be greater than the good of a few more organs obtained. But we do not yet need to strike this balance, because the prescription of a market solution appears to rest on a fundamental misdiagnosis.

Why Doesn't the Current System Provide More Organs?

The heart of the market proponents' proposals is that the organ-shortage problem will be cured by giving individuals and perhaps their families a financial inducement to provide organs. This diagnosis presumes that reluctant prospective donors and the families of newly dead persons are the principal obstacles to procuring more organs. But a more significant barrier prevents the recovery of more organs: health professionals.

Cohen himself admits that "the primary roadblock to organ retrieval was and remains the reluctance of medical professionals to, on the one hand, harvest the organs without consulting the next of kin, or on the other hand, to approach the next of kin with such a request."[49] If Cohen is correct on this point, then the remainder of his analysis is suspect. He proposes a cure—the market—for a problem he diagnoses as a lack of incentives for people to authorize the taking of organs. But he fails utterly to present a convincing case for why anyone would authorize organ donation in the current system, despite the fact that a majority of families who are asked say yes. To put it another way, he wants to provide incentives to people who may well not need them, knowing that other people—medical professionals—are the principal barrier to obtaining more organs.

Some evidence indicates that adding financial incentives would increase, possibly substantially, resistance among the professionals involved in identifying candidates for organ retrieval and talking with their families. Jill Altshuler and Michael Evanisko conducted a survey with health professionals likely to be involved in these tasks. They found very high support for organ donation among all the groups they surveyed, and a high degree of comfort in approaching families of prospective donors among most of the groups, ranging from 99 percent among organ-procurement coordinators to 80 percent for neurosurgeons and social workers and 59 percent for critical-care nurses. Still, every group expressed considerable uneasiness at the prospect of having to mention financial incentives. Only 20 percent of neurosurgeons said they were comfortable approaching families with this message, and even fewer nurses said they were comfortable.[50] Surely a portion of health professionals' reluctance to approach families about financial incentives is due to their recognition that money cheapens the event by attempting to transform a solemn social and biological occasion into a quasi business transaction.

If health professionals represent the primary barrier to increased organ donation, and if providing financial incentives may make these professionals more reluctant to approach families in distress, then a plan such as the one Peters proposes might well lead to a substantial drop, not an increase, in available organs. Whether the hostility of health professionals to financial incentives would be as devastating to the plans offered by Cohen and Hansmann is less clear. Cohen has no patience with them. Recall his claim: If a couple of disgruntled relatives deprived of a payoff were to file lawsuits against physicians who heeded other family members' objections, that would quickly dissuade other physicians from paying any attention to family wishes. Nonetheless, health professionals' reluctance to raise the issue of money for organs suggests that perhaps something that escapes the understanding of market proponents is at work.

A Preference for Gifts over Markets in Human Organs

It has not been easy for opponents of market schemes for human organs to articulate their case. In part, I believe, the difficulty may be caused by an undue willingness to accept how market proponents describe the circumstances of organ recovery, as if their descriptions were unquestionably accurate and thoroughly neutral, containing no value-filled presumptions. If we accept their descriptions and their characterizations of the terms of dispute—saving lives with more organs versus sentimental, probably neurotic, aversions to surrendering our own or our relatives' organs—discussion is over before it begins. But we have good reasons for not accepting the way market proponents want to frame the debate. Thus far I have tried to show how their descriptions are anything but neutral, unobjectionable, and accurate, notably, how they fail miserably to understand why people give organs without the prospect of financial reward. I now want to make a case briefly for framing the situation differently—as belonging in the realm of gifts and crucial human relationships.

The world of markets and contracts regulates a great many human interactions. But a prominent sphere of gifts also exists, intimately tied to establishing and maintaining important human relationships. The sphere of gifts differs from the sphere of markets in many ways. In markets, the contract specifies your obligations; once the contract is satisfied, your obligations and whatever relationship existed during the life of the contract may be terminated. In gift relationships, your obligations are never fully satisfied; each gift you receive creates certain obligations—to be a grateful recipient, to use the gift gratefully, and to reciprocate with another gift at an appropriate time. Although services, tangible items, or even money might be transferred in either markets or gifts, in the market the relationship exists in the service of the transaction; in gifts, the transaction is in the service of the relationship. Perhaps the simplest way to put it is to say that markets are principally about goods and money; gifts are about human relationships.

When a family member dies, we could take the market perspective on the body of the newly dead person and speak of salvaging the economic value from what will rapidly become useless rotting flesh. But this is not the only reasonable view. We could choose to take family relationships seriously at this time. If we did, we might find the survivors forced suddenly and drastically to redefine their relationship with the newly dead person. When we ask the family members if they will agree to donate the organs of their newly dead son or daughter, sister or brother, they might see this decision as one of the crucial, telling, and final acts with which they will accomplish that redefinition.

We can attach great importance to the family's struggle without becoming Pollyannaish about families. They may love the person who has just died, but they may feel a surge of other emotions as well: loss; anger at the person for leaving them or for doing something so risky that it caused his or her death; remorse for not having loved the person better; guilt for not having warned the person to avoid whatever caused his or her death. The fact that family members in all likelihood have a complex mix of emotions, not all laudable as Peters observed, does not lead inexorably to the conclusion that we should adopt a policy of appealing first to their mercenary instincts.

Why not assume that the family of a newly dead person has as powerful a moral claim to that person's body, based on their long-standing relationship with that person and on their need to work through their own acute grief and ambivalence, as an anonymous stranger who desires one of his or her organs? Whether or not the family owns the legal title to those organs, in light of the moral and emotional centrality of family relations, seems a trivial point. It is a point that gives Hansmann, who has the courage to deal with it openly, great trouble. He asks, What should be done when the family prevents organs from being taken despite the person's having received the ten-dollar discount on his or her health insurance? He sees three options: ignore the family, make them pay the market value of the harvested organs, or make them pay only a "refund, with interest, of the insurance premium reductions."[51] Hansmann believes that only the first two options respect the contract, but he realizes there "might be considerable pressure to accept the third." He recognizes that family relationships may have force here, but does not recognize why they might be important and legitimate considerations.

Human beings pursue relationships with other human beings because relationships have value and because a network of relationships is conducive to human flourishing. Gifts help establish and regulate those relationships. Despite ludicrous attempts to reduce such relationships and the norms governing them to economic principles, the market view fails to comprehend the significance—and the ethics—of gifts, just as it fails to comprehend what is important in social solidarity, community, family relationships, friendship, and love.

In his recent study of "acts of compassion," sociologist Robert Wuthnow explores how and why Americans show care for others.[52] In a culture that proclaims self-interest to be the only motive, caring for others is deviant behavior, unless it can be explained as just another form of self-interested action. Wuthnow demonstrates the shallowness of such a view. We now live, he observes, "in open networks of intimate associations and casual acquaintances," deriving most of our fulfillment from our closest relationships.[53] But our lives also intersect with many other people in "diffuse webs of association that tie us together. The caring we may show toward persons other than our intimate friends and family demonstrates our commitment to these larger networks."[54] Acts of compassion show "a commitment to those who may not be able to reciprocate, an acknowledgment of our essential identities as human beings, and a devotion to the value of caring itself."[55]

Wuthnow describes very well the function the compassionate life plays in modern society. It counters "our fears of the impersonality of modern life and the corruption and exploitation that can occur in a bureaucratized society" and "provides a way of expressing our concerns about materialism and its corrosive effects on human life. . . . It reminds us of our humanity and therefore of the deeper qualities that are essential to our common human existence."[56] Compassion reaffirms that "not all of life depends on efficient, large-scale organization and a productive economy. [Compassion helps to] create a space in which to think about our dependence on one another, the needs that can never be fulfilled by bureaucracies and material goods, and the joys that come from attending to those needs. Above all, compassion gives us hope—both that the good society we envision is possible and that the very act of helping each other gives us strength and a common destiny."[57]

Wuthnow's study helps answer the question of why people donate organs, the question that so befuddles market proponents. I have already described a family's decision to donate the organs of their just-deceased relative as a crucial event in the transformation of that family's relationship with the now-dead family member. Wuthnow helps us to understand why so many families see donation—an act of compassion—as an appropriate choice.

Proposals to use the market to procure transplantable organs have a certain superficial appeal to our preference for individual choice. But they miss virtually everything that is important in the setting in which such decisions are made: families struggling to come to terms with the death of someone who, for better or worse, has helped determine what gives meaning and form to their lives and their enduring relationships.

Families can and should be asked to donate the organs of their newly dead relatives. Indeed, I believe a strong case can be made that families have a moral obligation in some cases to do so.[58] But I do not think we aid families in such straits by inventing futures contracts or offering them a thousand dollars for organs. We are more likely to outrage them. Nor do I believe that we are likely to increase the supply of organs with enticements of discounts now or cash later. The economic analysis of organ recovery fails to comprehend the circumstances under which transplantable organs are recovered, the significance of the death to the surviving family of the newly dead, and the distorting impact of financial incentives on those crucial opportunities to begin to come to terms with the family's loss. A prescription based on a colossally faulty diagnosis could aggravate the problem.

Notes

1. See the chapters in this volume by Renée Fox, on the social meaning of organ transplantation, and Ruth Richardson, on the analogy of obtaining cadavers for dissection. Also see the chapter by Margaret Lock, who describes the Japanese aversion to commodifying organs.

2. Lloyd R. Cohen, "Increasing the Supply of Transplant Organs: The Virtues of a Futures Market," *George Washington Law Review* 58, no. 1 (1989): 1–51.

3. Henry Hansmann, "The Economics and Ethics of Markets for Human Organs," *Journal of Health Politics, Policy and Law* 14, no. 1 (1989): 57–85.

4. Thomas G. Peters, "Life or Death: The Issue of Payment in Cadaveric Organ Donation," *Journal of the American Medical Association* 265, no. 10 (1991): 1302–5.

5. Cohen, "Increasing the Supply," 24.

6. Ibid., 34.

7. Ibid.

8. Ibid., 50.

9. It seems ironic that Hansmann's plan would offer such a small amount of money, an amount we might well dub symbolic. The irony lies in the skepticism with which proponents of financial incentives regard what they call, disparagingly, merely symbolic concerns.

10. Hansmann, "Economics and Ethics of Markets," 69–70.

11. Ibid., 83–84.

12. Peters, "Life or Death," 1305.

13. See the chapters in this volume by Stuart Youngner, Renée Fox, and Ruth Richardson for discussions of the uses of language in organ transplantation.

14. *Webster's New International Dictionary of the English Language*, 3d ed., s.vv. "donor" and "donation."

15. Cohen, "Increasing the Supply," 11.

16. Hansmann, "Economics and Ethics of Markets," 70.

17. Ibid., 72.

18. Peters, "Life or Death," 1303.

19. In many discussions of noneconomic factors, economists often dismiss such concerns as aesthetic, and rely on *aesthetic*'s unfortunate connotations of "weak, arbitrary, or something relegated to a mere matter of taste," a difference that is unsettleable, perhaps trivial.

20. Cohen, "Increasing the Supply," 9–11.

21. Ibid., 12–13.

22. Hansmann, "Economics and Ethics of Markets," 67.

23. Peters, "Life or Death," 1303.

24. Ibid.
25. Cohen, "Increasing the Supply," 24 n. 82.
26. Ibid., 25.
27. Ibid., 25–26.
28. Hansmann, "Economics and Ethics of Markets," 69.
29. Ibid., 74.
30. Peters, "Life or Death," 1303.
31. Ibid., 1304.
32. Hansmann, "Economics and Ethics of Markets," 75.
33. Ibid.
34. Ibid.
35. Ibid., 76.
36. Ibid.
37. Renée C. Fox and Judith P. Swazey, *Spare Parts: Organ Replacement in American Society* (New York: Oxford University Press, 1992).
38. Ibid., 65.
39. Ibid., 72.
40. See the chapter by Margaret Lock in this volume for a discussion of this issue in Japanese culture.
41. Michael Walzer, *Spheres of Justice: A Defense of Pluralism and Equality* (New York: Basic Books, 1983).
42. Blaise Pascal, *The Pensées*, cited in Michael Walzer, *Spheres of Justice,* 18.
43. Thomas H. Murray, "On the Human Body as Property: The Meaning of Embodiment, Markets, and the Needs of Strangers," *Journal of Law Reform* 20, no. 4 (1987): 1055–88.
44. See Ruth Richardson's chapter in this volume for the remarkable parallels between historical policy debates (and debacles) over obtaining bodies for dissection and contemporary debates over obtaining organs for transplantation.
45. W. Prosser and W. Keeton, *The Law of Torts*, 5th ed. (St. Paul, Minn.: West Publishing, 1984), 63.
46. See the chapter by Renée Fox in this volume for a discussion of the moral significance of the newly dead human body.
47. See the chapter by Renée Fox in this volume for a discussion of gifts.
48. Renée C. Fox, "Regulated Commercialism of Vital Organ Donation: A Necessity? Con," *Transplantation Proceedings* 25, no. 1 (February 1993): 55–57.
49. Cohen, "Increasing the Supply," 14.
50. Jill S. Altshuler and Michael J. Evanisko, "Financial Incentives for Organ Donation: The Perspectives of Health Care Professionals," *Journal of the American Medical Association* 267, no. 15 (1992): 2037–38.
51. Hansmann, "Economics and Ethics of Markets," 65 n. 21.
52. Robert Wuthnow, *Acts of Compassion: Caring for Others and Helping Ourselves* (Princeton: Princeton University Press, 1991).
53. Ibid., 300–301.
54. Ibid., 301.
55. Ibid.

56. Ibid., 303–4.
57. Ibid., 304.
58. See Thomas H. Murray, "Are We Morally Obligated to Make Gifts of Our Bodies?" *Health Matrix: Journal of Law-Medicine* 1, no. 1 (1991): 19–29. This article attempts to distinguish the moral from the legal dimensions of organ donation, and it offers an argument that under certain circumstances we may have a moral duty to donate our own or our newly dead relative's organs and tissues, in the absence of any formal legal requirement to do so.

7 *Barry D. Kahan*

Organ Donation and Transplantation— A Surgeon's View

Personal Statement

The offer to participate in the Park Ridge Center discussions on organ transplantation raised considerable ambivalence in my mind. On the positive side, I had the impression that the effort might be fatuous without a clinician's input. My previous experience had revealed that many members of the group were relatively uninformed about the expanding need for and shrinking supply of organ donors, and particularly about the mechanics of the organ transplantation process. In addition, I anticipated that the sociocultural approach of the project might help uncover a "quick answer" to the public reticence to donate. I believed that, because of the participants' interdisciplinary backgrounds and varied yet knowledgeable perspectives on cultural issues, the group might strike a chord, possibly a magic jingle, whose timbre might generate public interest in organ donation. The parallel effort of the transplant community through the collaborative work of the Coalition on Donation and the Advertising Council was based on a similar supposition: We merely need to get the issue to the public in the proper form. Smokey the Bear is a well-accepted American cultural character; perhaps the "bouncing ball of sharing" could likewise be introduced into American iconography. My dream was that the group would unwittingly discover the American symbol for all that is altruistic in the organ donation process. On the negative side, I was apprehensive about the questions

126

raised by some members of the panel concerning current practices in organ transplantation.

The meetings revealed new conceptions of donation and transplantation processes and literary allusions to them. Could it be that never in thirty years had I made a connection between Mary Shelley's depiction of Dr. Franken-stein's actions and my practice of transplantation? Is there really a tyranny of technology? Are surgeons perceived as arrogant adventurers in this new land? I gradually came to understand that a difference exists between what I know defines a surgeon—that is, the shaping of the surgeon's mind through medical education and residency programs, as well as the excitement of discovery—and the opinions of the general public that are molded by the mass media.

The transplantation practice that the members of the group attacked was as foreign to me as it was to them: the surgeon was the swashbuckler, the pet of the media, the "fixer." Is this the image that has tarnished the public's perception of transplantation? Indeed, are the sociocultural impediments to donation intrinsic to our culture, or are they merely reflections distorted by the media's attempt to glamorize a specialty that is only emerging from its infancy? My contribution seeks to introduce the reader to the world of transplantation, a globe populated with many types of practitioners, regulated by unknowing but powerful forces, and imprecisely interpreted by media molders.

Although a decade ago I would have renounced the idea of a gatekeeper, the present confusion in transplant practice leads me to argue for an objective force to examine outcomes versus costs, limited supply versus unlimited demand, and clinical practice versus experimentation. I continue, however, to believe that overall the public has not lost confidence in transplant professionals and that we all have much to gain from careful consideration of the sociocultural themes revealed by the members of this panel.

The past three decades of the modern application of organ transplantation represent but one frame in the three-millennia movie encompassing mythic descriptions, surgical developments, and evolutions of immunological theory and clinical application. This single frame, entirely within the view of my personal experience, is worthy of further inspection because it includes the introduction of chemical immunosuppression. This conceptual leap in therapy together with the assistance of the public and its "id," the media and the federal government, markedly accelerated transplant technology transfer from the experimental arena to clinical practice. Although the medical and legislative communities accept the concept of brain death and provide financial resources to support the organ acquisition process, the public's response to calls for donation has unfortunately not matched these efforts. The limited number of donors has restricted the delivery of the lifesaving or life-enhancing technology of transplantation. Indeed, disquieting evidence indicates that the number of suitable donors is decreasing. Why has this adverse effect been produced in spite of the improved technology? How might the transplant community address these concerns?

The Transplant Surgeon

Several forces unique to the enterprise have an impact upon surgeons who specialize in transplantation. A scientific expertise in immunology distinguished most surgeons who entered this field thirty years ago. Their obsession with immunosuppression and postoperative care tended to surpass that of other surgical specialists, whose primary interests rested in the technical perfection of operative procedures. This concern resulted from a transplanter's experience that even technically perfect procedures were guaranteed successful only when grafts were donated by an identical twin sibling. Although Sir Peter Medawar, Nobel laureate in 1960 for his contributions in transplantation immunology, observed that the clinical success of organ transplantation far exceeded justifiable expectations considering its weak scientific underpinnings,[1] transplant surgeons had to accept the caveat that allograft rejection frequently vitiated technical efforts. However, even the most comprehensive knowledge of transplantation immunobiology did not confer clinical insight, a situation that has not improved in spite of three decades of intensive inquiry. Rejection processes remain multifaceted and unpredictable; in fact, not infrequently, even the "gold standard" of a tissue biopsy is inaccurate. Although legions of surgeons were vanquished by the uncertainties, imperfections, and frustrations of transplant practice in the 1960s and 1970s, a handful of workers sustained their interest through intense laboratory investigations.

Thus, by its very nature, transplantation is an investigative endeavor. However, because it frequently represents the only, or by far the best, treatment option, the procedures stipulated as proper for clinical research, as defined by the Belmont Report of 1978 (from the National Commission for the Protection of Human Subjects of Biomedical and Behavioral Research), tend to be relaxed. Initial clinical trials have generally been conducted in a therapeutic setting without preliminary Phase I studies, which assess toxicity, or Phase II trials, which establish the efficacy of the treatment. Can consent by the patient ever be fully "informed" if even the physicians do not fully understand the potential risks? Can a patient rationally assess the lethal risks of an experimental transplant procedure that offers only a modest, but also the sole, hope of benefit? Because surgeons empathize with the risks, they often treat their patients as colleagues by bringing them into the decision-making process and providing them with a high level of education, thereby sharing the burden of responsibility. Additionally, transplant physicians publicly honor their patients' courage in the media. This unique relationship comforts practitioners about their own uncertainties and therapeutic limitations. Fox and Swazey note that, "by honoring them, they [transplant physicians] offer patients symbolic compensation for their suffering and for medicine's current inability to dispel it."[2] Furthermore, this collaboration assuages the transplanter's concerns about the widespread sentiment in American society that clinical research involves misleading and exploitative physicians who act under the false pretense of aiding scientific progress.

Although some surgeons use animal models to demonstrate their scientific prowess, others challenge the limits of medicine and grasp personal prestige as "innovators" by claiming unprecedented, extraordinary benefits of new clinical treatments. This trailblazing represents an integral theme in American culture from the time of the pilgrims' journey to the American continent and the pioneers' venture across brutal terrain to establish lives out West.[3] Further, the presence of this theme in the transplant enterprise complements its team approach: a collaboration of individuals who—although from broadly varied backgrounds, "brought together by their suffering, competence, hope, courage, sense of adventure, quest for knowledge and meaning, and desire to serve— collaborate, in equality and trust, to realize distinctively 'human . . . noble,' melioristic goals."[4] Each success represents an individual patient's personal saga, an empiric adventure that establishes anecdotal guideposts for the team to use in addressing future patients. In contradistinction, a small cadre of "rigorous investigators"[5] emphasizes the uncertain and experimental aspects of new procedures or drugs more than the clinical urgency of their application. In the transplant arena, however, almost all work is experimental, because it generates new information as opposed to solely delivering treatment.[6] Indeed, according to such a view, even taking an aspirin may be considered experimental, because one does not always know if the drug will treat the condition.[7]

A rigorous design for clinical trials demands definition of inclusion-exclusion criteria, as well as a rigorous plan of therapy with well-defined end points. Because of the difficulties of applying clinical trial technology in transplantation, some members of the medical community have been reluctant to employ randomized studies. One of the most vocal opponents of randomized studies, distinguished transplant surgeon and clinical investigator Thomas Starzl asserts that "an insistence upon carrying out randomized trials before learning the optimal use of new therapeutic tools may discredit promising developments."[8] This statement may merely underscore the need for careful Phase I and Phase II trials that establish the guidelines for appropriate use of a new treatment, but Starzl claims that "a randomized trial is not an instrument of discovery, but rather a means of validation." He further cites Schneider's statement that "significance tests are more adapted to preventing progress than to achieving it,"[9] because ordinarily in randomized trials the significance tests "are concerned primarily with preventing erroneous rejection of a null hypothesis. Thus they reveal treatment differences at an error level of 5% only for very large deviations or with very large samples."[10] However, randomized trials can be justified if there is no evidence that one arm of the study is superior to another arm. A study can achieve appropriate power only if the effect of the intervention can be readily assessed; however, this represents a real challenge because the number of suitable transplant patients for any trial is limited and because the objective end points of patient and graft survival depend on so many variables other than the experimental protocol.

The potential of randomized clinical trials was demonstrated in 1983 by cyclosporine (CsA), a potent immunosuppressant which prevents or weakens rejection responses. Moreover, CsA represented the greatest boon to clinical transplantation since the introduction of azathioprine in 1964. The improved (albeit imperfect) results of regimens containing CsA were evident in a variety of treatment settings.[11] Its superior, reasonably reliable effects led to a precipitous knighting of CsA, in the belief that its vasculopathic side effects were intrinsically susceptible to solution—in due time. In short, the introduction of CsA brought transplant surgeons out of the cave and into the daylight. Unfortunately, it took a few years for our eyes to adjust and to see the long-term limitations intrinsic to the therapy.

As the success of transplantation improved, the demand grew not only for kidney transplants but also for heart, lung, and liver transplants. Unfortunately, rather than stimulating an intense and rigorous quest for even better regimens, the ease of CsA immunosuppression ironically released the frustrations of a "cult" committed to the mantra that *intense surgical effort* combined with *clinical acumen* could catapult transplantation from the discovery phase to the era of technology transfer. Fox and Swazey refer to this belief system as "ritualized optimism," claiming that it "blends scientific and clinical knowledge and judgment with a degree of optimism in the face of uncertainty that often seems to involve magicoreligious dimensions."[12] Surgeon Francis D. Moore has dealt even more harshly with this approach, saying that "it calls into discredit all of biomedical science, and it gives the impression that physicians and surgeons are adventurers rather than circumspect persons seeking to help the suffering and dying by the use of hopeful measures."[13] Those who had also studied immunology became a minority among primarily technical practitioners. The complexion of transplantation changed when considerations of quality were replaced by quantity, when imperfections were eclipsed by more spectacular technical feats ("stunts"), and when the aura of "good science" was exchanged for the halo of publicized "success."

The Media

Just as legends about transplantation offer rich allusions for literature, so personal health tragedies and the valiant efforts of medical professionals feed the media, who recognize in these modern circumstances a reawakening of our yearning for immortality. In "The Public, the Media, and the Professions," medical reporter J. Hollobon notes that "the very nature of newspapers guarantees their own shortcomings. Under the constant pressure of time and events, newspapers can rarely maintain the continuity required for 'education.' They are not designed to educate, but to inform and to entertain."[14] Unfortunately, members of the media are subjected to purposeful manipulation by a few patients who publicize their unsuccessful quests for extrarenal transplantation because they either lack financial resources or live in relative obscurity, and also by a few would-be surgical celebrities, cult members with pretensions to mythic status by virtue of legendary surgical stunts.

These "spin doctors" produced two spectacular press stories of 1992—the twelve-hour bridge of a pig liver into a dying woman prior to unsuccessful human organ replacement, and the short-term success of transplantation of a liver from a baboon infected with a broad spectrum of viruses into a patient who bore the human immunodeficiency virus. These "wizards" offered to prolong life regardless of the financial or spiritual cost; indeed, they claimed an ability to correct almost any disease state and agreed to repeat the transplant procedures as often as necessary to achieve their goal. Although some physicians felt that these attempts represented poor medical judgment, a flaw not unique to transplant surgeons, media loyalty seemed to be their special privilege. Perhaps because of their courage to do all that is necessary to preserve life, they embodied yet another popular American cultural theme—the survival instinct.

Although its initial response was awe, the American public (it now seems) was uneasy, sensing a failure to temper application of these new lifesaving therapies with humane and moral considerations.[15] Is this uneasiness responsible for the decreased level of consent for donation? The present cultural climate fosters the more frequent selection of euthanasia options by patients and their families (as evidenced by the considerable public sympathy for the practices of Jack Kevorkian) than of "heroic" measures like organ transplants. In addition, antipathy for organ donation has become a major tenet of the right-to-life movement. Thus, in my opinion, Medawar in 1968 put the transplant effort in perspective: "In the long run, the best quantitative measure of the success of clinical transplantation is the degree to which it does not receive publicity, that is, the degree to which we take its accomplishments for granted."[16] However, the media harnessed its affection for transplantation in order to proselytize the public to demand governmental support of the enterprise. This governmental intervention has at least reduced the number of carefully orchestrated media appeals by individual patients that result in unequal access to care, special recognition, and privilege.[17]

The Federal Government

The transplant enterprise has undergone unprecedented public scrutiny when compared with other medical procedures; for example, the moderately expensive procedure of coronary angioplasty was widely used within three years after its introduction, in spite of analyses that showed relatively modest long-term results.[18] In contrast, the federal government commissioned studies and held extensive hearings to assess transplant technologies, presumably because of the emerging federal participation in reimbursement. The government's commitment began with the congressional decision to ensure equitable access to dialysis and renal transplantation and to declare them both therapeutic procedures.[19] This legislation guided the lion of federal bureaucracy into the sheep's cage of immunological science. In retrospect, the resolution was amazing, not only because the government agreed to subsidize a surgical procedure regardless of the recipient's age or diagnosis, but also because the results were not worthy of, nor was transplantation in 1972 prepared for, this imprimatur. Not only were organ-recovery systems primitive, but the one-year success rates of transplantation were 60 percent at best, unless one administered intensive, frequently fatal, levels of immunosuppression.

Fortunately, the improved results obtained today under CsA therapy justify the confidence bestowed on the enterprise in 1972. The cost of the enterprise is high and is currently regulated only during the inpatient period under Diagnosis Reimbursement Guidelines, which set the fee paid by Medicare for the hospital costs incurred at the time of transplant. Recently, managed-care contracts have begun bundling entire one-year hospital and professional costs. However, in comparison with the ongoing expense of hemodialysis, any transplant that functions beyond two years yields cost savings for the overall Medicare End Stage Renal Disease Program. The governmental analysis of outcome based upon graft- and patient-survival rates for each transplant center depends upon information provided by the centers and is not verified by Health Care Financing Administration (HCFA) files. Seemingly innocent but certainly not insubstantial errors becloud the process. Indeed, a formal assessment of cost-benefit ratios awaits the development of algorithms that stratify important risk factors, such as recipient cardiovascular status and donor organ status.

Distinguished cardiac transplant surgeon Norman Shumway's declaration in a congressional hearing that heart transplantation is as therapeutic as kidney transplantation invoked the government's next foray into the transplantation arena.[20] The 1985 Batelle Report suggested that the funding requirements for heart transplantation did not exceed those of alternate medical therapies offered to end-stage cardiac disease patients. Government interest was justified by the 1991 estimate that heart transplantation, despite an average first-year cost of $170,000–$2,000,000, yielded a cost-effectiveness ratio of $32,000 per quality of adjusted life year (QALY).[21] Although improved, this value was still four to ten times higher than that of most other medical therapies,[22] but much lower than that of the artificial heart, which consumed a net cost of $299,000, for a cost-effectiveness ratio of $105,000 per QALY. The legislation entitling reimbursement for heart transplantation demanded that the recipient *already* be Medicare-eligible and that the procedure be performed at HCFA-designated transplantation sites, whereas the renal legislation conferred Medicare eligibility on potential recipients.

In its 1983 assessment of a National Institutes of Health Consensus Conference, HCFA proclaimed that liver transplantation is a technically feasible but extremely expensive and very complicated operation that can extend the lives of selected patients who suffer from a carefully stipulated cluster of diagnoses.[23] The regulations released in 1989 not only outlined a rigorous approval process for liver transplantation sites that would receive Medicare reimbursement but also stipulated appropriate diagnoses for Medicare-eligible potential recipients. As a result, they seem to have unintentionally shifted payment responsibility for the majority of liver transplant procedures to private insurers and to

Medicaid, thereby disenfranchising the uncovered majority of potential recipients.

With cost now the pivotal issue for the federal estate (considering prospects of universal health care), as it has long been for state governments, transplant procedures have been subjected to greater scrutiny. The Massachusetts Public Task Force highlighted this issue in 1985: "They [transplants] are extreme and expensive, potentially costing four to ten times as much as any other currently available medical procedure (based on comparative average fully allocated first-year survival costs); their introduction could distort the medical system to the detriment of higher-priority medical care; and organ transplantation has for the first time put rationing (by organ scarcity if not by ability to pay) on the public agenda."[24] The task force, then, recommended that organ transplant procedures not be performed if they diminish funds for higher-priority medical care and if the ability to pay remains an issue.[25] An even more radical approach to rationing health care by the state of Oregon excluded liver transplant payment for Medicaid recipients. Some physicians have suggested that the public distaste for organ donation is caused by high costs, repugnance for technology, or the sentiment that the procedure would not be available to the donor's family members if one of them were to require it.[26] Although the issue of accessibility might be addressed if a system of universal health care coverage were put in place, the squandering of resources may remain a nagging concern, particularly because everyone involved in the donation process, except the donor family, receives substantial payment.

The second arena of federal involvement in transplantation is the allocation of the restricted pool of donor organs. As early as 1969, ethicist Joseph Fletcher pondered the issue that today remains unresolved: "Shall machines or organs go to the sickest, or to the ones with the most promise of recovery; on a first-come, first-served basis; to the most *valuable* patient (based on wealth, education, position, what?); to the one with the most dependents; to women and children first; to those who can pay; to whom? Or should lots be cast, impersonally and uncritically?"[27] Moreover, organ transplantation is the only medical procedure that requires another human being to be a donor, thus creating a situation that involves the public from the standpoint of consent. With these issues in mind, four approaches to organ rationing have been proposed: (1) the market approach, (2) the selection committee approach, (3) the lottery approach, and (4) the customary approach.

The first, the market approach, advocates that "if you can pay, you can have it," thereby placing a high value on individual rights and a low value on equality and fairness. In the United States, the use of paid, living, unrelated donors, which are a major donor source in many countries including India and the Philippines, was prohibited by the National Organ Transplant Act of 1984, as was brokerage in organs. This action resulted from the increased activity in organ commerce during the early 1980s, as described by David Lamb in *Organ Transplants and Ethics*.[28] In the United States people were placing advertisements in newspapers, offering kidneys at prices of $5,000–$160,000. In fact Dr. H. Barry Jacobs attempted to establish an International Kidney Exchange that would buy and sell kidneys. The National Kidney Foundation denounced this plan as "immoral and unethical." During a 1983 congressional session, then–Tennessee representative Albert Gore Jr. also opposed the plan: "People should not be regarded as things to be bought and sold like parts of an automobile."[29]

The second method, the selection committee approach, is based on achieving the best outcome for the organ, thus also tending to result in favoritism and inequality.[30] Despite the rejection of a selection committee approach, socioeconomic factors undoubtedly influence access to transplantation. Wealthy individuals "know the system . . . they seek out evaluation for transplantation more effectively, and in so doing they access the system more readily than the poor and disadvantaged."[31]

The lottery approach, a third possibility, allows everyone an equal opportunity but does not utilize medical criteria; it can therefore become a mindless endeavor. Finally, the customary approach allows physicians to select recipients on the basis of medical criteria of clinical suitability, broaching the area of social worth.[32] However, it does not assume absolute equality. For example, one "medical" criterion is that the recipient has adequate family support for posttransplant care,[33] a policy the Massachusetts Public Task Force labels as discriminatory against those without families or with estranged families.[34]

The National Organ Transplant Act of 1984 established a national network, currently designated the United Network for Organ Sharing (UNOS), to encourage donation and ensure equity of organ distribution and expertise of transplant centers. Unfortunately, inadequate financial resources have prevented the Office of Transplantation at the Health Resource Services Administration (HRSA) from effectively implementing these goals. The as-yet-unresolved, but critical, issue is whether the slight decline in donation rates is due to a conscious decision against the process or simply to a lack of knowledge about it. Do some segments of the population perceive inequities in organ allocation? Do the poor refuse donation because they are convinced that, if they needed an organ transplant, it would not be available for them?[35] The issue of better public education is being addressed by an advertising campaign sponsored by the Coalition on Donation, which is a joint effort of transplantation centers, donor agencies, and scientific societies.

Several scholars have theorized that two key factors may limit the size of the donor pool: the number of donors who are medically suitable may be lower than first estimated, and a family's decision to donate may be influenced by the manner in which the request for organ donation is managed.[36] At the present time, the law requires that hospitals approach potential donor families for consent regarding organ retrieval, a process termed *required request*. Some groups believe that minority coordinators can address the special demands of their own racial groups, whose needs the organ donation process may ignore. Most transplanters see the major obstacle to organ donation as an inaccessibility to potential donor families, which could be overcome by "required referral," the Prottas solution.[37] Lack of access continues, however, despite required request, perhaps because many neurosurgeons are unwilling to "give up" on brain-dead patients, or because many nurses hold superstitious beliefs about donation, as described by physician Stuart Youngner, which lead them to resist donor referral ("shielding").[38]

Youngner proposes several interrelated reasons that many health professionals disregard required-request laws. For one, society reinforces the concept of organ donation as an act of spiritually uplifting gift giving, but retrieving these organs from a recently expired patient evokes far different emotions. Fears are resurfacing in society about medical science and the proper treatment of dead bodies, including a sense of repulsion at the notion of cutting them up and pulling them apart. Moreover, many health care professionals are confused about the definition of brain death, and they are uncomfortable with attempts to change the definition of death so that it may include anencephalic newborns or patients who are persistently in a vegetative state. Youngner believes that these "dark sides" of the donation process "fan the flames of suspicion [of the medical community] and paranoia" and that a "rebound effect will further reduce the number of actual organ donations."[39]

A growing, vocal group links payment to success in organ retrieval, calling for "rewarded gifting." This controversial plan would require a change in the law. Tom Peters, a transplant surgeon in Jacksonville, Florida, has recommended a thousand-dollar bounty to the family who gives consent for organ donation.[40] Would it be unreasonable for him to try the experiment locally? One can't help wondering if a recipient's chances for posttransplant survival might increase if the patient bore financial responsibility for his or her transplant, because a personal commitment to a goal has been shown to be stronger when the individual has a financial investment in achieving that end. Such a resolution would also provide an outlet from the debtor-creditor relationship that is especially manifest in live donations.[41] This aspect of financial incentives is further considered in Thomas Murray's chapter in this volume.

The Gatekeeper

Is it possible to establish gatekeepers to assess the quality and costs of transplant services as well as to ensure equal access to them?[42] The popular aversion to gatekeepers emanates from the historical precedent of committees that chose which end-stage renal disease patients were offered dialysis therapy. The gatekeeper function is now viewed by embittered medical and societal communities as similar to that of the *gauleiter* of concentration camps—to decide for others between life and death. Because patient plight drives the entire transplant process, it seems inhumane to prohibit a person from any treatment that may restore life or health. Fox and Swazey note that the situation has progressed to the point where physicians cannot deny a transplant to a patient, even one who is unlikely to benefit from the procedure, despite the complications and suffering it may produce. And yet these authors designate the physician as the final, albeit often powerless, gatekeeper in the organ exchange process.[43] One precept to guide us through this controversy is that the primary goal of gatekeeping as a screening process is to optimize the patient's chances for survival and to offer him as enduring, active, and meaningful a posttransplant life as possible without inflicting undue physical, psychic, or social harm.

Some members of the public cite instances of poor judgment by individual surgeons to argue that organ transplantation should be regulated in the same fashion as research, for its basic intent remains to garner new knowledge as well as to benefit patients. This group further demands that the social, ethical, financial, and resource allocation issues of transplantation be reviewed in a special process involving respected authorities from both a spectrum of disciplines and the community, not unlike the panel that drew up guidelines for the use of human research subjects.[44] This approach is unrealistic, however, because of the restricted spectrum of knowledge of medical professionals outside the transplant field. The disquieting conclusion is that only the profession has the expertise to serve as the gatekeeper. Perhaps the assistance or closer involvement of federal and nonfederal groups would inspire better analytic functions of peer review.

Some scholars are adamant that the medical community on both the local and national levels should accept the burden and responsibility of watching over colleagues.[45] For several reasons, the logical premise that the profession would undertake this task has failed. First, transplant surgeons are concerned that questioning any element of the field will sabotage the overall enterprise. Second, transplant surgeons are afraid of litigation instigated either by their colleagues for allegedly libelous statements or by embittered patients. In 1965 medical malpractice suits were infrequent; today, however, they are commonplace, and they add to the burden of rising health care costs. Third, transplant surgeons must remember that the *reviewer* of today is the *reviewee* of tomorrow because of the relatively small expert group. In his 1975 inaugural presentation to the American Society of Transplant Surgeons, Starzl addressed this concern:

Progress consists of a series of great and small revolutions against authority. A great advance necessitates the overthrow of an established dogma, and when that occurs the advance itself becomes the new dogma to which advocates flock. It is natural for those disciples to become *protectors* of the status quo instead of *improvers* of the status quo, guardians of the past instead of seeders of the future. To make matters formal, they might even consider creating a society which, if unaware of the dangers, could be the means by which the next stages of development were blocked.[46] (emphasis added)

Fourth, transplant surgeons recognize that criticism is frequently ignored. For example, the censure of cluster transplants by Dr. Francis Moore, formerly chief of surgical services at Peter Bent Brigham Hospital in Boston, had no effect on the enthusiasm for the procedure. Fifth and most important, few guidelines for clinical investigation objectively establish efficacy or assess outcome.

In light of these five factors, many would suggest that the gatekeeper be the agency that pays for the procedure. The "green screen" is not unique to transplantation; it is known that indigent patients are also far less likely to undergo coronary artery bypass grafting.[47] Is this inequity of access acceptable? Is it reasonable that each state has different aid programs—some with no coverage, others with funds for medicines and for transportation?

In the United States an attitude pervades that all people are entitled to health care and that in a country as affluent as the United States no one should be left untreated. Sociologist Roger Evans and others have claimed, however, that individuals must first care for their own health in a responsible manner by eating properly and exercising routinely, because often those who are in need of health care services have neglected to care for themselves appropriately.[48] N. Bell has suggested that if everyone has a right to health care, then appropriate contracts should be drafted to ensure that individuals keep their end of the bargain by caring for themselves properly.[49] Contract violations would be difficult and costly to enforce, but such a system might prove more efficacious than the present arrangement. The question then becomes this: What course will be taken for those who do not keep up their end of the bargain yet still require medical treatment?

Comment

The transplant process involves the surgeon, the public, the government, and the media in a synergistic relation that has intensified in the way a mild wind escalates into a hurricane. Now the only constraints are organ-donor availability and payment for the procedure. Whether the lack of donors reflects pubic reluctance regarding transplant practices or more subtle, superstitious, or operational obstacles is unclear. The field does, however, need a gatekeeper, a function probably best served by the profession, to establish recipient eligibility and restore parity between the extreme demand and limited supply. The development of this gatekeeper function will require intense study and utilization of the skills of those individuals who are familiar with supply and demand issues from the standpoints of economic and business theory.

Notes

The author is deeply indebted to Jennifer Senft for editorial assistance and to Melinda Mosheim for research assistance.

1. Peter Medawar, *Memoir of a Thinking Radish: An Autobiography* (Oxford: Oxford University Press, 1986).

2. Renée C. Fox and Judith P. Swazey, *The Courage to Fail: A Social View of Organ Transplantation and Dialysis* (Chicago: University of Chicago Press, 1974), 107.

3. Fox and Swazey, *Courage to Fail*.

4. Fox and Swazey, *Courage to Fail*, 381.

5. A. Cournand, "Chairman's Introductory Remarks," *Proceedings of the National Academy of Sciences USA* 63 (1969): 1018. See also Fox and Swazey, *Courage to Fail*.

6. Fox and Swazey, *Courage to Fail*.

7. Fox and Swazey, *Courage to Fail*.

8. Thomas E. Starzl, "Protecting the Patient's Interest," *Kidney International* 28, no. 17 (1985): S-31–33, quotation from S-32.

9. Ibid., S-33.

10. Starzl, "Protecting the Patient's Interest," S-33.

11. Canadian Multicentre Transplant Study Group, "A Randomized Clinical Trial of Cyclosporine in Cadaveric Renal Transplantation: Analysis at Three Years," *New England Journal of Medicine* 314 (1986): 1219–25.

12.   Renée C. Fox and Judith P. Swazey, *Spare Parts: Organ Replacement in American Society* (New York: Oxford University Press, 1992), 107.

13.   Quoted in Fox and Swazey, *Courage to Fail*, 189.

14.   J. Hollobon, "The Public, the Media, and the Professions: Perceptions of Reality," *Transplantation Proceedings* 22, no. 3 (1990): 1050–51.

15.   Fox and Swazey, *Spare Parts*.

16.   Quoted in Fox and Swazey, *Courage to Fail*, 74.

17.   T. Cooper, "Survey of Development, Current Status, and Future Prospects for Organ Transplantation," in D. Cowan, J. Kantorowitz, J. Moskowitz, and P. Rheinstein, eds., *Human Organ Transplantation: Societal, Medical-Legal, Regulatory, and Reimbursement Issues* (Ann Arbor: Health Administration Press, 1987), 18–26.

18.   B. P. Healy, "Organ Transplantation: Future Directions for Federal Policy," in Cowan et al., *Human Organ Transplantation,* 193–200.

19.   End Stage Renal Disease Act, Sec. 2991 of the Social Security amendments of 1972, Public Law 92–603.

20.   Quoted in Cowan et al., *Human Organ Transplantation,* 20.

21.   Fox and Swazey, *Spare Parts*, 152.

22.   George Annas, "Part 2: Background on Issues: Excerpts from the Report of the Massachusetts Task Force on Organ Transplantation," in Cowan et al., *Human Organ Transplantation,* 203–50.

23.   Annas, "Background on Issues."

24.   George Annas, "Organ Transplants: Are We Treating the Modern Miracle Fairly?" in Cowan et al., *Human Organ Transplantation,* 166–70, quotation from 169.

25.   Annas, "Organ Transplants."

26.   Arthur L. Caplan, "Problems in the Policies and Criteria Used to Allocate Organs for Transplantation in the United States," *Transplantation Proceedings* 21, no. 3 (1989): 3381–87.

27.   Quoted in Annas, "Organ Transplants," 232.

28.   David Lamb, *Organ Transplants and Ethics* (London: Routledge, 1990).

29.   Quoted in Lamb, *Organ Transplants,* 134.

30.   Annas, "Background on Issues."

31.   Anthony P. Monaco, "Transplantation: The State of the Art," *Transplantation Proceedings* 22, no. 3 (1990): 898.

32.   Annas, "Background on Issues."

33.   Fox and Swazey, *Courage to Fail*.

34.   Annas, "Background on Issues."

35.   Caplan, "Problems in the Policies."

36.   James A. Cutler, Susan D. David, Christina J. Kress, et al., "Increasing the Availability of Cadaveric Organs for Transplantation: Maximizing the Consent Rate," *Transplantation* 56 (1993): 225–28. See also R. W. Evans, C. E. Orians, and N. L. Ascher, "The Potential Supply of Organ Donors: An Assessment of the Efficiency of Organ Procurement Efforts in the United States," *Journal of the American Medical Association* 267 (1992): 239; United States Department of Health

and Human Services, *Organ Transplantation Issues and Recommendations: Report of the Task Force on Organ Transplantation* (Washington, D. C.: U. S. Government Printing Office, 1986); Howard M. Nathan, Bruce E. Jarrell, Brian Broznik, et al., "Estimation and Characterization of the Potential Renal Organ Donor Pool in Pennsylvania," *Transplantation* 51 (1991): 142; and R. Neal Garrison, Frederick R. Bentley, George H. Raque, et al., "There Is an Answer to the Shortage of Organ Donors," *Surgery, Gynecology, and Obstetrics* 173 (1991): 391.

37. Jeffrey M. Prottas and Helen L. Batten, "Neurosurgeons and Human Organs," *Health Affairs* 1989: 125.

38. Stuart J. Youngner, "Organ Retrieval: Can We Ignore the Dark Side?" *Transplantation Proceedings* 22, no. 3 (1990): 1014–15.

39. Ibid., 1015.

40. Thomas G. Peters, "Life or Death: The Issue of Payment in Cadaveric Organ Donation," *Journal of the American Medical Association* 265, no. 10 (1991): 1302–5.

41. R. G. Simmons, S. D. Klein, and R. L. Simmons, *Gift of Life: The Social and Psychological Impact of Organ Transplantation* (New York: John Wiley and Sons, 1977).

42. Annas, "Background on Issues."

43. Fox and Swazey, *Courage to Fail.*

44. D. Cowan, "Regulation of Medical Practice," in Cowan et al., *Human Organ Transplantation,* 105–30.

45. Cowan, "Regulation of Medical Practice."

46. Thomas E. Starzl, *The Puzzle People* (Pittsburgh: University of Pittsburgh Press, 1992), 134.

47. David S. Gaylin, Philip J. Held, Friedrich K. Port, et al., "The Impact of Comorbid and Sociodemographic Factors on Access to Renal Transplantation," *Journal of the American Medical Association* 269, no. 5 (1993): 603–8.

48. Evans et al., "Potential Supply of Organ Donors."

49. N. Bell, "The Scarcity of Medical Resources: Are There Rights to Health Care?" *Journal of Medical Philosophy* 4 (1979): 158–69.

8 *Margaret Lock*

Deadly Disputes: Ideologies and Brain Death in Japan

Personal Statement

I first became interested in definitions of death when doing research in Kyoto in 1988 on an entirely different theme. I noticed that a large amount of media time was being devoted to the subject of brain death and organ transplants and that the Japanese public was regularly being polled as to what it thought about this issue, a situation that continues today. Clearly in that technologically sophisticated, highly literate, economic superpower something is causing alarm that has apparently not touched the North American imagination. I have carried out anthropological research in Japan for twenty years into matters relating to the body in health and illness, but the "brain-death problem," as it is called in Japanese, provides one of the best lenses through which to view contemporary Japanese culture and society while it struggles with the search for a cultural identity in late modernity.

This particular debate, however, provides another, even more important, challenge: Most anthropologists today, including me, are extremely sensitive about how we represent the "exotic other," and with this in mind I am exceedingly grateful for having been included in the group convened at the Park Ridge Center, not only because of the highly stimulating interdisciplinary company I enjoyed at our meetings, but also because it rapidly became clear to me that probably the most important question to ask is not, Why have the

142

Japanese refused to accept brain death as the end of life? but, Why did North America and most of Europe accept the quiet remaking of death with so little public fuss? North American practices should not be taken as the gold standard for what is natural and inevitable with respect to biomedical technology. The "gift of life" is at first glance an exceedingly seductive metaphor, but the goal of anthropology should be not only to represent how others differ from us but also to use this knowledge to interrogate ourselves. To dismiss the Japanese as irrational or inscrutable would be to miss the point entirely. We must engage emotionally with them in order to expose our own tacit knowledge: failure to do so means that we are simply dabbling in voyeurism, when what we should be doing is searching for the basis of our shared humanity. In the time between writing this chapter and its publication, I started research in Montreal on the same topic and have found that the situation is not as different from Japan as one might expect. Not everyone, including one or two people who have received organ transplants, is satisfied that brain death is the end of life.

The highly stylized Japanese dramatical form known as Noh has been a forum since the fourteenth century for an exploration of the relationship between the world of spirits and earthly life. A conservative tradition to say the least, it is very rare indeed for anything written later than the mid-nineteenth century to enter the consecrated canon that is actually performed in public. However, in 1991 a play entitled *The Well of Ignorance*, the creation of an eminent Tokyo immunologist, Tomio Tada, was premiered at the National Noh theater to a standing-room-only crowd.

The play is about a fisherman knocked unconscious in a giant storm and taken for dead. The wealthy father of a young woman who is very ill summons a traditional Chinese-style doctor who removes the fisherman's heart and uses it to save the woman's life. The ensuing drama focuses on both the plight of the donor of the heart, who remains hovering in the world of restless spirits, neither alive nor dead, and the guilt that racks the young woman for having caused this misery. The narrative in Noh is furnished by a chorus of chanters accompanied by traditional musical instruments, and it is through them that the spirit of the fisherman describes the removal of his own heart: "When I was barely hanging on to life, the doctors decided to come at me with blades and scissors. They opened my chest and took my beating heart out and I heard the sounds of snipping and cutting. But my body was totally frozen, and no voice came out when I screamed! Am I living, or am I dead?"

In characteristic Japanese form, the ambiguity is unresolved by the end of the play; the spirit remains suspended, restless, mutilated; and the young woman's efforts to purify herself at the village well prove fruitless: it dries up, according to the frightened villagers, because of a curse. Tada claims that he personally has no objection to organ transplants. But despite his lifelong interest in Noh, the inertia he had to overcome to have the drama produced in public and the powerful emotional responses he set out to create in the audience belie his words, especially since his play is about the most controversial of bioethical issues in Japan today. In choosing the medium of Noh rather than the contemporary theater, Tada was able to give the drama mythological dimensions, to infuse it with mystical and nostalgic associations. The play can be read simply as an allegory for the current national debate in Japan about the acceptability of the brain-death standard. At the same time, particularly because use is made of the Noh tradition, I believe that it represents much more than this, for it is designed to unify the audience subtly by drawing on and rekindling their sensitivity to qualities widely considered to be uniquely Japanese, including shared attitudes about the relationship of the natural to the cultural domain.

At present, Japan and North America differ remarkably with respect to organ transplant technology: Whereas in America nearly two thousand heart transplants took place in 1990, for example, in Japan there were none. This situation is associated with a second contrast between the two societies: In North America debate about the recent remaking of death in order to carry out heart, liver, and lung transplants is confined largely to the pages of professional journals and academic conferences. Moreover, this debate is happening *after* transplants have been routinized and, more recently, human organs have been recognized as a scarce commodity. Media attention and overt public participation are minimal in the debate, particularly when compared with the furor over abortion.

In Japan the debate about what constitutes death and the implications associated with redefining it in order to implement transplant technology have been major items of national dispute over the past twenty-five years. Public opinion has been systematically monitored and made use of in supporting arguments both for and against changing the definition of death. The result to date is that organ transplants from a brain-dead donor remain unacceptable medical practice in Japan.

These differences obviously cannot be attributed to lack of technology or skills or to a shortage of economic resources. So culture *must* be at work, we assume, and the tendency is to ask what it is about Japanese but *not* North American culture that could account for this discrepancy. This question seems particularly pertinent because Japan utilizes complex medical technology more than any other nation in the world does. What widely shared knowledge do the Japanese possess, therefore, that makes them resist the technologically aided extension of human life? Is the difference to be found at the level of attitudes toward the mastery of nature or, more specifically, in a concern about tinkering with the bodies of the dying and the dead? Is Japan perhaps not as secular and rational, not as "modern," as its outward trappings would lead us to believe? Are the Japanese unable to objectify the body in the way we assume that North Americans do? An assumption implicit in this line of interrogation is that something is inherently odd about not striving to "save" lives in a secular society with neither economic nor technological constraints. Hence, scrutiny of the relics of tradition lurking in Japanese modernity, survivals from an archaic past, is used to account for this anomaly.

Some Japanese commentators themselves take up the question of tradition, but usually with the intent of embracing it wholeheartedly as a positive force. They draw explicitly on what is labeled as unique to Japan and contrast it favorably with a perceived cultural vacuum in the contemporary West that facilitates an easy implementation of medical technology without careful consideration of ethical and moral implications. These commentators are explicit that Japan should not simply ape the West but should strive to create a contemporary moral order grounded in the culture of tradition.[1]

In contrast with these commentators, most of whom are conservative in orientation, the majority of Japanese dismiss arguments that reify the Japanese tradition. Further, they go on to state that culture, that is, the "culture of tradition," is of little or no importance in accounting for the present impasse in the debate over medical technology versus ethics. One forceful line of criticism is directed, for example, at medical knowledge and practice. Such criticism suggests that brain death is not easily ascertained and, moreover, that, even when correctly determined according to currently accepted diagnostic standards, this does not signify that the brain is entirely dead.[2] Other analysts instead give pragmatic reasons regarding why the nation is embroiled in the present debate about death; some implicate the way in which medical practice is institutionalized in Japan, describing politics and power relations between the professions and between the medical world and the public.[3] Other explanations, articulated less often, refer to the impact of social organization on the dispute, in particular the fact that the family, not the individual, constitutes the primary social unit in Japan.[4] It is pointed out, moreover, that gift giving is formalized as an integral part of virtually all Japanese social relations, with obvious implications for anonymous organ donation. Those people who produce political and societal explanations, though they generally agree on the origins of the conflict, nevertheless remain divided over whether brain death signals the end of life. In contrast, those who argue for the importance of defending Japan's unique heritage are adamantly opposed to accepting brain death as death.

Taking yet another tack, we can argue that culture influences the production of scientific discourse,[5] with the result that in this particular instance, biomedical understanding of brain activity in Japan may be somewhat different from that in North America, with significant implications for discussion about the end of life. Some highly visible Japanese commentators have essentially made this position integral to their arguments, as we will see. Yet other commentators claim that neither tradition, nor politics, nor social organization, nor medical knowledge is of much import, and they believe it merely serendipitous that Japan is not in the same position as North America today. This group assumes that the particular circumstances of the first and only heart transplant conducted in Japan (described later in this chapter) affected subsequent history, creating a public furor that could not be quietly ignored. The only heart transplant to be carried out in Japan to date certainly would have been contentious in any cultural setting, but the question remains regarding why, after twenty-five years, the debate it triggered rages on.

Thus far, very little empirical evidence has been amassed to corroborate any of the arguments outlined above.[6] The debate is essentially one of ideological clashes in which the suffering of patients does not figure very prominently; relatively little concern has been shown for those patients whose lives might have been extended had transplant technology been made available to them. Neither have questions been asked regarding why brain death, much more than, for example, abortion, reproductive technologies, or the human genome project, has become and remains such a contentious issue in Japan.

In this chapter I will elaborate on the competing discourses outlined above, not by way of dismissing them as so much cultural flotsam, whether that of tradition or of contemporary Japanese social and professional life, but as a way of reflecting on the current North American situation. To regard the Japanese situation as one of cultural lag and the North American one as the product of rational technological progress is entirely inappropriate. Decisions to implement biomedical technology are intimately associated with the cultural construction of bodily knowledge and practice just as deeply as disputes are about their nonimplementation: Value judgments cannot be avoided, whether the argument is for or against technological innovation. To dismiss the Japanese case as backward, or as an anachronism, is to miss an excellent opportunity to examine the impasse we have reached in North America, where we are now told that we have an organ shortage and are confronted with pressures to redefine death yet again in order to meet what is thought of as the unfulfilled needs of waiting patients.

The Japanese Debate: Doctors under Observation

Shortly after the world's first heart transplant was conducted in South Africa, two or three attempts were made to carry out the same procedure in other locations, including Sapporo, Hokkaido, in 1968. The Sapporo procedure, like similar procedures in other parts of the world, initially produced an accolade from the media and was heralded as a dramatic medical triumph. However, several months later, the physician in charge, Dr. Wada, was arraigned on a charge of murder and acquitted only after six years of wrangling. The majority of Japanese now believe that the patient whose heart was removed was not brain dead and that the recipient, who died two and a half months after the operation, was not sufficiently in need of a new heart to have undergone the procedure in the first place. As part of the current national debate about organ transplants, discussion of the case was formally reopened in 1991. The chairman of the Japan Medical Association, testifying before a government committee, reported that twenty-three years ago, right after the removal of the supposedly defective heart from the recipient patient, it had been tampered with, indicating that the involved doctors may have tried to exaggerate the degree of its deterioration.[7] In retrospect, the case is considered a barbarous piece of medical experimentation carried out by a doctor who, significantly, had received a good portion of his training in America.

There have been other cases connected with organ transplants in which the Japanese medical profession has not shown up in a good light. One involved a highly controversial kidney and pancreas transplant at Tsukuba University in which organs were removed from a young mentally retarded woman diagnosed as brain dead, but neither she nor her parents had given permission for her to be a donor.[8] In another instance, in 1989, a doctor at the Hamamatsu National Medical School hospital was arrested for swindling more than twenty million yen ($180,000) from a patient by offering to find a donor for a kidney transplant the patient needed. The patient died one day after handing the money over, having been told by the doctor that the large fee was necessary as recompense *(sharei)* to the organ donor.[9] It is illegal to buy and sell human organs in Japan, but since the Japanese have a long-standing custom of giving substantial presents to doctors to ensure good medical care, especially during surgery (a custom one Japanese doctor who resides in America described to me as bribery), many people believe that commercialization of human organs is a possibility and perhaps already a reality.

In 1991, a team of physicians appeared in a newspaper photograph defiantly lined up side by side, having decided to go public, months after the actual event, about a kidney transplant they had conducted using a brain-dead donor.[10] It is estimated that more than two hundred kidney transplants from brain-dead donors, usually close relatives of the recipients, have been carried out in Japan, but details of these procedures are rarely made public.[11] In a recent case, a patient was declared brain dead by a medical team, and his kidneys were removed for donation. It was later revealed that, although the family had given assent, they were not informed at the time that their relative was brain dead and that his heart was still beating. When confronted with the situation, one of the surgeons involved stated, "It didn't even occur to me to tell the family that I was removing the organs after their relative was pronounced brain-dead. They were eager to donate his kidneys and the chances of success are higher with fresh organs, so I went ahead with it."[12]

More recently, in full view of the nation while it watched on television, police entered Osaka University Hospital to issue a warning to surgeons that they should not remove the liver of a patient. In this case, the fifty-one-year-old man had provided in his will that his organs could be made available for transplants, and approval had also been obtained from his family. After being hit by a car, the man was taken in an unconscious state to a nearby hospital and then transferred to the Osaka University Hospital so that his liver and other organs could be removed after he had been declared brain dead by three independent teams of doctors. The police declared that an autopsy was legally necessary after a car accident. They also reminded the doctors that brain death is not legal in Japan, and they warned the physicians to wait until the man's heart had stopped beating. Television viewers were treated to the sight of police marching purposively around hospital corridors and defiant doctors shutting doors in the face of both television cameras and the police. By the time the liver was removed, it had degenerated badly and was beyond use, but the kidneys and pancreas were extracted and transplanted. At the time of this incident, it was revealed that this was not the first case where police had intervened and prevented physicians from removing organs from brain-dead donors.

Contested Definitions of Death

The first definition of brain death was formulated by the Japan
Electroencephaly Association in 1974. Probably in response to the much-
publicized case of the mentally retarded patient at Tsukuba University,
the Life Ethics Problem Study Parliamentarians League, composed
of twenty-eight Diet members and forty-five other professionals, was
established in 1985; after one year, this group endorsed the need for
legislation about brain death.[13] In the same year, the Ministry of Health
and Welfare set up the Brain Death Advisory Council, the final report of
which contained the definition of brain death currently in use in Japan.[14]
This report makes explicit, however, that "death cannot be judged
by brain death." Nevertheless, the diagnosis is frequently applied,
although it remains unclear whether treatment of patients is affected
once one is given this diagnosis.[15]

The report spurred other involved groups to make pronouncements
about their position in the debate. In January 1988, after two years of
meetings by a working group, the directors of the Japan Medical Association voted unanimously to accept brain death as the termination of
human life. Despite this decision, a lack of agreement remains among the
representatives of medical specialties and also among individual physicians, who are deeply divided on the issue. The politically active Japan
Association of Psychiatrists and Neurologists, for example (some of the
sixty-nine hundred members of whom are responsible for making brain-
death diagnoses), fears that, if brain death is equated with death, this will
lead down the slippery slope for the handicapped, mentally impaired,
and disadvantaged, who may face premature diagnoses rooted in a
greedy desire to get at their organs. The association's 1988 report states
that it is difficult to decide when the brain function is irreversibly lost.[16]

Some physicians have joined members of the public to form the highly
visible Patients' Rights Committee, whose interests range well beyond
the question of brain death. Under the leadership of the flamboyant
Dr. Honda from the prestigious Department of Internal Medicine at
Tokyo University, this group has recently filed several lawsuits charging
murder when organs have been removed from brain-dead patients; one
such lawsuit was in connection with the Tsukuba University case described above. Another involved a Niigata hospital, where the kidneys
of a brain-dead patient were removed; and in a third, a recent case,
a doctor who is also a Buddhist priest turned off the respirator of a
comatose woman and removed the kidneys and corneas in accordance
with a living will and with the consent of the family.[17] The public
prosecutor's office has thus far not reached a decision in connection

with any of these cases, but has thrown two of them out of court, stating that there is no public consensus in Japan about how to define death.[18] Feldman believes that, because complaints made by the Patients' Rights Committee remain unresolved after almost seven years, doctors hesitate to forge ahead with transplantation.[19]

As a result of the unresolved debate, copiously documented by the media, the government felt compelled in late 1989 to set up the Special Cabinet Committee on Brain Death and Organ Transplants in order to bring about closure. This committee, composed of fifteen members from various walks of life, was charged with making a report to the prime minister by 1991, and its very formation signaled to the public that the government was ready to support a formal move to make brain death the termination of life. The group was so deeply divided that for a while it appeared that it would never produce anything more than an interim report. But in January 1992, a final report was delivered. In principle, the members should have reached consensus, but this they could not achieve. The majority position is that brain death is equivalent to human death, that organ transplants from brain-dead donors are acceptable, and that the current definition of brain death as formulated by the Ministry of Health is appropriate. The minority position made it clear that they wish to have the social and cultural aspects of the problem fully debated; in their opinion the debate thus far has been largely confined to "scientific" information, which they believe is inadequate.[20] The public has been kept fully apprised of who has appeared before the committee. It is evident that many who testified, including certain scientists and doctors, have argued against the acceptance of brain death; nevertheless, the majority of the committee eventually moved to support its approval.[21]

Meantime, the Japan Federation of Bar Associations (Nichibenren) maintained its position that brain death should not be accepted as the termination of life. In an earlier report it had expressed concern for the "sanctity of life," and about possible medical "experimentation." It also pointed out that unforeseen consequences in connection with inheritance claims may surface and that a lack of public consensus on the issue exists.[22] In addition, the day following the announcement of the cabinet committee, the Ministry of Justice, the National Police Agency, and the public prosecutor's office all reiterated their continued resistance to brain death.[23]

The Patients' Rights Committee, lawyers, the police, many authors of newspaper articles and books on the subject of brain death, and even a good number among the medical profession appear to be publicly contesting the authority of transplant surgeons. What they usually cite as their principal cause for concern is a lack of trust in the medical teams who will make decisions about cases of brain death; they believe that, in the rush to retrieve organs, the process of dying will be curtailed or even misdiagnosed. The opposition is explicitly opposed to the secrecy and arrogance of some members of the medical profession, and they point out that patients and their families are vulnerable to exploitation when left in physicians' hands.

Certain of these same opponents of brain death are also pushing for informed-consent procedures, together with a frank disclosure and discussion of diagnoses with patients, neither of which activity is by any means routinely established in Japan. This contest, although at one level a debate about the accuracy and replicability of scientific decision making, also challenges the hegemony of invested authority—authority exerted in what is characterized by several challengers as a traditionally Japanese way, whereby subjects are rendered passive and expected to comply to medical regimen without question.

One national newspaper, the *Asahi Shinbun,* recently described the medical world as "irritated" with government dithering, because doctors sense that their international reputations as outstanding surgeons are withering on the vine. At the annual meeting of the Japan Medical Association (JMA) held in Kyoto in 1990, which I attended, two plenary sessions and several smaller panels were given over to brain death and organ transplants. The principal presenters of papers were physicians who had lived and worked for some time in the United States and who had practiced transplant surgery while there. Aside from the scientific part of their presentations, every one of them strongly asserted that Japanese medicine is suffering because of the national uproar over brain death. They all showed slides of themselves standing, usually in surgical garb, side by side with American transplant surgeons and happy, lively patients who had recently received organ transplants. These presentations at the JMA represented one of the few occasions, until very recently, when attention was focused on the situation of patients whose lives might be prolonged, however temporarily, by transplant procedures.[24]

In the meantime, doctors have been trying to salvage what they can by working to perfect artificial organs. They have also been experimenting, watched closely by the media, with live liver donations from parents to children, of which more than 150 have been carried out. A development that received extensive television coverage was the participation by a Japanese doctor in a surgical team in America that transplanted a baboon liver into a human patient.

Reaching Public Consensus

Taking place in concert with government and professional discussion and extensive media coverage is the most persistent search for a national consensus *(kokuminteki gôi)* among the Japanese public that has taken place to date on any subject. At least twelve national surveys about brain death and organ transplants have been done between 1983 and 1994. Over the years, the number of people who accept the concept of brain death has increased from 29 percent to approaching 60 percent.[25] A recent poll conducted by the special cabinet committee produced a remarkable 79 percent response rate. In that poll, taken among three thousand respondents over age twenty, 72 percent stated that they have an "interest" in organ transplants and brain death. However, as with all the previous surveys, a paradox emerged in that more people approved of organ transplants from brain-dead patients than accepted brain death as a definition of death. In this particular poll, 55 percent accepted the idea of organ transplant from brain-dead patients, 14 percent were opposed, and 30 percent were undecided. However, only 51 percent of men and 39 percent of women agreed that brain death is the end of life, although nearly 50 percent of all respondents stated that even if brain death is not recognized in Japan, provided both the potential donor and the family have given consent, a major transplant would be acceptable.[26] Members of the Japanese public are perhaps indicating that, even though they themselves are not eager to participate in this particular medical technology, they are willing to let others do so should they so choose.

Those who oppose brain death usually draw on opinion polls to support their argument, since it has been frequently reiterated that public consensus must be reached before brain death can be nationally recognized. Nevertheless, one is left with the feeling, voiced by many members of the Japanese public, that the whole exercise of repeatedly surveying the nation is essentially a farce and that the idea of trying to achieve a simple consensus on such an inflammatory subject is without meaning. One piece of evidence has emerged regularly from the opinion polls, however: Those who oppose the acceptance of brain death as the definition of death repeatedly state that they take this position because they do not trust the medical profession.

Media Constructions of Death

In December 1990 Japanese national television (NHK) presented a three-hour Saturday evening prime-time program on the subject of brain death and organ transplants. This two-part program, one of several on this subject, was devised and moderated by the nationally recognized Takashi Tachibana, a journalist with the newspaper the *Yomiuri Shinbun*. The first hour and a half was devoted to a film made largely in America about the harvesting and dispersal of organs on a nationwide basis. The second half was given over to a roundtable discussion among six "experts," three for and three against the acceptance of brain death as the end of life. I have discussed this program with a good number of Japanese who saw it, and even those who are naturally skeptical about media presentations thought it was a balanced discussion. In my opinion, however, it was clearly biased, but perhaps not intentionally so. Tachibana does not accept brain death as the end of life, and he has written numerous articles and two books to explain why he takes this position;[27] although he tried, I believe, to remain neutral, the stamp of his interests is clear.

To the background of sweet music, viewers are introduced at the beginning of the program to a lively, beguiling Japanese child who was born from a brain-dead mother and who, we are told, symbolizes the fact that new life started from what is thought of by some to have been a dead body. The audience is then taken to North Carolina, where a young man, badly injured in a car accident, was pronounced brain dead and transported to another hospital where his heart was about to be removed when he "came back to life." He lived for another six days before death was finally established. This section of the program ends with a close-up of a large ornamental cross attached to the outside of the hospital and a pan of a nearby graveyard, filled with crosses and with a view of the hospital behind it.

In the next scene, an American doctor states that it is difficult to diagnose brain death, that a clear legal definition is not possible, and that if the guidelines are too lenient, one is in danger of misdiagnosing certain cases; on the other hand, with too stringent a diagnosis, many organs "go to waste." Later in the program, Willard Gaylin, a psychiatrist and president emeritus of the Hastings Center in New York, described the "excitement" he experienced when he first realized that what he terms *neomorts* could be used for testing new drugs, for dissecting in medical schools, and for "recycling body parts into other people." Earlier in the program, he had vividly described how neomorts are still warm and breathing but nevertheless legally dead. Following Gaylin's description, yet another American doctor made clear that, in his opinion, not only brain-dead bodies but also people in so-called persistent vegetative states will be recognized as dead before too long. The camera then moves to a Japanese ward full of patients diagnosed as being in a vegetative state *(shokubutsu ningen)*. Viewers are shown how some of these patients respond to human communication by subtle movements of their bodies and are informed that, in another institution, thirteen out of thirty patients in a vegetative state made some significant recovery after constant intensive treatment, sometimes to the point of being able to speak again.

Together, these scenes and others like them in the program, including several from Europe, give an impression that brain death is not easily diagnosed and that, in any case, brain-dead patients are in some clear sense living. Further, a continuum exists between brain death and other states, so that no easy black-and-white, Western-style dichotomy can be made between the living and the dead unless one waits patiently for further proof in the form of whole-body death, at which time vital organs such as the heart, liver, and lungs would no longer be fit for transplantation.

Viewers are then taken into a surgical unit in Florida, where they see in graphic detail, accompanied by an anxiety-producing funereal sound track, the dismemberment of a young woman whose blonde hair in one well-angled shot is displayed through the drapes. They learn that seventeen kinds of organs are taken from her, starting with the heart and ending up with large sections of bone, joint, and muscle tissue and are then shown several cartons of dismembered body parts, stored in dry ice, being wheeled out for computer-organized distribution around the United States. The audience is told that as a result of this seven-hour "operation" parts of this twenty-one-year-old will "continue to live in seventy other people." What is left of the body, tidied up by the nursing staff and ready for burial, is then shown.

One other theme that raises its ugly head in this program is the question of the sale of organs.[28] Although no direct reference is made to the selling of organs in the United States (although books and newspaper articles in Japanese sometimes cite cases of this),[29] viewers are told about Brazilian children who are illegally taken to Europe for possible slaughter and sale of their organs and are shown a line of people in India waiting to sell one of their kidneys, for which they will receive the equivalent of five years' income.

At its end, the program introduces a professor at Tohoku University in Japan who found, when he transplanted brain cells between mice, that he could restore some of the brain functioning that he had previously destroyed in the recipient mice. This experiment indicates, viewers are told, that a brain-dead person could perhaps be returned to life as a result of future developments in medicine. It is emphasized throughout this part of the program that *because* death cannot be readily defined, the brain-death debate must inevitably be linked to ethics and religion. An implicit but clear contrast is set up between America, the pragmatic land of Christianity (symbolized by crosses on hospitals and in graveyards), where altruistic giving is part of the cultural tradition and where black-and-white decisions are reached quite easily, and Japan, which is somehow closer to nature, does not think in oppositional dichotomies, and is less willing to tinker with larger-than-human forces.

In the roundtable discussion, the lawyer and two doctors made a narrowly construed argument that brain death means the irreversible stoppage of brain functioning that can be rationally and systematically deduced with accuracy when certain procedures are correctly applied. Those making the argument for brain death as death returned again and again to universal scientific standards as the basis for decision making; they were explicit that what they termed emotional arguments (by which they apparently meant references to values and cultural difference) should be kept out of the discussion; and they pointed out that in America the donation of organs had been set up on a "rational" basis in which people are free to refuse to participate.

In contrast, the three opposed speakers repeatedly stated: that the religious background of the problem must be considered; that emotional matters and scientific theory should not be separated but, on the contrary, united; that an examination of the "truth" must be accompanied by "feelings" as well as logic; and that the "social concept" of death must be considered. One of the speakers taking this line was the conservative philosopher Takeshi Umehara, who, characteristically, made several deliberately inflammatory statements. He pointed out that the "Japanese people" dislike transplantations because they do not like "unnatural" things, that they had never in the past accepted "extreme" Chinese customs such as foot binding and the eunuch system, and that, in a similar vein, contemporary Japanese "hate" homosexuality and the use of drugs. He then laid blame for the sorry state of the "West" at the feet of René Descartes, who had focused attention on the brain as the center of the living person, but went on to point out that humans everywhere are unique, rational beings. While "Western modernism" makes "us Japanese happy in one sense," he stated, at the same time it has "destroyed our surroundings and nature." If this discussion had taken place one month later, Umehara might have seized upon the opportunity to mention that a recent Japanese recipient of a kidney from "foreign" parts died of AIDS contracted from the donated kidney.

A perusal of the vast popular literature and media presentations in Japanese on brain death shows that no simple ideological dichotomies can be made between those for and against its acceptance as death.

While those of a conservative, traditionalist persuasion are unanimously opposed, they are joined by others who are politically left wing, such as the producer of the television program, Tachibana, and by a good number of the medical profession, both young and old, including some surgeons. Those who are politically active on behalf of the handicapped and the mentally ill are also opposed to its acceptance and, as we have seen, so too are many lawyers, people concerned about patients' rights, and the police. Advocates for acceptance include a good number of intellectuals and professionals, among them physicians who have spent some years in the West, but they are joined by many others, including several patient groups, supporters of those who are potential recipients of organs.

What is striking to an anthropologist is that it is mostly the culture and values of the Other which are scrutinized. We hear and read a lot about Christianity (but nothing of Judaism), about rationality, about the brain as the center of the body, about altruism, and about individuality but, despite a call to move the discussion beyond the scientific realm, Japanese traditions and values are rarely examined more than peremptorily. Among the more than twenty physicians I have interviewed on the subject, only three focused spontaneously on cultural features in order to explain why the brain-death "problem," as it is known, is of such importance in contemporary Japan. One of them, a neurosurgeon opposed to the acceptance of brain death as the end of life, described *obon*, a major annual festival in which the dead return to earth and after several days of ritual celebrations go back again to their repose, their departure symbolized by thousands of tiny paper boats that are floated downstream. When asked, he asserted that these beliefs will continue to be of great significance to younger Japanese in the future. Another, a physician who practices herbal medicine, talked about the concept of fate, and explained how life is understood in Japan as something larger than that of individual people; he emphasized that one's body is a parental gift and that the lives of individuals belong, not to them, but to their family. However, these kinds of responses, drawing heavily on the Japanese cultural and philosophical tradition to buttress arguments against brain death, are, I believe, in the minority.

When I first started to consider the brain-death debate, I was struck by the many features of Japanese culture that could work against its acceptance as death, several of which have also been commented on by the Japanese anthropologist Emiko Namihira.[30] That there has never been a philosophical thrust to separate mind and body is obviously significant, as is, no doubt, the fact that traditionally the spiritual center of the body was found in the metaphorical space known as *kokoro*, located in the region of the thorax. This concept remains important in everyday language, all kinds of educational endeavors, the martial arts, and traditional art forms.

Much is made in North American bioethics of individualism and autonomy. In Japan, personhood is not seen as residing in a unique, bounded individual but, instead, as residing at the center of a network of obligations; it is constructed out-of-mind, beyond body, in the space of ongoing human relationships. The person in Japan is a dialogical creation, therefore, and what one does with one's body and what is done to it are by no means an individual affair.[31] Moreover, the ancestors remain as a presence in the Japanese cosmos and, for many people, continue to participate in their daily lives. Even among those who have ostensibly cast aside this tradition, the majority remain aware that, according to Buddhist tradition, the process of dying is not complete until services held on the seventh and forty-ninth days are performed. Furthermore, a large number of Japanese still go through the very long Buddhist-orchestrated process, which continues over many years, of converting their dead relatives into ancestors.[32]

The idea of having a deceased relative whose body is not complete prior to burial or cremation is associated with misfortune, because in this situation suffering in the other world never terminates. Furthermore, Confucianism, the ethical tradition on which Japanese social life was grounded for many hundreds of years, prohibited all tampering with dead bodies. In addition, Shinto, the indigenous religion of Japan, regards all contact with death as ritually polluting.

Of course, many people today categorically reject these beliefs as old-fashioned; any essentialist argument to the effect that Japanese tradition effectively curtails the acceptance of brain death as the end of life would be entirely out of place. However, this tradition is actively drawn on by politicians, educators, cultural commentators, and others in the construction of contemporary Japanese identity, individual and national, and contrasted favorably with a West believed to be lacking in a sound moral order. Undoubtedly, the force of specific elements of Japanese tradition, coupled with a widespread concern about both a perceived loss of spiritual values as a result of rapid modernization and a rampant spread of excessive individualism (an import from the West about which many people are highly ambivalent), contributes to the present impasse. Ideologues can draw readily, therefore, on cultural difference to buttress their arguments, which resonate to some extent with the concerns of their audience, despite many peoples' self-conscious denial of their cultural heritage as being of much importance and their focus instead on political and social explanations.

A large number of educated people in Japan, very sensitive to ideological posturing, fear that open acknowledgment of cultural difference as the prime reason for the brain-death debate will place them in the same camp as chauvinistic, nationalistic thinkers, and therefore they reject such arguments *in toto*. Others share a largely tacit understanding that to acknowledge Japanese tradition as influential would in effect be to say that the Japanese are superstitious and irrational—a position with which most people disagree, although some physicians in their frustration have no trouble in accepting this argument. Thus, to acknowledge a cultural contribution to the brain-death debate is not easy, for it implicitly sides with nationalism and the power of tradition over economic and scientific progress, both of which in Japan are clearly among the most advanced in the world today. As an outsider I am perhaps more at liberty than many Japanese to argue for what I see as the contribution made by the culture of tradition to the brain-death debate, although I am acutely sensitive to the dangerous direction this line of argument can so easily take.

Turning to institutional organization, another sphere of culture, the structure of hospital life in Japan has a role to play in the debate. Japanese families are deeply involved in the nursing of their dying relatives in many hospitals, and upon death they wash, lay out, and dress the corpse. Therefore, the Japanese have much more familiarity with the dying process than many northern Europeans or North Americans have, and many Japanese are exceedingly alert regarding how "alive" a brain-dead body appears to be. Sensitive about family concerns, most doctors are exceedingly reluctant to approach next of kin in Japan, especially women, to ask for permission to remove organs, and it would be entirely inappropriate to pass this task on to a junior doctor or a nurse. In this situation, doctors on occasion, having established ahead of time that relatives agree in principle to the donation of organs, simply go ahead and remove kidneys without the brain-dead state of the patient being made explicit to the family.

The formal obligation system upon which the exchange of gifts is based in Japan, while it has no direct bearing on the definition of death, presents a major impediment to an easy acceptance of organ transplants. Although gift giving is central in Japanese culture, it is inevitably carried out within an established framework of ongoing reciprocity. The idea of receiving an anonymously donated organ is not easy for most people to accept, since the question of repayment then looms large. Nor is it easy to accept the idea of receiving an organ from someone designated as an outsider. Culturally constructed boundaries between self and other, between those who are designated as inside the family and those who are distinguished as outsiders, are finely tuned in Japan with many ramifications in daily life. Many people instinctively think of the donation of organs to or from persons outside the family as unnatural. Perhaps it should not come as a surprise that Tomio Tada, the immunologist whose Noh play opened this chapter, thinks of immunology as the science of "self and other."[33]

Finally, because giving gifts to physicians is an established part of the system whereby doctors are encouraged to do their best for patients, the fear that many organs will not be freely donated but will be bought and sold, despite a comprehensive socialized health care system, is of great concern to many people. An effort is made by some commentators in Japan to divorce the brain-death debate from transplant technology, and to focus attention overwhelmingly on possibilities for misdiagnosis of the death of the potential donor. Nevertheless, in addition, concern about the institutionalization of transplant technology and its possible abuse clearly is a major contributing force in the brain-death problem. However, antipathy to organ transplants is very difficult to express openly, since it suggests that Japanese are unwilling to be altruistic, that they do not care for the plight of their neighbors. As with the brain-death debate itself, it is much easier to focus on the shortcoming of doctors as the root of the problem.

The Second Iwakura Mission

In the television program, Takashi Tachibana pointed out that, when considering a subject as difficult as death, it is important to examine how other countries have managed the problem. In 1988, two years before the NHK television program aired, members of the Japanese Diet had already expressed an opinion similar to that of Tachibana: One mandate of the special cabinet committee was to travel widely, not only throughout Japan but also in Europe, America, Australia, and Thailand, in order to study the situation in those countries. This committee was explicitly requested, therefore, to reach an agreement about what would be best for Japan in light of a long and close scrutiny of the Other. (This plea calls to mind the Iwakura mission of more than 100 years ago, which constituted the formal ending of 250 years of self-imposed isolation in Japan. Its task was to examine the democratic process, the school system, the armed forces, the legal and medical systems, and the treatment of women in Europe and America.)

Of all the countries the cabinet members visited, the one that captured the most media attention was Denmark, because brain death was accepted there only in July 1990. Until that time, patients had to go abroad for transplants, as some Japanese do at present. Prior to the acceptance of the brain-death standard, the Danes held more than two hundred public hearings, and the government generated a large amount of publicity on the subject. This experience led some members of the Japanese committee to state that, despite all that had been published thus far, the Japanese still had not engaged in enough public discussion. The committee was also impressed with the trust shown in doctors, particularly in the European countries they visited, a situation they contrasted with that of Japan.

Nationalism, Modernity, and the Other

Many Japanese people believe that fairly soon brain death will be legally recognized as death, that the inspection trips abroad and the search for a national consensus are simply placatory exercises before those in power go ahead and facilitate organ transplants. At the suggestion of the Ministry of Health and Welfare, the Japanese Association for Organ Transplants was established in 1992 in order to centralize and standardize transplant procedures.[34] Although it is reasonable to assume that rather few organs will be donated to a central bank, this step indicates a forward move on the part of the government. Several hospitals have reported that they are ready to undertake transplants on a regular basis as soon as the way is clear to do so, and recently, in the spring of 1994, a bill was submitted to the Diet to begin the legislative process to make brain death the legally accepted end of life.

Allowing one's dead relatives to be cut up is genuinely repulsive for many Japanese, while others are willing to donate parts of their own bodies or of their close relatives to save the lives of others. When limited to the question of medical procedures, clearly what most worries those both for and against redefining death are the reports published with monotonous regularity about an unprofessional medical world. The section on the NHK program that showed Indians selling their kidneys and the fantasy that has appeared in more than one article in Japan about poor black Americans selling their dead children to hospitals[35] reveal a deep-seated fear in Japan: Should brain death be accepted as death, the buying and selling of organs will be established rather rapidly as a matter of course, to the detriment of all concerned. Repeatedly, people I have interviewed, including physicians, have made unsolicited statements to the effect that doctors are not to be trusted; that what passes for *omoiyari* (sympathy and consideration) is unqualified paternalism; and that medical ethics has no meaning because very few people seriously question the power of the medical profession, which essentially looks after its own. Medicine used to be thought of as a benevolent art—*i wa jin jitsu nari*. Today, everyone knows the pun in which medicine is now characterized as a money-making art—*i wa kin jitsu nari* (although the income of Japanese physicians lags well behind that of Americans).

The media and Japanese citizens have taken on this secret medical society, which for the first time is being frontally attacked about many aspects of its current behavior, ranging from a resistance to informed consent to performing unnecessary hysterectomies for profit.[36] The medical world has been exposed to public scrutiny in a way it never before experienced, and opposition to brain death represents in part a flamboyant expression of a major ideological struggle over relationships of power in modern Japan, especially between the medical profession and its clientele. Paradoxically, while North America is cited as a negative example to bolster arguments against accepting brain death as the end of life, it is drawn upon by a wide range of people as a model for emulation when it comes to the handling of relationships of power. Japan, in contrast, is denigrated as feudalistic and backward.

It has been suggested that if the original Japanese heart transplant, now known simply as the Wada case, had not flared up into a legal battle, the entire brain-death debate may never have erupted, and the Japanese medical world would simply have gone ahead with relatively little opposition, as occurred in North America. But the Wada case was initially lauded, and its quackery exposed only at a later date, after other cases had come under scrutiny and participants in the debate had for the most part taken sides. Brain death is obviously a sensitive topic, especially because it was inflamed by the Wada case. Moreover, the redefinition of death and the remaking of the human body, at the nub of the debate, take on metaphoric significance and trigger a cascade of wide-ranging ideological responses. Contemporary Japan, like North America, is in theory a rational and secular society. Appellations such as tradition, culture, and religion smack of superstition and premodern sentimentality to a very large number of people. But the waters are muddied because until recently, although not outwardly in support of the theory that with modernization all societies will eventually become essentially the same (that is, convergence theory), Japan has nevertheless thought of itself as catching up. That era is now clearly past, and the Japanese are taking a leadership role in the modern world order, in a climate where it is increasingly recognized that modernization can take more than one form, and much can be learned from the Japanese experience. The result is that Japan continues to be set off from the West, and repeatedly described by both inside commentators and outside observers as different.

Historically, Confucianism, although mandated by heaven, was predominantly a secular and highly rational system of ethics. Imported from China in the sixth century, it failed to come fully into its own in Japan until the sixteenth century, after which time it held sway for more than 250 years. Although both Buddhism and Shinto have been powerful religious forces throughout Japanese history, the secular tradition of Neo-Confucian behavioral norms dominated both political and daily life until the end of the last century, and its stamp is still very evident in many areas of Japanese society. At the core of Confucian ethics is a preordained social hierarchy, but one in which benevolence and mutual reciprocity are central. I think it safe to say that the majority of Japanese today believe intuitively that the ethic of individualism has gone too far in America. Deification of the individual was never part of the process of secularization in Japan; in contrast, society was deified, and social interests inevitably took, and usually continue to take, precedence over individual needs. The very notion of individual rights is tainted with an aura of selfishness, and the idea of a thoroughly autonomous individual is patently absurd to most Japanese (as indeed it is for many Westerners).

The present dilemma for liberal-minded thinkers in Japan is how to dispose of the remnants of patriarchal and patronage thinking without drawing on a language that single-mindedly pursues the entrenchment of individual autonomy and rights, that is, how to create a meaningful social contract in late modernity that follows neither the authoritarianism of Confucianism nor the perceived anomie of individualism. This is the context in which the argument about brain death is taking place, and as in the West, it is an overwhelmingly secular argument from which representatives of religious organizations are, for the most part, remarkably absent.[37]

Although overtly about scientific progress, the legitimation of scientific knowledge, the status of the medical profession, and patient well-being, the debate is also concerned with Japan's self-image as an advanced society, with what the outside world thinks of Japan, and with the question of continuity and the value of tradition, although these topics are not always made explicit. At a metalevel, the current angst is, therefore, a manifestation of the ceaseless, restless, contradictory argument about Japan and the West, tradition and modernity. As one pediatrician put it, "Why should we mindlessly imitate Westerners? We would only be turning ourselves into white Westerners with Asian faces."[38] Of course, a good deal of genuine passion does go into the contested meanings of death, but because those meanings are often framed in the language of difference, painful comparisons that reach way beyond individual deaths become evident. At stake are questions about progress, internationalization, scientific and technological expertise, and the relationship of the state, professional bodies, and the media to society at large and to individuals.

The posing of these questions is in turn a manifestation of the struggle by people from a whole range of political persuasions to create a moral framework for late modern and postmodern Japan that is not simply a cardboard copy of the West. In entering the debate, traditionalists rub shoulders with those who are promoting further reform toward social equality and the empowerment of individuals: Physicians who believe that their authority should not be subjected to questioning find themselves in the same camp as the mentally impaired. And patients' rights advocates who are striving for more autonomy for the person in the street find themselves cheering on the police while they extend the hand of the law.

Meanwhile, as the debate drags on, very little is heard from patients and their families, whether they be potential organ donors or receivers, although a woman whose daughter will soon require a liver transplant, when interviewed by *Newsweek* for its Japanese edition, complained, "Why do we have to suffer just because we have the misfortune to be Japanese?"[39] Individual and family suffering is largely pushed to one side and only rarely appears as part of the argument. Similarly, any serious examinations of subjective feelings about tampering with the newly dead, the sanctity of the body, or the limits of scientific exploration are effectively displaced onto the Other and transformed into an ambivalent and ideological portrayal of what is purportedly happening in the West.

In North America today the talk is of rewarded gifting and organ wastage, signs of the urgent need to procure ever more organs in a steady move toward the large-scale commodification of human parts.[40] In our haste, we hear little of the flow of organs from the poor to the rich, from the Third World to the First World, and even less of possible atrocities involved, despite some suggestive newspaper articles. Leon Kass has described this process as a "coarsening of sensibilities and attitudes," and adds, "there is a sad irony in our biomedical project, accurately anticipated in Aldous Huxley's *Brave New World:* We expend enormous energy and vast sums of money to preserve and prolong bodily life, but in the process our embodied life is stripped of its gravity and much of its dignity. This is, in a word, progress as tragedy."[41]

Although the remaking of death has not captured the North American imagination in the same way as that of the Japanese, research has shown that North Americans, like the Japanese, are not entirely at ease with the transformation and have concerns about premature diagnoses of death.[42] Our inability to bring ourselves to refer simply to "death," and our continued talk about "brain death," are indications of the ambiguity and uncertainty involved, as is the language of health professionals which suggests that patients die twice.[43] Perhaps the difference is one of emphasis, since both the Japanese and North American public are apparently sensitive to the risks patients face as a result of the competitive and at times ruthless pressure for advancement of medical knowledge. In North America, although members of the public are less well informed than the Japanese are about the issues around brain death, they have had the opportunity to learn more than the Japanese have about the dangers inherent in, for example, uncontrolled use of reproductive technologies.

After all, the issues involving anticipated danger produce the national debates. In North America, our history has taught liberal-minded thinkers to be exceedingly wary of technologies such as enforced abortion and the manipulation of genes that can open the door to eugenics. Japan, a remarkably homogeneous society, has harbored few fears to date around these issues, although one or two radical commentators, among them feminists, are beginning now to sound the alert. Few people in North America sensed any danger in connection with reformulating death in order to carry out organ transplants; the desire to save lives has apparently overridden most concerns about the remaking of death. Nationalistic feelings around the moral worth of giving to needy others coupled with the heroics of saving lives have dominated North American discussions, and it must be stated emphatically that, as a result, many people enjoy full and productive lives for many years after undergoing major organ transplants. In Japan, where Buddhism has encouraged a special fascination with death, both with respect to its meaning and form and to the belief that an innocent gift does not exist, the setting was ripe for the brain-death debate to erupt, and for its easy embellishment into nationalistic cant by those so inclined.

Perhaps few specific lessons can be transferred directly from Japan to North America, particularly since the Japanese debate is by no means sensitive to the suffering of individuals. Nor can the clock be reversed so that we North Americans can put ourselves in the same position as that of the Japanese. Nevertheless, some reflection is in order regarding why most people in North America apparently accept medical judgment about the redefining of death when they dispute medical judgment in so many other realms today, why those who have resisted the remaking of death have captured so little national attention, and why the suffering of the donor is so easily eradicated from our discourse while we dwell exclusively on the restoration (resurrection?) of the organ recipient. Until we allow ourselves to confront death as something other than failure, as has increasingly been regarded in post-Enlightenment history, the remaking of death will remain marginal among biomedical debates. Perhaps this is the most important lesson to be gleaned from Japan.

Notes

The research on which this paper is based was funded by the Social Science and Humanities Research Council of Canada, grant number 410-93-0544.

1. Takeshi Umehara, "Nôshi, Sokuratesu ne to wa hantai guru" (Socrates and his companions would have been against brain death), *Bungeishunju* 12 (1990): 344–64.

2. Takashi Tachibana and Tonegawa Susumu, *Seishin to bushitsu* (Spirit and substance) (Tokyo: Bungei Shunka, 1990); and Takashi Tachibana, *Nôshi* (Brain death) (Tokyo: Nihon Hôsô Shuppan Kyôkai, 1991).

3. Jiro Nudeshima, *Nôshi, zokiishoku to Nihon shakai* (Brain death, organ transplants and Japanese society) (Tokyo: Kôbundo, 1991).

4. Masahiro Morioka, *Nôshi no hito* (Brain dead people) (Tokyo: Fukutake Shoten, 1991).

5. Bruno Latour and Steve Woolgar, *Laboratory Life: The Social Construction of Scientific Facts* (Beverly Hills, Calif.: Sage, 1979); Margaret Lock, *Encounters with Aging: Mythologies of Menopause in Japan and North America* (Berkeley: University of California Press, 1993); and Peter W. G. Wright and Andrew Treacher, eds., *The Problem of Medical Knowledge: Examining the Social Construction of Medicine* (Edinburgh: University of Edinburgh Press, 1982).

6. Jiro Nudeshima, *Nôshi*, in an exception.

7. "Cover-up Suspected in First Heart Transplant," *Mainichi Shinbun* (newspaper), 31 March 1991.

8. "Organs Removed from Woman without Consent," *Mainichi Daily News*, 24 December 1984.

9. "Jin ishoku o chûkai' to sagi" (Medication of kidney transplant and fraud), *Asahi Shinbun* (newspaper), 23 April 1989.

10. "Kidney Transplant from Brain-Dead Man Revealed," *Mainichi Daily News*, 30 May 1991.

11. It is not essential to use a brain-dead donor for a kidney transplant, but physicians judge at times that there is a better chance of a successful transplant if the organ is "fresh."

12. "Family Not Told of Donor's Brain Death," *Mainichi Daily News*, 31 May 1991.

13. Eric A. Feldman, "Over My Dead Body: The Enigma and Economics of Death in Japan," in N. Ikegami and J. C. Campbell, eds., *Containing Health Care Costs in Japan* (Ann Arbor: University of Michigan Press, in press).

14. The criteria for determining brain death as set out by Kôseishô (the Ministry of Health and Welfare) are as follows:

1. deep coma
2. cessation of spontaneous breathing
3. fixed and enlarged pupils

4. loss of brain stem reflexes

5. flat brain waves

6. numbers 1–5 must continue for a least six hours

Children under six are not subject to the criteria. The presence of two physicians with no vested interest in the retrieval of the patient's organs in addition to the patient's attending physician are required to make the diagnosis, Kôseishô, Tokyo, 1985.

15. Gen Ohi, Tomonori Hasegawa, Hiroyuki Kumano Ichiro Kai, Nobuyuki Takenaga, Yoshio Taguchi, Hiroshi Saito, and Tsunamasa Ino, "Why Are Cadaveric Renal Transplants So Hard to Find in Japan? An Analysis of Economic and Attitudinal Aspects," *Health Policy* 6 (1986): 269–78.

16. "Giron fûjûbun to hihan no kenkai" (Insufficient debate is the critical opinion), *Asahi Shinbun* (newspaper), 17 October 1991; Masaya Yamauchi, "Transplantation in Japan," *British Medical Journal* 301 (1990): 507.

17. "53 sai josei 'sengensho' ikasu" (Written declaration of 53-year-old woman restores life), *Yomiuri Shinbun* (newspaper), 18 October 1992.

18. Taro Nakayama, *Nôshi to zôki ishoku* (Brain death and organ transplants) (Tokyo: Saimaru Shuppansha, 1989).

19. Feldman, "Over My Dead Body."

20. Kantô Chiku Kôchôkai (Kanto region public hearing), *Rinji nôshi oyobi zôkiishoku chôsa kai* (Special hearing on brain death and organ transplants) (1992); "Nôshi ishoku yonin o saigo tôshin" (Final report approves of brain death, organ transplants), *Yomiuri Shinbun,* 23 January 1992.

21. "'Nôshi ishoku' michisuji nao futômei" (Brain death and organ transplants, the path to follow is still unclear), *Nihon Keizai Shinbun* (newspaper), 23 January 1992.

22. "'Nôshi wa shi to mitomeru.' Nichibenren ikensho rincho o hihan jinken shingai no osore" (Recognition of brain death as death: Fear of violation of human rights in the opinion of the Japanese Confederation of Lawyers), *Asahi Shinbun,* 21 September 1991.

23. "'Nôshi wa hito no shi,' tôshin" (Brain death is death, says report), *Asahi Shinbun,* 23 January 1992.

24. See also Shumon Miura, "Attitudes towards Death," *Japan Echo* 18 (1991): 67; "Zôki ishoku no saizensen" (The frontline in transplants), *Newsweek Nihon Han* (Japanese ed.), 25 February 1993.

25. "Nôshi o dô handan?" (What is the judgment about brain death?), *Nihon Keizai Shinbun,* 16 May 1994.

26. "55 Percent Approve of Transplants from Brain-dead," *Mainichi Shinbun,* 16 October 1991.

27. Takashi Tachibana, *Nôshi.*

28. See the chapters in this volume by Renée Fox and Thomas Murray for discussion of this issue in the United States.

29. K. Amano, "Nôshi o kangaeru, zôki ishoku to no kanren no naka de" (Thoughts on brain death in connection with organ transplants), *Gekkan Naashingu* 15, no. 13 (1987): 1949–53; Shohei Yonemoto, *Inochi saisentan: Nôshi to*

zôki ishoku (The leading edge of life: Brain death and organ transplants) (Tokyo: Yomiuri, 1985).

30. Emiko Namihira, *Nôshi, zôki, ishoku, gan kokuchi* (Brain death, organ transplants, and truth telling about cancer) (Tokyo: Fukubu Shoten, 1988).

31. Margaret Lock, *East Asian Medicine in Urban Japan: Varieties of Medical Experience* (Berkeley: University of California Press, 1980).

32. Robert Smith, *Ancestor Worship in Contemporary Japan* (Stanford, Calif.: Stanford University Press, 1974).

33. Tomio Tada, *Meneki no imi ron* (The meaning of immunity) (Tokyo: Seidosha, 1993).

34. Nôshi ishoku yônin o saigo tôshin (Final report approves of brain death), *Yomuiri Shinbun*, 23 January 1992.

35. K. Amano," Nôshi o kangaeru."

36. Shizuko Sasaki, "Guaranteeing Medical Integrity: Unnecessary Hysterectomies in Japan," paper presented at the AM International Conference on Health Law and Ethics, Sydney, Australia, August 1986.

37. Helen Hardacre, "Response of Buddhism and Shintô to the Issue of Brain Death and Organ Transplants," *Cambridge Quarterly of Healthcare Ethics* 3 (1994): 585–601.

38. "Zôki ishoku no saizensen," *Newsweek Nihon Han.*

39. Ibid.

40. See the chapters in this volume by Renée Fox and Thomas Murray.

41. Leon Kass, "Organs for Sale? Propriety, Property, and the Price of Progress," *Public Interest*, April 1992, 65–84, at 83.

42. J. F. Childress, "Ethical Criteria for Procuring and Distributing Organs for Transplantation," in J. F. Blumstein and F. A. Sloan, eds., *Organ Transplantation Policy: Issues and Prospects* (Durham, N. C.: Duke University Press, 1989); Renée Fox and Judith P. Swazey, *Spare Parts: Organ Replacement in American Society* (New York: Oxford University Press, 1992).

43. S. J. Youngner, M. Allen, E. T. Bartlett, et al., "Psychosocial and Ethical Implications of Organ Retrieval," *New England Journal of Medicine* 313 (August 1985): 321–24; also see Stuart Youngner's chapter in this volume.

9 *Elliot N. Dorff*

Choosing Life: Aspects of Judaism Affecting Organ Transplantation

Personal Statement

I am a Conservative rabbi and a professor of philosophy, and my interest in organ transplantation derives from both parts of my professional life. My doctoral dissertation was on ethical theory, and during the last twenty years I have written extensively on the theory and practice of ethics within Judaism, with special attention to bioethics. My willingness to join a project on organ transplantation, therefore, was in part motivated by the opportunity it presented to extend my knowledge and thought to an important area of medical ethics that I had not explored before with sufficient thoroughness.

The expertise brought by the other members of the team in anthropology, literature, sociology, philosophy, and religion, in addition to medicine, made this an especially attractive invitation for me. It indicated from the outset a recognition that organ transplantation is not simply a matter of exchanging parts of a machine but also involves our deepest feelings, our broadest conceptions, and our core values. This vision coincided nicely with the rabbinic part of me: As a rabbi I have taught and counseled significant numbers of people about issues in bioethics, and I have found that Jewish concepts and values become very important to them, even people who are not otherwise religious in their practice, when they contemplate matters of life and death.

The experience of working with the group that has produced this volume confirmed the visions of its organizers. Stories, films, art, customs, and folklore from around the world richly illuminated our discussions of what it means to be embodied or to have a body (which expression you use is itself an interesting philosophical question) and the implications of transferring part of one's body to another. The promise of saving people's lives through organ transplantation is, for Judaism and many other traditions, of supreme importance, but that does not diminish, much less eliminate, the human dimension of this whole process.

The discussion that honed the chapters of this book proved beyond a shadow of a doubt that the various faculties we have as human beings are integrated within us, that we are not separate minds, bodies, and souls, but rather thoroughly blended mixtures of all three, such that each affects the other in significant ways. If people are to become more willing to donate or receive organs in the future, then attention must be paid to this combination of factors. Moreover, if society is to permit and even encourage and financially support organ transplantation, it must take into account the moral, social, aesthetic, and religious components of the matter in shaping social policy on this issue. From my own perspective, the value of saving lives, so paramount in Judaism, ultimately overcomes objections to organ transplantation per se. Still, deeply human factors shape our understanding of our bodies and of the divine image in which we are all created, and transplantation efforts must preserve the dignity and respect that God's creation demands.

Organ transplantations have become possible only in the second half of the twentieth century. It should not be surprising, then, that classical Jewish sources written hundreds, if not thousands, of years ago have nothing specifically to say about transplantation. For a living tradition like Judaism, however, that only means that concepts, values, practices, and laws from the past must be applied to this new technological possibility, just as they are to many other new realities.

The Status of Organ Donation in Jewish Law

Before describing the rich background in concepts and folklore that affects Jews' response to organ transplantation, we shall briefly review what contemporary rabbis have been saying about the issue in their decisions designed to guide Jewish practice. We shall then probe the larger conceptual framework that prompts rabbis to rule this way and leads lay Jews to accept their rulings only in part.

Two principles undergird Jewish legal discussions of organ transplants from living donors. When interpreting Leviticus 18:5, which says that we should obey God's commands "and live by them," the rabbis of the Talmud deduce that this means we should not die as a result of observing them. The tenet that emerges is *pikkuah nefesh,* the obligation to save people's lives. This tenet is so deeply embedded in Jewish law that, according to the rabbis, it takes precedence over all other commandments except those prohibiting murder, idolatry, and illicit sex. That is, if one's choice is to murder someone else or give up one's own life, one must give up one's own life. The same priorities would hold if a king, for example, were to force a Jew to bow down to idols or to commit acts of incest or adultery. If, however, one were to need to violate the Sabbath laws or steal something to save a life, then one is not only permitted but commanded to violate the laws in question to save a life.[1] Another talmudic precedent establishes that saving one's own life takes precedence over saving anyone else's.[2]

In applying these precedents to the case of living donors, contemporary rabbis have generally permitted, but not required, such donations. Rabbi Immanuel Jakobovits, former chief rabbi of the British Commonwealth and author of the first comprehensive book on Jewish medical ethics, is typical. He has ruled that a donor may endanger his or her life or health to supply a *spare* organ to a recipient whose life would thereby be saved as long as the probability of saving the recipient's life is substantially greater than the risk to the donor's life or health. "Since the mortality risk to kidney donors is estimated to be only 0.24% and no greater than is involved in any amputation, the generally prevailing view is to permit such donations as acts of supreme charity but not as an obligation."[3]

With regard to deceased donors, another principle enters the picture, that of *kavod ha-met,* the honor of the dead person. The body, even though dead, continues to be God's creation, and therefore Jewish funeral rites ensure that it be handled and ultimately buried with dignity. Even though a cadaveric donation inevitably involves mutilating the body, saving a person's life (*pikkuah nefesh*) is so sacred a value in Judaism that it is construed to be an honor to the deceased person (*kavod ha-met*) to use his or her bodily parts in that way. That is certainly the case if the person completed an advance directive, either orally or in writing, indicating willingness to have portions of his or her body transplanted; but even if not, the default assumption is that a person would be honored to help another live.

Some rabbis insist that the person to be saved be immediately present and that the transplant be necessary to save nothing less than the person's life.[4] However, with the advent of organ banks, most rabbis, including Orthodox ones, would permit transplants if it were known that the body part will eventually, but definitely, be used for purposes of transplantation. Moreover, most would permit invading the deceased's body to save or improve a person's health as well as his or her life, as, for example, in a cornea transplant to restore sight in one eye when the recipient's other eye is functioning. Thus, the Rabbinical Assembly, the organization of rabbis of the Conservative movement, the largest denomination in American Judaism, approved a resolution in 1990 to "encourage all Jews to become enrolled as organ and tissue donors by signing and carrying cards or drivers' licenses attesting to their commitment of such organs and tissues upon their deaths to those in need."[5]

The Value of the Body

Why, then, do many Jews hesitate to do what their rabbis encourage them to do? Part of the reason comes from the very concepts that undergird the rabbis' rulings, and part stems from official and folk beliefs about death and what follows it. We shall turn first to the relevant beliefs officially held in Judaism, and then we shall look at popular stories and superstitions that influence Jews' reactions to transplantation at least as much.

Pikkuah nefesh, the principle invoked in the formulation of the law, is, in turn, based upon two underlying concepts: (1) The human being is the integrated product of all human faculties, and so the body has the same worth as does the mind, the emotions, and the will. (2) As creator of all human beings, God owns our bodies and allows us to use them during the lease of our lifetimes, but that privilege comes with obligations of care that continue after death. Western philosophical thought and Christianity have been heavily influenced by the Gnostic and Greek bifurcation of the body and the soul (or the mind). In those systems of thought, the body is seen as the inferior part of the human being, either because it is the part we share with animals, in contrast with our distinctively human minds (Aristotle), or because the body is the seat of our passions and hence our sins (Paul in Romans, Galatians, and Corinthians).

While some Jewish thinkers were influenced by these views,[6] classical rabbinic sources do not share this understanding of the human being. One's soul is, in some senses, separable from the body,[7] but it is never depicted as superior to the body. Indeed, one rabbinic source speaks of the soul as a guest in the body here on earth, and thus the body must be respected and well treated.[8] Moreover, for the rabbis, sin is impossible without the complicity of *both* the body and the soul, and so while either might blame the other, God judges the person as one

integrated whole.[9] Thus, concentration on study of the Torah, the most
honored of the activities of the soul, can actually lead a person to sin if
not accompanied by work with one's body: "An excellent thing is the
study of Torah combined with some worldly occupation, for the labor
demanded by both of them causes sinful inclinations to be forgotten.
All study of Torah without work must, in the end, be futile and become
the cause of sin."[10]

The body is respected in the Jewish tradition, not only because it
houses and interacts with the soul, but also because a person's body, for
the Jewish tradition, is as much God's creation as one's mind, emotions,
and will are. As such, the classical rabbis considered the body a good
thing. It is, in fact, God's masterpiece, proving his infinite goodness
and boundless wisdom, and the rabbis wax eloquent in admiring its
intricate construction. The body could, of course, be used for ill purpose
in the process of sinning, but in that it was no different from the mind,
emotions, or will. Conversely, just like them, the body could be used to
carry out God's will.[11] The body continues to belong to God after death,
and so the honor due the dead body (kavod ha-met) is only in part respect
for the person who has died; it is also appropriate care for the creation
and property of God.

If the body is honored to this extent in Judaism, and if it is considered
to be God's property even in death, one can easily understand why
many Jews would hesitate to mutilate it, or allow one's own body
to be mutilated, even when it is for the noble purpose of helping to
save someone else's life. In the case of living donors, fear for one's
future health and longevity—no matter how much the doctors assure
the potential donor that it would be safe to donate—and psychological
worries about invading the integrity of one's body inevitably play an
important role. But those are not the only factors for Jews. The value of
one's body as part of God's creation and the continued divine ownership
of one's body generate deeply rooted attitudes and behaviors that are
hard to overcome, even when presented with the opportunity of saving
someone else's life.

The Ontic Status of the Dying and the Dead

Another factor deeply embedded within the Jewish tradition that im-
pedes cadaveric organ donations is the Jewish developmental concept
of dying and death. That is, for Judaism, death does not occur in one,
definite, clearly recognizable moment; rather, it is a process that begins
before a person's heart and lungs stop functioning and continues well
after that time.

Criteria for Determining Death in Jewish Medical Decisions

The previous sentence may seem surprising in light of recent rabbinic decisions concerning the accepted signs of death. All the early rabbinic responsa on autopsies, dissection, and transplants concerned people who were indisputably dead by the traditional criteria of death, namely, cessation of breath and heartbeat. Even after those criteria are met, traditional Jewish law as practiced among Eastern European Jews (Ashkenazim) and their descendants requires that relatives wait up to an hour before initiating burial procedures, for fear that physicians have inadequate knowledge to distinguish definitively between death and a fainting spell or swoon.[12] Presumably, those wishing to invade the body for purposes of autopsy, dissection, or transplant would similarly have to wait until then.

This delay, though, is much too long for those wanting to transplant the dying person's heart, so when heart transplants became possible, rabbis, following the lead of the medical community, turned to cessation of brain-wave activity as the criterion for pronouncing a person dead. As early as 1969, Rabbi Jack Segal submitted a responsum to the Conservative movement's Committee on Jewish Law and Standards, urging the adoption of the 1968 Harvard criteria as the new standard for determining the moment of death within Jewish law. Subsequently, in 1975 and 1976, Rabbi Seymour Siegel, then chairman of that committee, and Rabbi Daniel Goldfarb wrote articles endorsing the new criteria in use by the medical community. In turn, that position was formally adopted by the committee when it approved responsa on end-stage medical care by Rabbis Elliot Dorff and Avram Reisner in 1991.[13] The Reform movement officially adopted the Harvard criteria (presumably, as modified by the medical community) in 1980.[14] Orthodox rabbis have differed with each other vigorously over the last two decades concerning the adoption of the brain-wave criterion for death, but the Chief Rabbinate of the state of Israel accepted it for heart transplants under specified conditions in 1968 and reaffirmed this decision in a formal responsum in 1987.[15]

The Gradual Process of Dying

This increasing specificity in defining death in the context of organ transplantation belies the complicated process by which most people die. While accidents can kill healthy people instantaneously, most people die of chronic, rather than acute, illnesses.

The gradual way in which people die has had an effect on the willingness of some Jews to donate organs. Like other people, Jews may worry that, if it is known that they have agreed to donate one or more of their organs, the medical team caring for them will not try as hard to save their life and may, some suspect, even have a vested interest in their death. Similarly, Jews, like others, may simply not want to contemplate their mortality, for that makes them afraid or sad. Discussions about donating organs after death, then, are avoided as part of a general aversion to talking about anything that assumes their death.

Other Jews' refusal, though, stems from both official and folk beliefs concerning the death of the body and its aftermath. Turning to the official beliefs first, Jewish sources depict the process of coming into life in stages,[16] and they similarly describe the process of leaving life in stages. Specifically, when first diagnosed with an irreversible, terminal disease, the person is a *terefah*.[17] For technical reasons regarding the rules of evidence and because the *terefah* is considered as if already dead (*ke gavra ketilla hashiv leih*), one who kills a *terefah* is exempt from capital punishment; this killing, however, is forbidden, and other extralegal punishments imposed by God or the king apply.[18]

Put another way, the Talmud establishes the general principle of the sanctity of every human life by posing the rhetorical question, "How do you know that your blood is redder? Perhaps the blood of the other person is redder!"[19] As Rabbi Joseph Babad says, the provision in Jewish law exempting the killer of a *terefah* from the death penalty effectively makes the *terefah* an exception to this tenet of the equality of all human lives; that is, a *terefah*'s blood *is* less red than that of a viable human being.[20]

When one is about to die, one is a *goses*. A *goses* "brings up a secretion in his throat on account of the narrowing of his chest."[21] Rabbinic sources describe the life of a *goses* like that of a flickering candle, such that even moving the person to prevent bed sores is prohibited lest the motion bring on death. Even then, the patient is to be treated as a living person in all respects.[22] Since Jewish law permits medical inaction (passive euthanasia) once a person becomes a *goses*, however, there has been intense interest in defining the moment of the onset of that category.

The most stringent contemporary rabbis, the ones who permit medical inaction least often, are those who define it as the stage within three days of death.[23] More liberal rabbis, who want to expand our ability to withhold or withdraw medical therapies and let nature take its course, have expanded it to as much as a year and/or changed the relevant issue in defining *goses* to the incurability of the disease.[24] I have argued elsewhere, though, that the sources' analogy of a *goses* to a flickering candle, such that even moving the patient becomes life-threatening, suggests that a *goses* is literally in the last hours of life and that the legal category of *terefah* applies much more appropriately to the critical medical decisions that we find ourselves increasingly called upon to make.[25] Whether to withhold or withdraw medications, machines, and perhaps even artificial nutrition and hydration is most commonly asked about people who could live days or even months or years on such support; by the time a person's life is "a flickering flame," there is little to decide, even with modern medical technology.

Death and Thereafter

However one defines *goses*, the moment of death comes next, defined traditionally as the cessation of breath and heartbeat. As we have seen, though, contemporary rabbis have confused the issue by determining that cessation of all brain-wave activity can count instead, and even under the old definition, one was not certifiably dead until an hour had passed after no heartbeat or breath could be detected. The moment of death, then, is anything but clear in Jewish sources.[26]

Even after one or more of these criteria for death have been met, though, the story is not over. Early rabbinic sources speak of death as "the going out of the soul," but rabbinic lore maintains that the association between body and soul is not altogether severed until three days after death. During that time, according to the classical rabbis, the soul hovers over the grave, hoping to be restored to the body. It departs only when the body begins to decompose and the face changes in character. This, it was believed, is why mourners' grief often reaches its emotional climax on the third day after a loved one's death.[27] It is only after the three-day period that the soul begins its journey in the person's life after death.

This belief did not alter Judaism's insistence on immediate burial of the body. It did, however, serve to disallow evidence on the identity of a person when the body was viewed more than three days after death.[28] It also motivated the permission, notwithstanding the ban on heathen practices, to watch graves for three days in case the interred body is still alive, "for once it happened that they watched one who thereupon continued to live for twenty-five years and another who still had five children before dying."[29]

The story does not end even there. According to some rabbinic sources, at least, for the first twelve months after death the soul retains a temporary relationship to the body, coming and going until the body has disintegrated. This explains, for the rabbis, why the prophet Samuel could be raised from the dead within the first year of his demise in the story of the witch of En-dor. During this year, people's souls—or, according to another view, only the souls of the wicked—are in a kind of purgatory, after which the righteous go to paradise (Gan Eden) and the wicked to hell (Gehinnom). The actual condition of the soul during that time is unclear. Some sources see it as being quiescent, but most seem to ascribe it full consciousness, with one even saying that the "only difference between the living and the dead is the power of speech." A series of disputes surround the question of how much the dead know of the world they leave behind.[30]

During the Middle Ages, these beliefs in continuing life after one physically dies were amplified considerably, especially in folklore and superstition. According to such sources, people's ghosts live a very full life. They gather nightly by the light of the moon, converse with one another or pursue their studies (the Jewish emphasis on education persists even in ghost stories!), adjudge disputes between the latest arrivals and older members of the spirit community, and pray.

Spirits also complain to the living, usually in dreams, when their bodily existence has been affronted in some way. Grave tampering will almost surely bring the ghost of the person buried to haunt the offenders and even innocent family members at night.

The spirits' concern with the state of their bodies on earth, though, is not only a residual expression of interest in their earthly existence; according to many legends, the spirits of people who have died retain their bodily forms. Consequently, spirits also torment the living when the clothes in which they were buried are inadequate for their spiritual existence. For example, a girl whose father had been too poor to provide her with a burial shroud could not come out into the open to gather with the other spirits and begged that her nakedness be clothed; another spirit, who had been buried with the sleeve of his shroud torn, said that he was ashamed before the others to appear in that disgraceful state. Visits of this nature were repeated until the grave was opened and the defect remedied.

In biblical times, people were buried in their normal clothes, but the ostentation that custom produced led to the rabbinic ruling that everyone—rich or poor, young or old, male or female—must be buried in plain linen shrouds.[31] Even in such humble clothing, though, concern for modesty and honor in one's attire persisted. If the spirits were worried about being properly clothed, they worried even more about the integrity of their bodies—a direct argument against donating any of one's bodily parts for fear of subsequent wrath from one's own spirit.

That was no small matter, for dead spirits were known for their angry and threatening ways. They were, after all, members of the unknown and uncanny spirit world, and they possessed much power. In extreme cases, one needed to extricate spirits that took possession of a person, as in the popular Yiddish story and play *The Dybbuk*. A medieval source provides the formula for attempting to do this:

> With the consent of the celestial and earthly tribunals I conjure you in the name of the God of heaven and of earth, and by all the holy Names, that you desist from pursuing any human, whether man or woman, adult or child, near or far, and that you do them no harm with your body or your spirit or your soul. Your body must lie in its grave until resurrection; your soul must rest in that place where it belongs. I command this upon you with a curse and with an oath, now and forever.[32]

Such texts of exorcism bespeak the genuine concern of Jews not to offend the spirits. Mutilating the body in which the spirit formerly existed was one sure way to ask for trouble.

The Implications for Organ Transplantation

Judaism, then, perceives dying as extended over several phases; it has a basic diffidence with regard to our ability to define the moment of death exactly; and it has official and popular beliefs in spirits who live on after death. Given these features of Judaism, one can understand how it is that some Jews, at any rate, would be wary of agreeing to donate their organs. The medical community and, indeed, Jewish law may define you as dead, but other elements within the tradition would undercut your certainty.

Beyond this uncertainty, one must remember, too, the strong emphasis Judaism puts on life. Jewish law requires that Jews take steps to preserve their life and health, and they must live in a town with a physician so that they can get professional help when they are sick.[33] The push to cure is so strong in Judaism that you violate Jewish law if you give a dying person any inkling that you doubt his or her ability to continue living.[34] Indeed, this precept leads a minority of rabbis to oppose hospice care, since such care is based on the premise that the person acknowledges the inevitability and imminence of death and acquiesces to it.[35] A much stronger strain within the tradition cites the need to bolster patients' hope as overriding the requirement to tell them the whole truth about their medical condition.[36] The Jewish emphasis on life also prompts the rule that places preservation of life above all but three other duties. More pervasively still, a hearty attachment to this life undergirds the strong activist tendencies of Judaism to make this world a better place and even the traditional toast Jews use—*Le hayyim*, "to life!"

No wonder, then, that despite the ability of transplantation to save another person's life, some Jews have difficulty agreeing to donate their organs. Everything in the tradition urges them to hold on to life as long as possible, and so they never contemplate their own death and the ways they could contribute bodily to someone else's life. Moreover, they have no clear conception of when they are "really" dead such that they can legitimately give up their body parts. Finally, popular beliefs in an existence of spirits after death—but spirits who look like the embodied people they were in life—might make them hesitant to allow their bodies to be altered prior to that spiritual existence.

Bodily Existence after Death

If a person's after-death existence in the form of a spirit might deter organ donation, beliefs about bodily resurrection pose an even greater deterrence. In most biblical literature, people after death go down to the dark realm of the dead, where they presumably no longer have independent existence as persons. "The dead cannot praise You, nor any who go down into silence," the Psalmist reminds God. Job and Ecclesiastes know of the doctrine of the resurrection of the dead but deny it; it is only the Book of Daniel, chronologically the last book of the Hebrew Bible (c. 150 B.C.E.), that affirms this tenet.[37]

In the last two centuries before the common era and the first five of the common era, ideas about what happens after death were hotly debated. Members of some Jewish groups, especially the Sadducees, continued to deny any particular existence of individuals after death. Some Jewish groups supported the idea of the immortality of the soul, while others affirmed resurrection of the dead.

The Pharisees—that is, the rabbis who shaped the Jewish tradition—affirmed both, even though those doctrines are, on some readings at least, mutually contradictory. After all, if the person dies in all respects, resurrection must occur for there to be any future life. On the other hand, if the soul lives on eternally, the need for resurrection is questionable for, by hypothesis, the person continues to live, albeit in a disembodied form. Most rabbis nevertheless combined these views, affirming that the soul, after death, continues on with God until messianic times, when it is rejoined with the dust of the earth in resurrection. The Pharisees held this belief so strongly that they claimed that a Jew must not only believe the doctrine but also aver that it is rooted in the Torah—where, as we have said, the idea of resurrection never occurs.[38]

That the Pharisees even entertained the idea that the soul could exist on its own may seem surprising in light of the rabbis' view, explained earlier, that the body and soul are an integrated whole. As I noted there, however, that belief did not prevent the rabbis from imagining a separate existence for body and soul. For one thing, the phenomenon of sleep[39] suggested to them that one's life can be at least temporarily separated from one's body. For another, as Genesis 2:7 states, "The Lord God formed man (Adam) from the dust of the earth. He blew in his nostrils the breath of life, and man became a living being." Following this, the rabbis maintained that God created a formless glob of matter—in Hebrew, a *golem*—from the earth and threw life breath into it.[40] Among the mystics of the seventeenth and eighteenth centuries, this assertion became the basis of many golem legends, according to which the speech of certain rabbis actually had the power to create such shapeless beings. For our purposes, though, God's joining of the body with its life breath at its creation, as described by the Genesis verse, suggested to the rabbis that God would rejoin the two during resurrection as well.

This graphically physical depiction of resurrection helps to explain why the traditional rabbinic belief in bodily resurrection is, for some Jews, the source of an important objection to organ donation. They believe that the body must be buried with all its parts so that they will all be there when it comes time for resurrection. This belief is deeply ingrained in the folk religion. During the many times that I have spoken to Jewish audiences about providing for the transplantation of one's organs after death, someone almost inevitably asserts the belief that Jews may not donate their organs to others because that would prevent their bodily resurrection.

Rabbis' and other religious Jews' raising of this point may not be surprising, but most often this idea comes from Jews who are otherwise totally secular in their thought and actions. Similarly, this issue came up in Israel in 1977, when the Labor Party failed to form a coalition with the religious parties, in part because of Orthodox objection to autopsies. In one exchange, a writer in the *Jerusalem Post* interviewed an Orthodox rabbi in Tel Aviv, and began his questions with this one: "Is it true that the Orthodox are against post-mortems because when the 'dead are resurrected' *(tehiyat hametim)*, those who lack parts (or organs) from their bodies cannot rise from the grave?" The rabbi answered, "There is no truth in all this. It is some sort of mysticism to which we do not subscribe. When the dead arise, nobody will be excluded, even if parts or all of his body are missing." He then explained that Orthodox objections to autopsies were based instead on fear of unnecessarily desecrating the body.[41]

Medieval Jewish philosophers, while not addressing organ donation per se, provided some important arguments against the need to keep the body intact. Saadia Gaon (892–942 C.E.), for example, pointed out that if one believes that God created the world from nothing, one certainly should also believe that God can revive the dead, for that involves only the comparatively easier task of creating something out of something that has existed already but is now disintegrated: "We know of no Jew who opposes this doctrine, or finds it difficult from the point of view of his Reason that God should revive the dead, since it has already become clear to him that God created the world *ex nihilo*. He can find no difficulty therefore in believing that God should, by a second act, create something from something disintegrated and dissolved."[42]

Maimonides (1135–1204 c.e.) took a different tack. Like many of the Neoplatonists and Neo-Aristotelians of his time, he denigrated the body. As a result, he actually mocked his co-religionists who looked forward to a bodily resurrection:

Concerning this strange world to come, you will rarely find anyone to whom it occurs to think about it seriously or to adopt it as a fundamental doctrine of our faith, or to inquire what it really means, whether the world to come is the ultimate good or whether some other possibility. Nor does one often find persons who distinguish between the ultimate good itself and the means which lead to the ultimate good. What everybody wants to know, both the masses and the learned, is how the dead will arise. They want to know whether they will be naked or clothed, whether they will rise in the same shrouds with which they were buried, with the same embroidery, style, and beauty of sewing, or in a plain garment which just covers their bodies. Or they ask whether, when the Messiah comes, there will still be rich men and poor men, weak men and strong men, and other similar questions.[43]

Such literal understandings of bodily resurrection, according to Maimonides, are childish, taught by the sages to encourage the masses to obey God's commandments in hopes of a future physical reward or in fear of future physical punishment. The truth, for Maimonides, is that after death the soul continues on without the body, and its pleasures are the vastly more enduring and important pleasures of the spirit. In line with such thinking, he quotes this talmudic passage: "In the world to come there is no eating, drinking, washing, anointing, or sexual intercourse; but the righteous sit with their crowns on their heads enjoying the radiance of the Divine Presence."[44]

Such philosophic views, however, have not penetrated the beliefs of most Jews who believe in resurrection. For them, bodily resurrection continues to be a living element of their faith, and Saadia's argument, which most do not know in any case, has not relieved their anxiety over what will happen to them if they give up some parts of their bodies for organ donation.

The Jewish Duty of Helping and Giving to Those in Need

We have seen a number of factors embedded deeply within the Jewish psyche that impede Jews' willingness to donate their organs. They should not, however, be exaggerated. A *Los Angeles Times* poll taken in December 1991, for example, found that 67 percent of Christians and 45 percent of those with no religious affiliation believed in life after death, but only 30 percent of Jews said that they did. In explaining their position, most Jews claimed that we just do not know enough, or that people live on in the influence they have on the lives of others, especially their children, or that there is nothing after death. Even fewer Jews believed in a devil or in a hell to which sinners are condemned: 58 percent of Christians believed in those doctrines, but only 4 percent of Jews did.[45] Of the 30 percent of Jews who believed in a life after death, of course, only some would worry that, if they were not buried whole, they would suffer handicaps in an afterlife.

Moreover, several features of Judaism, rooted just as deeply within the tradition, impel other Jews to sign up as organ donors and require those who do not do so to think twice about their decision. Chief among these, of course, is the imperative to save the lives of others (*pikkuah nefesh*). Two other parts of the tradition, however, while legally not directly relevant to organ donation, form some of the psychological background that would incline people favorably toward organ transplantation.

One is the Torah's command not to stand idly by the blood of one's neighbor (Leviticus 19:16). As is generally the case, rabbis have interpreted this command, as they do all others, to delineate specifically what it requires of Jews, and they have included quite a bit. Ransom of captives and saving drowning persons are two clear examples of what this law has been interpreted to require.[46] In practice, though, the verse has been used widely within the tradition to motivate action to help others well beyond what is legally demanded by the law, even according to the rabbis' broad interpretations. One must come to the rescue of others, even at some risk to oneself—a resounding imperative that clearly would prompt some Jews to consider applying it to organ transplantation as well.

Another pervasive feature of Jewish consciousness, while not legally connected to organ transplantation, undoubtedly has an effect on it psychologically. Judaism includes a highly developed set of laws that require Jews to help those in need. When that is done through financial support, the term used is *zedakah*. When one helps in other ways, the term is *hesed*.

In English we usually call such actions charity, but that term misrepresents the two Jewish concepts involved. *Charity* comes from the Latin word meaning affection or love, and it indicates an act done out of such love, a supererogatory act, one done above and beyond the call of duty. Therefore people who give charity are to see themselves, and are to be seen by others, as unusually good.

Within Judaism, in contrast, the Hebrew word used for monetarily helping others in need is *zedakah,* coming from the root meaning "justice." That is, for Judaism, helping others is part of one's duty to God and to one's fellow human beings. One can feel good about helping others, but only because one has fulfilled one's duty, not because one has exceeded what can legitimately be expected of people. *Zedakah may* be given out of love as well as out of duty, but it *must* be given whether one wants to or not.[47]

Hesed, meaning originally "an act done out of loyalty to one's fellow," came to mean also acts of kindness, care, and concern. As such, acts of *hesed* are not as mandatory as are acts of *zedakah,* but they have a degree of obligation to them beyond that connoted by the English word *charity,* as the following makes clear:

"To walk in all His ways" (Deuteronomy 11:22). These are the ways of the Holy One: "gracious and compassionate, patient, abounding in kindness and faithfulness, assuring love for a thousand generations, forgiving iniquity, transgression, and sin, and granting pardon . . ."(Exodus 34:6–7). This means that just as God is gracious and compassionate, you too must be gracious and compassionate. "The Lord is righteous in all His ways and loving in all His deeds" (Psalm 145:17). As the Holy One is righteous, you too must be righteous. As the Holy One is loving, you too must be loving.[48]

"Follow the Lord your God" (Deuteronomy 13:5). What does this mean? Is it possible for a mortal to follow God's Presence? The verse means to teach us that we should follow the attributes of the Holy One, praised be He. As He clothes the naked, . . . you should clothe the naked. The Bible teaches that the Holy One visited the sick . . . ; you should visit the sick. The Holy One comforted those who mourned . . . ; you should comfort those who mourn. The Holy One buried the dead . . . ; you should bury the dead.[49]

As we have seen, rabbis have ruled that donating an organ to a person who needs one is *not* required of a healthy person because of the danger involved. One's own life comes first; the obligations of *zedakah* or *hesed* do not override that. When the danger is not great, however, then people *may* donate an organ, and it is, in those circumstances, an honored, godly thing to do. It is done *lifnim meshurat ha-din,* beyond the letter of the law, but in the spirit of its values.[50] According to these concepts, then, people are certainly encouraged to make arrangements to donate their own organs when they die, and family members are urged to agree to this and to make such arrangements on their own in the absence of an oral or written directive by the deceased to that effect, for then no danger threatens the donor, while the transplant may enable another person to live.

Thus, while *zedakah* and *hesed* cannot be construed to require organ donation from the living as a matter of Jewish law, they influence Jewish life so thoroughly that they inevitably constitute part of the psychological background that prompts Jews to think seriously about donating, at least in death. The concepts underlying the obligations to help those in need, after all, are among the most central and powerful in the Jewish tradition. They include the meaning, privileges, and responsibilities of membership in a community; compassion for fellow human beings; obedience of God's commandment to care for others and to act to help them; the need to preserve the dignity of God's creatures; the obligation to live up to the Covenant with God, including the promises and expectations inherent in that relationship; and the mandate to aspire to holiness.[51] No wonder, then, that these obligations occupy a central place in the minds of Jews who are at all connected to the tradition, and no wonder that they are one important factor—as the theological and psychological background, even if not as the legal basis—in Jews' attitudes toward organ transplantation.

The Jewish Imperative to Donate

Jews may fail to sign the back of their driver's license or some other legal instrument for the donation of organs for any of a variety of reasons, some of which relate to Judaism and some of which do not. Many people, from all sorts of backgrounds, are afraid to contemplate their own death. Others have psychological difficulty with the notion that their body's integrity will be compromised or that part of their body will exist in some other person. Still others have simply never heard about the possibility of donation or the reasons for it.

Along with these and other reasons that inhibit the general population from agreeing to donate, Jews might have some special reasons. Respect for the body as God's property and for the deceased person prohibits, in a few Orthodox rabbis' interpretation of Jewish law, all but those organ transplants that are immediately lifesaving. The concerns of other Jews stem from their folk beliefs regarding the dying process and life after death.

All these factors should not obscure the fact, however, that Judaism's overarching command to save life and limb has prompted almost all rabbis who have written on this subject to permit and, indeed, to urge Jews to make provision for donating bodily parts. Where little or no danger to the recipient is involved—as in blood and bone-marrow donations—Judaism imposes a duty even on people who are not family of the person in need. Kidneys and any other organs (for example, part of one's liver) cannot be demanded because of the risks involved for the donor, but it certainly is an honored act within Judaism for a person to save another's life by being such a donor.

When it comes to deceased donors, the overwhelming number of rabbis who have written about this see organ donation not only as permitted, but indeed, as commanded. The imperative to save lives supersedes the normal prohibitions against invading the integrity of the corpse out of honor for it, and it even more definitely supersedes any worry about the condition of one's body in a life after death. The biblical command not to stand idly by the blood of one's neighbor also plays a role here, and so does the Jewish conception of sharing and giving as acts of justice, not charity.

This chapter has not dealt with the hard decisions society must make in allocating its resources. The need to save lives does not automatically mean that organ donation should be the only, or even the primary, way we do this. Preventive medicine and, for that matter, provision of food, clothing, and shelter to those lacking them may arguably take precedence over organ donation, if only because we can save more lives using those measures than we can through organ transplantations.

The clear mandate of the Jewish tradition, however, is that if organ donation can be done, both medically and financially, Jews must lend a hand in seeing to it that it is done. Thus, in our day, when medicine is at once so promising and yet so morally perplexing, these famous words from the Torah have new and deep significance: "I call upon heaven and earth to witness against you this day: I have put before you life and death, blessing and curse. *Choose life*—if you and your offspring would live—by loving the Lord your God, heeding His commands, and holding fast to Him . . ."(Deuteronomy 30:19–20).

Notes

In the following, M. = Mishnah (edited c. 200 C.E.); T. = Tosefta (edited c. 200 C.E.); J. = Jerusalem (Palestinian) Talmud (edited c. 400 C.E.); B. = Babylonian Talmud (edited c. 500 C.E.); M.T. = Moses Maimonides' *Mishneh Torah* (1177 C.E.); S.A. = Joseph Karo's *Shulhan Arukh* (1565 C.E.).

The Mishnah, the Tosefta, the Jerusalem Talmud, and the Babylonian Talmud are all, in turn, divided into sections called tractates (for example, *Yoma, Sanhedrin, Berakhot*), and each tractate is divided into chapters and specific laws.

References to the Mishnah, Tosefta, and Jerusalem Talmud, therefore, appear with the tractate name, chapter, and law number, for example, M. *Sanhedrin* 4:5 (that is, chapter 4, law number 5). Since the pagination of the first printed edition of the Babylonian Talmud became standard, references to it are by tractate and folio page, for example, B. *Sanhedrin* 35b (that is, page 35, on the second side of the tractate's page). Most pages of the standard, printed editions of the Babylonian Talmud contain, in addition to the Talmud text itself, the commentary of Rabbi Shelomo Yitzhaki ("Rashi," 1035–1104 c.e.) and the questions and answers of some of the rabbis in the generations which succeeded him, the Tosafot. References to comments of Rashi or the Tosafot will cite them, the page of the Talmud on which they are commenting, and often the first Hebrew words of the particular comment to which the person writing the citation wants to make reference, for example, Rashi, B. *Sanhedrin* 2a, s. v. (that is, the comment beginning with the words) *gezelot vehavalot*. The same style is used for other commentators on the Talmud, but sometimes their comments are numbered, and so the citation will generally cite the number and sometimes the beginning words of the comment to make sure that everyone knows which comment is intended.

In addition to the literature described in the previous paragraph, which is organized by topic, another genre of rabbinic literature developed in the first five centuries of the common era that was organized according to the order of the Bible, that is, the Midrash—or the interpretations of biblical verses. Interpretations of the legal verses of the Torah are contained in the *Mekhilta* (on Exodus), the *Sifra* (on Leviticus), and the *Sifre* (on Numbers and Deuteronomy). Interpretations of the nonlegal verses are found primarily in the collections known as *Genesis Rabbah, Exodus Rabbah,* and so on, where *Rabbah* means "expanded," or "great." Thus *Genesis Rabbah* is the biblical book of Genesis expanded with rabbinic homilies and commentary, and so on for the rest of the books of the Torah and the Five Scrolls read in the synagogue at various times of the year (Song of Songs, Ruth, Lamentations, Ecclesiastes, Esther). References to the Midrash are usually to the chapter and section of the particular book of Midrash (for example, *Genesis Rabbah* 29:4) or, if the book of Midrash is divided only into chapters, by the section of the book of the Torah in which the comment appears and the chapter of that section of Midrash, for example, *Tanhuma*, Vayikra (the name of a section of the Torah) 6 (chapter 6). Sometimes, though, midrashic sources are instead cited according to the biblical verse which is being interpreted, for example, *Song of Songs Rabbah* on Song of Songs 4:2, *Mekhilta* on Exodus 19:15.

The two most prominent codes are the *Mishneh Torah* (or *Yad Ha-Hazakah*), written by Moses Maimonides, and the *Shulhan Arukh* by Joseph Karo. Maimonides' code is divided into sections of laws, and those, in turn, are divided into chapters and specific laws. References to it therefore look like this: M. T. (or Yad) *Laws of Murder* 4:7 (chapter 4, law number 7). The *Shulhan Arukh* is divided into four books, which, in turn, are divided into chapters and specific laws. The four books are: *Orah Hayyim, Yoreh De'ah, Even Haezer,* and *Hoshen Mishpat.*

References to it therefore look like this: S. A. *Orah Hayyim* 139:6. These codes quickly developed a number of commentaries, and those are referenced by the commentary and the place in the code on which the commentator is making a point, for example, *Kesef Mishneh* to M. T. *Laws of Murder* 4:7, *Taz* to S. A. *Orah Hayyim* 5:2. Because he indicated where Eastern European practices differed from the Mediterranean ones in Karo's code, Rabbi Moses Isserles' commentary to the *Shulhan Arukh* is the most important and is actually inserted into the printed text of the *Shulhan Arukh* itself as glosses (printed in different typeface for clarity of identity).

Because the *Shulhan Arukh* became quite authoritative, later books of rabbinic rulings were often organized by its order. So, for example, Rabbi Moses Feinstein, a twentieth-century rabbi, wrote many volumes of responsa, each divided into the topics covered by the four divisions of the *Shulhan Arukh*. Thus references to his responsa will look like this: *Iggerot Moshe* (the name he gave to his books of responsa), *Yoreh De'ah* 2 (volume 2), #174 (responsum number 174). Other rabbis, though, organize their responsa simply by volume number and responsum number within the volume, for example, Eliezer Waldenberg, *Responsa Tzitz Eliezer* (the name he gave to his volumes of rulings) 13 (volume 13), #89 (responsum number 89).

1.   B. *Yoma* 85a–b (with Rashi's explanatory comments there); B. *Sanhedrin* 74a–b; *Mekhilta* on Exodus 31:13; and, for a general discussion of this topic, see Immanuel Jakobovits, *Jewish Medical Ethics*, 2d ed. (New York: Bloch, 1972), 45–98.

2.   B. *Bava Metzia* 62a.

3.   Jakobovits, *Jewish Medical Ethics*, 291; see also 96–98. This is the generally held opinion regarding living donors not only for Orthodox rabbis, some of whom he references, but also for Conservative and Reform rabbis. For Orthodox opinions, see the responsa (judicial opinions) of Moshe Feinstein, *Iggerot Moshe*, Yoreh De'ah 229 and 230 (Hebrew); Eliezer Waldenberg, *Tzitz Eliezer*, vol. 9, no. 45, and vol. 10, no. 25 (Hebrew); Obadiah Yoseph, *Dinei Yisrael*, vol. 7 (Hebrew). For a Conservative position (the only one I know of to date on living donors), see my *"Choose Life": A Jewish Perspective on Medical Ethics* (Los Angeles: University of Judaism, 1985), 23. For Reform positions, see Solomon B. Freehof, *New Reform Responsa* (Cincinnati: Hebrew Union College Press, 1980), 62ff. Solomon B. Freehof, *Current Reform Responsa* (Cincinnati: Hebrew Union College Press, 1969), 118–25; and Walter Jacob, *Contemporary American Reform Responsa* (New York: Central Conference of American Rabbis, 1987), 128–33.

4.   This is the position of J. David Bleich, *Judaism and Healing* (New York: KTAV, 1981), 132, 166–67; see generally 129–33, 162–68.

5.   *Proceedings of the Rabbinical Assembly* 52 (1990): 279. Provision for organ donation is also included in the new (1994) advance directive edited by Rabbi Aaron Mackler and published by the Rabbinical Assembly after being approved by the Conservative movement's Committee on Jewish Law and Standards. That, in turn, was based on the joint approval of organ transplantation by Rabbis

Elliot N. Dorff and Avram Reisner, who wrote the validated responsa for the Conservative movement on matters at the end of life. See Elliot N. Dorff, "A Jewish Approach to End-Stage Medical Care," *Conservative Judaism* 43, no. 3 (spring 1991): 3–51; and Avram Reisner, "A Halakhic Ethic of Care for the Terminally Ill," *Conservative Judaism* 43, no. 3 (spring 1991): 52–89. A similar stance can be found in the work of another Conservative rabbi, David M. Feldman, *Health and Medicine in the Jewish Tradition* (New York: Crossroad, 1986), 103–8.

For a summary of Orthodox positions, see Jakobovits, *Jewish Medical Ethics*, 278–91; and Fred Rosner, "Organ Transplantation in Jewish Law," in Fred Rosner and J. David Bleich, eds., *Jewish Bioethics* (New York: Sanhedrin Press, 1979), 358–74.

For a Reform position on this, see Solomon B. Freehof, "The Use of the Cornea of the Dead," *C.C.A.R.* [Central Conference of American Rabbis] *Yearbook* 66 (1956): 104–7; Solomon B. Freehof, "Surgical Transplants," *C.C.A.R. Yearbook* 78 (1968): 118–21 (both these last two responsa are reprinted in Walter Jacob, ed., *American Reform Responsa* [New York: Central Conference of American Rabbis, 1983], 288–96); Solomon B. Freehof, "Donating a Body to Science," *Reform Responsa* (Cincinnati: Hebrew Union College Press, 1960), 130–31; Solomon B. Freehof, "Bequeathing Parts of the Body," *Contemporary Reform Responsa* (Cincinnati: Hebrew Union College Press, 1974), 216–23.

In a March 1986 responsum, the Central Conference of American Rabbis as a body officially affirmed the practice of organ donation, and in 1992 the synagogue arm of the Reform movement, through its Committee on the Synagogue as a Caring Community and its Committee on Bio-Medical Ethics, published a manual for preparing for death that specifically includes provision for donation of one's entire body or of particular organs to a specified person, hospital, or organ bank for transplantation and/or for research, medical education, therapy of another person, or any purpose authorized by law. The manual is Richard F. Address, ed., *A Time to Prepare: A Practical Guide for Individuals and Families in Determining One's Wishes for Extraordinary Medical Treatment and Financial Arrangements* (Philadelphia: Union of American Hebrew Congregations Committee on Bio-Medical Ethics, 1992).

Although somewhat dated, a good summary of the positions of all three movements, with relevant quotations from responsa and other official position statements, can be found in Alex J. Goldman, *Judaism Confronts Contemporary Issues* (New York: Shengold Publishers, 1978), 211–37.

6.   Philo and Maimonides in the *Guide* (but not nearly as much in his law code, the *Mishneh Torah*) are probably the prime examples of Jewish thinkers who espoused a soul-body or mind-body dichotomy, largely because of Greek influence. See, for example, Philo, in Hans Lewy, Alexander Altmann, and Isaak Heinemann, eds., *Three Jewish Philosophers* (Philadelphia: Jewish Publication Society of America, 1960), pt. 1, esp. 42–51, 54–55, and 71–75; he calls the body a "prison house" (72). See also Maimonides, *Guide of the Perplexed*, trans. Shlomo Pines (Chicago: University of Chicago Press, 1963), 532–34, pt. 3, chap. 33, where he maintains that one of the chief objects of the commandments is "to make man

reject, despise, and reduce his desires as much as is in his power." For in the attempt to satisfy his bodily desires, "in the manner of fools, man loses his intellectual energy, injures his body, and perishes before his natural time; sighs and cares multiply; and there is an increase of envy, hatred, and warfare for the purpose of taking what another possesses."

7. So, for example, the departure of the soul during sleep and its return upon waking is articulated in the first words that one is supposed to say when one regains consciousness: "I am grateful to You, living, enduring Sovereign, for restoring my soul (my life breath, *nishmati*) to me in compassion. You are faithful (trustworthy) beyond measure" (see, for example, *Siddur Sim Shalom: A Prayerbook for Shabbat, Festivals, and Weekdays* [New York: Rabbinical Assembly and United Synagogue of America, 1985], 2–3). Similarly, a daily morning prayer in Jewish liturgy depicts God as the one who each day "returns life-breaths [*neshamot*, plural of *neshamah*] to dead corpses," with the stark redundancy of that phrase emphasizing that the body without consciousness is indeed dead. Cf. Genesis 2:7; B. *Ta'anit* 22b; *Genesis Rabbah* 14:9. At death, also, some sources depict the soul as departing from the body and returning to it at the time of resurrection, while other sources maintain that the soul cannot exist apart from the body. Cf. B. *Berakhot* 18b–19a; B. *Haggigah* 12b; B. *Ketubbot* 77b, as against, for example, *Tanhuma*, Vayikra 11.

8. *Leviticus Rabbah* 34:3.

9. B. *Sanhedrin* 91a–b. See also *Mekhilta*, Beshalah, Shirah, ch. 2 (edited Horowitz-Rabin, 1960, 125); *Leviticus Rabbah* 4:5; *Yalkut Shimoni* on Leviticus 4:2 (no. 464); *Tanhuma*, Vayikra 6. The very development of the term *neshamah* from meaning "physical breath" to "one's inner being" bespeaks Judaism's view that the physical and the spiritual are integrated.

10. M. *Avot* 2:1. See B. *Berakhot* 35b, especially the comment of Abayae in response to the earlier theories of Rabbi Ishmael and Rabbi Simeon bar Yohai.

11. See B. *Berakhot* 61a–b; B. *Sanhedrin* 38a; *Genesis Rabbah* 1:3; *Exodus Rabbah* 24:1; and *Numbers Rabbah* 18:22 for examples of the rabbis' praise of the body. See B. *Sanhedrin* 91a–b; B. *Shabbat* 152b; and *Genesis Rabbah* 67:3 for examples of the interaction of body and soul in determining the virtuous or sinful nature of a person. See also A. Cohen, *Everyman's Talmud* (New York: E. P. Dutton, 1949), 67–78, 88–95, on these topics.

12. This is based on Moses Isserles's comment in S. A. *Orah Hayyim* 330:5 (and see the comment of the Magen Avraham there, no. 11) in which he disagrees with the Talmud and Joseph Karo, ibid., that surgeons should cut open a woman who has died during childbirth as soon as her breath and heartbeat have ceased in an effort to save the fetus. Isserles is concerned that in the laudable attempt to save the fetus, the woman, who by hypothesis is hovering over the moment of death, will be killed by the surgery rather than by natural causes, making the surgeon a murderer. The resultant custom in Jerusalem during the first half of this century was not to remove a corpse for burial until at least twenty minutes, and, according to some, for as much as an hour after cessation of breath and heartbeat. See Jakobovits, *Jewish Medical Ethics*, 126–29;

Bleich, *Judaism and Healing,* 146–57, esp. 152–53. Since lack of medical knowledge prompted this ruling, and since sphygmomanometers and electrocardiograms can now determine lack of blood pressure and heart function definitively, most contemporary sources would now claim that Isserles's concern can be met and that we can rest assured that we know exactly when a person has died. This is certainly behind the chief rabbinate's decision to permit heart transplants, described below.

13.　Jack Segal, "Judaism and Heart Transplantations," in the Rabbinical Assembly Archives, vol. Y (4 August 1969): 90–92; quoted in Goldman, *Judaism Confronts Contemporary Issues,* 229–30. That book presents, on pp. 211–37, a good overview of the positions on organ transplantation of all three movements up to its publication date in 1978. Seymour Siegel, "Fetal Experimentation," *Conservative Judaism* 29, no. 4 (summer 1975): 39–48; Siegel, "Updating the Criteria of Death," *Conservative Judaism* 30 no. 2 (winter 1976): 23–30; Daniel Goldfarb, "The Definition of Death," *Conservative Judaism* 30, no. 2 (winter 1976): 10–22; Seymour Siegel, "The Ethical Dimensions of Modern Medicine: A Jewish Approach," *United Synagogue Review* (fall 1976): 4. No mention of these articles is included in the "Index to Law Committee Responsa," published in *Conservative Judaism* 34, no. 1 (September/October 1980): 43–54, and so the first official endorsement of the new criteria for the Conservative movement came in the committee's approval in December 1990 of the responsa by Rabbis Elliot N. Dorff and Avram Reisner (see note 5 above), both of which assume and explicitly invoke the new medical definition.

14.　Walter Jacob, Leonard S. Kravitz, W. Gunther Plaut, Harry A. Roth, Rav A. Soloff, and Bernard Zlotowitz, "Euthanasia," in Jacob, ed., *American Reform Responsa,* 273–74.

15.　For a summary of some of the varying Orthodox opinions on this subject up to 1978 in America, England, and Israel, see Goldman, *Judaism Confronts Contemporary Issues,* 223–29. Rabbi Immanuel Jakobovits, immediate past chief rabbi of the British Commonwealth, has accepted heart transplants since 1966. In Israel, Ashkenazic chief rabbi Issar Yehudah Unterman permitted heart transplants in 1968 ("Points of Halakhah in the Question of Heart Transplantation," address to the Congress of Oral Law, Jerusalem, August 1968; discussed and cited in Fred Rosner, "Organ Transplantation," in Rosner and Bleich, eds., *Jewish Bioethics,* 367–71; a subsequently published essay by Rabbi Unterman, "The Problem of Heart Transplantation from the Viewpoint of Halakhah," can be found in *No'am* 13 [1970]: 1–9), and the Sephardic chief rabbi at that time, Rabbi Yitzhak Nissim, endorsed that responsum.

On the other hand, Rabbi Moses Feinstein, president of Agudat Harabanim, the Union of Orthodox Rabbis of America, and the rabbi whose responsa shaped right-wing Orthodox practice in North America throughout his life, issued a strong prohibition against heart transplants, claiming that they involve a double murder (the donor and the recipient) and that physicians who perform them are "evil" (*Hapardes* 43, no. 6 [March-April 1969]: 4; see his collection of responsa, *Iggerot Moshe, Yoreh De'ah,* pt. 2, no. 174, 286–94 [New York: Balshon 1973]).

His son-in-law, Rabbi Moses Tendler, and Dr. Fred Rosner, however, report subsequent conversations with him in which Rabbi Feinstein "clarified" his position this way: If the donor is absolutely dead by all medical and Jewish legal criteria, then heart transplantation is permissible, a view he seems to take in his responsum concerning the signs of death *Iggerot Moshe, Yoreh De'ah*, pt. 2, no. 146, 247–52; see Rosner, "Organ Transplantation," 370. Rabbi J. David Bleich (*Judaism and Healing*, 146–57) categorically denies the acceptability of brain-death criteria to determine death, and in his article "Time of Death Legislation" (*Tradition* 16, no. 4 [summer 1977]: 133), he claims that, in oral communications with him, Rabbi Feinstein "in no way is prepared to accept any form of 'brain death' as compatible with the provisions of Halakhah."

In any case, the Chief Rabbinical Council of the state of Israel reaffirmed the acceptability of heart transplants in a responsum issued in 1987. That responsum has been translated by Yoel Jakobovits, "[Brain Death and] Heart Transplants: The [Israeli] Chief Rabbinate's Directives," *Tradition* 24, no. 4 (summer 1989): 1–14.

For other Orthodox opinions, see Rosner, "Organ Transplantation," and Goldman, *Judaism Confronts Contemporary Issues*, both cited earlier in this note.

16.   Specifically, (1) the first forty days of gestation, when the fetus is "simply water" (B. *Yevamot* 69b; B. *Niddah* 15b, 17a [which speaks of the first trimester], 30a–b); (2) the remainder of pregnancy, when the fetus is "like its mother's thigh" (B. *Hullin* 58a; cf. B. *Gittin* 23b); (3) from the time that the head emerges (M. *Oholot* 7:6; T. *Yevamot* 9; B. *Sanhedrin* 72b) or "its greater part" (J. *Shabbat* 14:4; J. *Sanhedrin*, end) until thirty days after birth, during which time killing the child is murder, but full mourning rites are not held for a child who dies in that time since, in view of the high rates of infant mortality until recently, he or she is not yet considered an established life (*bar kayyama*) (B. *Niddah* 44b; S. A. *Yoreh De'ah* 344:8); and (4) from the thirty-first day after birth on, when the child is a full-fledged human being for all purposes. On this topic generally, see David Feldman, *Birth Control in Jewish Law* (New York: New York University Press, 1968), subsequently published under the title *Marital Relations, Birth Control, and Abortion in Jewish Law* (New York, Schocken, 1970), chaps. 15 and 16, esp. 266.

17.   The death of a *terefah* is usually expected within twelve months (M. *Yevamot* 16:4; commentary of Nahmanides to *Yevamot* 120b, s. v. *"umi matsit"*; commentary of Rashba to *Yevamot*, no. 230, s. v. *"umi matzit"*; commentaries of *Maggid Mishneh* and *Kesef Mishneh* to M. T. *Laws of Divorce* 13:16; S. A. *Even Haezer* 17:32), as is the death of an animal in that condition (B. *Hullin* 58a M. T. *Laws of Slaughter* 11:1; S. A. *Yoreh De'ah* 57:18). However, with regard to human beings, the condition is defined by medical evidence of terminality, not by time, as Maimonides says: "[A person is a *terefah* when] it is known for certain that he had a fatal organic disease and physicians say that his disease was incurable by human agency and that he would have died of it even if he had not been killed in another way" (M. T. *Laws of Murder* 2:8). See also Tosafot to B. *Gittin* 57b, s. v. *"venikar bemokho"*; Tosafot to B. *Eruvin* 7a, s. v. *"kegaon shidra"*; *Kesef Mishneh* to M. T. *Laws of Divorce* 13:16; Tosafot Yom Tov to M. *Yevamot* 16:4, all of whom assert that a human *terefah* may live longer than twelve months.

18. B. *Sanhedrin* 78a, and cf. Rashi there. M. T. *Laws of Murder* 2:8, cf. 2:2–5 and *Laws of Kings* 9:4. Note that, as Maimonides records there (*Laws of Murder* 2:6), the case of a *terefah* is exactly parallel to an infant in the first thirty days after birth; it is forbidden for one to murder either, but if one does, one is exempt from the capital punishment prescribed for murder. See Daniel Sinclair, *Tradition and the Biological Revolution: The Application of Jewish Law to the Treatment of the Critically Ill* (Edinburgh: Edinburgh University Press, 1989), 22–35, 57–59.

19. B. *Sanhedrin* 74a.

20. *Minhat Hinukh* no. 296, s. v. *"vehinei beguf hadin."* See also my discussion of the ruling of Rabbi Menahem Meiri along these lines in a case of siege (in his commentary on B. *Sanhedrin* 74a) in Dorff, "A Jewish Approach to End-Stage Medical Care," 22–24.

21. S. A. *Even Haezer* 121:7, gloss; and S. A. *Hoshen Mishpat* 211:2, gloss.

22. On the category of *goses*, including its definition, the requirement to treat a *goses* as a fully living person, and the permission (and, according to the first of these sources, the requirement) to stop medical interventions once this state has occurred, see *Sefer Hasidim* (attributed to Rabbi Judah the Pious of the thirteenth century), nos. 234, 723; S. A. *Yoreh De'ah* 339:1, gloss. On the image of a *goses* as a flickering candle, see M. *Semahot* 1:4, cited in many later sources including B. *Shabbat* 151b and the commentaries *Siftei Kohen* and *Be'er Hetev* to S. A. *Yoreh De'ah* 339:1.

23. Cf. Bleich, in Bleich and Rosner, eds., *Jewish Bioethics*, 34, and the contemporary rabbis he cites in note 120; Bleich, *Judaism and Healing*, 141–42. The main classical sources Bleich cites for this ruling are *Perishah, Tur, Yoreh De'ah* 339:5, and the ruling in S. A. *Yoreh De'ah* 339:2 that one must begin observing the laws of mourning three days after the onset of *gesisah*.

24. For example, among Orthodox rabbis, see Eliezer Waldenberg, *Responsa Tzitz Eliezer* 13, no. 89, and 14, no. 80; Immanuel Jakobovits, *Jewish Medical Ethics*, 124 and n. 46. Among Conservative rabbis, see Goldfarb, "The Definition of Death"; Siegel, "Updating the Criteria of Death," 23–30; and their subsequent discussion, *Conservative Judaism* 30, no. 2 (winter 1976): 31–39; and Reisner, "A Halakhic Ethic," esp. 56–58. I also originally adopted this approach in my monograph *"Choose Life": A Jewish Perspective on Medical Ethics*, 19–21; reprinted, in part, in my article, "Rabbi, I'm Dying," *Conservative Judaism* 37, no. 4 (summer 1984): 37–51, esp. 45–48. Because it is inappropriate to describe or treat most people with terminal illnesses as if they were "flickering candles," however, I have adopted and applied the legal category of *terefah* instead; see next note.

25. Elliot N. Dorff, "A Time to Live and a Time to Die," *United Synagogue Review* 44, no. 1 (fall 1991): 21–22; Dorff, "A Jewish Approach to End-Stage Medical Care," esp. 19–26.

26. In this volume, see Laurence O'Connell's discussion of the different contexts and multiple meanings of the concept and "lived" experience of death.

27. *Genesis Rabbah* 100:7, *Leviticus Rabbah* 18:1; *Ecclesiastes Rabbah* on Ecclesiastes 12:6; J. *Moed Katan* 3:5.

28. S. A. *Even Haezer* 17:26, based on M. *Yevamot* 16:3. See *Genesis Rabbah*

65–20 and *Ecclesiastes Rabbah* on Ecclesiastes 12:6 for a specific linkage of this law to the belief in the soul's association with the body for three days.

29.   The quotation is from M. *Semahot* 8:1; the practice is permitted in S. A. *Yoreh De'ah* 144:3. Some moderns, however, maintain that this applied "only in ancient days when they used to place the dead in sepulchral chambers which could be uncovered to reveal the corpse" (*Perishah, Tur, Yoreh De'ah* 339:5). See also gloss on the Rosh, *Moed Katan* 3:39 in the name of *Or Zarua*.

30.   The story of Saul and the witch of En-dor: I Samuel 28. The doctrine of twelve months: B. *Shabbat* 152b–153a; *Tanhuma*, Vayikra 8. The soul after death is quiescent: B. *Shabbat* 152b. The soul is fully conscious: *Exodus Rabbah* 52:3; *Tanhuma*, Ki Tissa 33; B. *Berakhot* 18b–19a; B. *Ketubbot* 77b, 104a. The quotation comes from *Pesikta Rabbati* 12:46. The disputes about how much the dead know about the living: B. *Berakhot* 18b.

31.   II Samuel 3:31; B. *Mo'ed Katan* 27a; M. T. *Laws of Mourning* 4:2. Jewish law follows the dictate of Rabbi Judah, president of the Sanhedrin in the late second century, but apparently the use of plain linen shrouds was already customary in the early first century, as the New Testament Book of John (19:40) attests.

32.   The last several paragraphs are based on Joshua Trachtenberg, *Jewish Magic and Superstition: A Study in Folk Religion* (Philadelphia: Jewish Publication Society, 1961), 61–68. See notes 5–8 on pp. 284–85 of Trachtenberg's book for the original sources of these and related practices.

33.   Maimonides provides a clear and detailed summary of the obligations inherent in the duty to take care of one's health (M. T. *Laws of Ethics* [Hilkhot De'ot], chaps. 3–5), but, as usual, Maimonides' discussion there is based on many talmudic precedents. The duty to live in a town with a physician: J. *Kiddushin* 66d; B. *Sanhedrin* 17b. For a general perspective on Judaism and health care, see my article "The Jewish Tradition," in Ronald L. Numbers and Darrel W. Amundsen, eds., *Caring and Curing: Health and Medicine in the Western Religious Traditions* (New York: Macmillan, 1986), 5–39.

34.   *Ecclesiastes Rabbah* on Ecclesiastes 5:6; S. A. *Yoreh De'ah* 338:1, 2.

35.   J. David Bleich, "The Jewish Entailments of Valuing Life," *Sh'ma*, 16 November 1990: 1–3.

36.   A good summary of traditional opinions on this issue can be found in Basil Herring, *Jewish Ethics and Halakhah for Our Time* (New York: KTAV and Yeshiva University Press, 1984), chap. 2. See also Seymour Siegel, "Some Reflections on Telling the Truth," *Linacre Quarterly* (August 1977): 229–39.

37.   Psalms 115:17. Job 7:6–10; 14:12, 14; 16:22; cf. also 10:20–22; 14:1–2; 17:13–16; 26:5–6. Ecclesiastes 3:19–22; 9:4–6, 10; 11:8; 12:7. Daniel 12:2. Isaiah 26:19 also apparently affirms resurrection of the dead, but scholars construe that as a verse imported into the Book of Isaiah in a much later period. On this topic generally, see *Encyclopedia Judaica*, s. v. "death."

38.   The immortality of the soul was apparently first affirmed in a Jewish source in 4 Maccabees 9:8; 17:5, 18. Resurrection, on the other hand, is affirmed in 2 Maccabees 7:14, 23. Both of these are books of the Jewish Apocrypha coming from the Second Temple period. On the rabbis' insistence that Jews believe not

only that there is a world to come but also that it is stated in the Torah, see M. *Sanhedrin* 10:1; B. *Sanhedrin* 90b–91a. That the Sadducces did not believe this, we learn from Flavius Josephus, The *Jewish War*, book 2, secs. 162–66. On these topics generally, see *Encyclopedia Judaica*, s. v. v. "death—in the Talmud and Midrash" and "afterlife." Louis Finkelstein has claimed that the second blessing of the Amidah, a group of blessings said by traditional Jews three times a day while standing, is deliberately ambiguous in order to accommodate both immortality of the soul and resurrection; it blesses God for being the one who "gives life to the dead." See Louis Finkelstein, *The Pharisees* (Philadelphia: Jewish Publication Society of America, 1966), vol. 1, 145–59 (esp. 158–59), and vol. 2, 742–51 (esp. 750–51).

39. *Genesis Rabbah* 14:9; see also note 7 above.

40. *Genesis Rabbah* 14:8.

41. Macabee Dean, "A Matter of Life and Death," *Jerusalem Post*, 24 June 1977, 6 (magazine section).

42. Saadia Gaon, *Book of Doctrines and Beliefs*, book 7, sec. 1, in Lewy, Altmann, and Heinemann, eds., *Three Jewish Philosophers*, pt. 2, 155–56.

43. Moses Maimonides, *Commentary on the Mishnah, Sanhedrin*, chap.10, in Isadore Twersky, trans., *A Maimonides Reader* (New York: Behrman House, 1972), 403–4.

44. Ibid., 410ff. The talmudic citation is from B. *Berakhot* 17a. In his *Commentary on the Mishnah*, Maimonides affirmed both the immortality of the soul and the resurrection of the body, but by the end of his life, when he wrote the *Guide of the Perplexed*, he made no mention of resurrection at all, concentrating solely on the eternality of the soul. See *Guide* 2:27, 3:54.

45. Cited in Allen S. Maller, "Gilgul, Dybbuks, and the Afterlife," *Heritage*, 20 March 1992: 5. His statistics were based on a *Los Angeles Times* poll taken on 14 and 15 December 1991 in the San Fernando Valley area of Los Angeles. The results of that poll were reported, in part, in the *Los Angeles Times*, 5 January 1992, Valley section (Valley edition), but the *Times* made the full data available to Rabbi Maller, a professional sociologist, for his article in *Heritage*.

46. B. *Sanhedrin* 73a.

47. For a general description of Jewish law and institutions with regard to helping the poor, see my paper, "Jewish Perspectives on the Poor," in Gary Rubin, ed., *The Poor among Us: Jewish Tradition and Social Policy* (New York: American Jewish Committee, 1986), 21–55.

48. *Sifre Deuteronomy*, Ekey.

49. B. *Sotah* 14a. In this passage, I have left out the biblical prooftexts that the Talmud uses to demonstrate that God has clothed the naked, visited the sick, and so on.

50. For a discussion of how Judaism treats obligations beyond the letter of the law, see my article "The Interaction of Jewish Law with Morality," *Judaism* 26 (fall 1977): 455–66.

51. I discuss at some length how all these concepts impinge on the Jewish duty to help others in my article "Jewish Perspectives on the Poor," 23–31.

10 *Wendy Doniger*

Transplanting Myths of Organ Transplants

Personal Statement

In 1971 my father died. He and my mother shared a rationalist worldview that excluded religious rituals of any kind. (I have no idea where, if anywhere, any of my grandparents are buried; my parents never mentioned or visited their graves, if graves there were.) My mother had my father cremated, as he had stipulated in his will, and she put the box containing the urn of his ashes into the front coat closet in our family home. When I literally stumbled on it one day and asked what it was, she replied, "Oh, that's Daddy." This troubled me, and continued to trouble me over the years, but I could mount no argument to persuade my mother to do anything about it, and no one else in the family seemed to mind.

Then, twenty years later, in 1991, my mother died, and was, as was stipulated in her will, cremated. Now there were two boxes of ashes, but there was also no one left to object to my wish to do something about them. I spoke to my two brothers, and they agreed with me that we would all feel better if we could purchase a family plot and bury the two urns of ashes there under a small, inscribed stone. Arrangements were made, and we met on the appointed day at the cemetery. It was raining, as it always does at funerals in myths (and in movies, which are much the same thing). While we waited for the rabbi to consecrate the grave (which was not what we wished, but a requirement

194

of the cemetery), cars began to draw up. My younger brother had casually mentioned to one of my father's nephews that we were burying the ashes at last, and the word had spread. Suddenly, one by one, every single living relative of my father appeared at the grave, uninvited (after all, it was, technically, our mother's funeral, not our father's). We were so happy to see them, and they to be with us.

That story about death illuminates the contrast between what Freud has called, on the one hand, the primary process, the unconscious mind, the latent level and, on the other hand, the secondary process, the conscious mind, the manifest level. For twenty years, everyone in my family had felt very uncomfortable (on the latent level) about the disposition of my father's ashes, but no one was allowed to say anything about it, because in our family we did not (on the manifest level) care about such things. And alongside that story that I know personally, I could set hundreds of similarly illuminating stories about the manifest and the latent that I know professionally, for I have spent some thirty-five years studying other peoples' myths, which often touch otherwise inaccessible parts of the human spirit and thus offer vivid manifestations of many latent ideas.

In his chapter in this volume, Stuart Youngner has pointed out the importance of excavating ideas that function on the latent level from under the public discourse, which functions primarily on the manifest level. The present chapter is my attempt to join him in that enterprise by bringing into the conversation a number of myths about human identity, the body, death, and organ transplants.

The Relevance of Myth

For many centuries, mythological texts have provided a kind of virtual reality testing ground for organ transplants: though it has become physically possible to do such operations only in recent decades, people have imagined, for a very long time indeed, the sorts of problems that might arise if one could do such things. And now that we find that such problems do, in fact, arise when we do, in fact, transplant part of one person's body into another person's body, these myths may serve as a source of both warning and hope. They warn us about the deep, often very dark, feelings that are evoked by such a process, feelings about the simultaneous sanctity and polluting power of dead bodies, racist fears of the bodies of strangers, and sexual fears about the bodies of our intimate partners. But, on the brighter side, some of these myths offer us positive images of organ donation that might be useful to both donors and recipients. Indeed, these images might furnish the magic mantras that one transplant surgeon, Dr. Barry D. Kahan, urged me to find for him to persuade potential donors to overcome their "irrational" resistance or to help recipients bear the traumas, both physical and mental, of preoperative anxiety and postoperative endurance.

In this enterprise I would argue, as I have argued elsewhere, that it is possible for people from one culture to find personal meaning in the myths of people from another culture.[1] I think certain myths have a universal human meaning, a meaning that transcends and supplements the local, cultural meanings of the myths. Other peoples' myths may function (to borrow a formulation from anthropologist Clifford Geertz) as both models of and models for real-life situations in cultures far removed from their place of origin: As models *of*, myths tell us that people who seem very unlike us share many of our feelings about certain subjects that are difficult for us to express; as models *for*, some of them might help people of our culture construct new ways of thinking about their bodies.

Just as it is possible to transplant an organ from one body to another, so it is possible to transplant a myth from one culture to another. In both cases, there is trauma and loss, but there is also survival. Myths, like all things in constant use, get broken and fixed again, lost and found again, and the one who finds them and fixes them, the handyman who recycles them, is what the French structural anthropologist Claude Lévi-Strauss calls a *bricoleur* and what we used to call a rag-and-bones man. The rags and bones of the stories, the units, or *mythemes*, are recycled to make new stories, just as body parts are recycled in transplant operations. In the ecology of narratives, recycling is a very old process indeed.

But we must use these myths with considerable caution, for shoals lie hidden under the surface of these exotic waters. For instance, there is a danger that ancient, sacred myths, created and validated by successive generations of individuals or by a priesthood with certain goals, might be conflated with modern "myths," or quasi myths, created by the media (or the medical profession, or the anti-medical lobby), which have very different sorts of goals. These two bodies of thought work in very different ways, and it is not easy to transform the first sort into the second sort, though people often try. I will be concerned here primarily with the first sort, ancient myths, and only secondarily with their reflection in the second sort, modern media myths.

In this chapter, I will be able to touch upon only a few of the insights that are available to us in the mythologies of the world, primarily in the mythologies of India (with which I am most familiar). I will begin with texts about the dismemberment of humans at their death and go on to texts about living human donors who give parts of the body, particularly eyes, legs, hearts, and heads. I will conclude with a discussion of the implications, for organ transplant, of the doctrine concerning the transfer of karma at death and during life.

Myths about Human Dismemberment at Death

One of the earliest texts to describe human dismemberment is contained in the *Rig Veda*, composed in northwest India around 1000 B.C.E. It is a funeral hymn that describes the fate of a man after death by instructing the dead man himself about the ultimate dispersal of his body:

May your eye go to the sun, your life's breath to the wind. Go to the sky or to earth, as is your nature; or go to the waters, if that is your fate. Take root in the plants with your limbs.[2]

Yet another funeral hymn seems to imply that the body is kept intact in heaven. The hymn again addresses the dead man:

Go forth, go forth on those ancient paths on which our ancient fathers passed beyond. . . . Unite with the fathers, with Yama [king of the dead], with the rewards of your sacrifices and good deeds, in the highest heaven. Leaving behind all imperfections, go back home again; merge with a glorious body.[3]

But, despite this "glorious body" with which the dead person unites, another hymn expresses concern that the old body be preserved, and confidence that this will be so. The hymn begins by addressing the funeral fire, Agni (cognate with the Latin *ignis* and the English *ignite*):

Do not burn him entirely, Agni, or engulf him in your flames. Do not consume his skin or his flesh. When you have cooked him perfectly, only then send him forth to the fathers.[4]

The fire is not supposed to destroy the body, but rather to restore it. Speaking to the dead man, the hymn says:

Whatever the black bird has pecked out of you, or the ant, the snake, or even a beast of prey, may Agni who eats all things make it whole.[5]

This is only an apparent contradiction. The actual corpse must be preserved as intact as possible, even though it is going to be cremated, because the cremation fire transmits a kind of hologram image of the corpse to heaven, where it is reconstructed as if from a diagram. Yet whatever flaws remain in the body, despite all reasonable precautions, will be mended in the heavenly body (a body that may then be naturally recycled).

In contemporary conflicts about transplant surgery, medical arguments in favor of recycling parts of the human body are often strongly opposed by religious (or quasi-religious) arguments in favor of preserving the human body intact after death. Yet the ancient Indians seemed to resolve the two points of view: the body was kept as intact as possible only until cremation, and then it was understood to be supernaturally restored and naturally recycled. We might be able to take something from this paradigm, but then again we might not, for Indian thought in general has always been able to hold contradictory ideas in suspension in ways that have made little sense to the Western Enlightenment tradition.[6]

The Upanishads, composed a few centuries after the *Rig Veda*, describe a more detailed path for the general dispersal of the body after death:

Those who worship in the village, concentrating on sacrifices and good works and charity, are born into the smoke [of the funeral fire], and from the smoke into the wind, and eventually into the moon, the food of the gods. When they have dwelt there for as long as there is a remnant (of their karmic merit),[7] then they return along that very same road that they came along, back into wind, and when one has become wind he becomes smoke, and when he has become smoke he becomes mist; when he has become mist, he becomes a cloud, and when he has become a cloud, he rains. These are then born here as rice, barley, plants, trees, sesame plants, and beans. It is difficult to move forth out of this condition; for whoever eats him as food and then emits him as semen, he becomes that creature's semen and is born.

But those who worship in the forest, concentrating on faith and asceticism, are born into the flame, and from the flame into the day, and from the day into the fortnight of the waxing moon, and from the fortnight of the waxing moon into the six months during which the sun moves north; from these months, into the year; from the year into the sun; from the sun into the moon; from the moon into lightning. There a Person who is not human leads them to the ultimate reality. This is the paths that the gods go on.[8]

We should note an important change since the *Rig Veda*. Dismemberment and reconstitution (re-memberment, as it were) are still assumed to take place, but now they are regarded as unfortunate: It is better not to enter the smoke at all, but to go into the flame, never to return to a body; for dangerous traps await those who do transmigrate.

The negative Upanishadic attitude toward re-memberment into the elements has prevailed and persists in India to the present day, where it was brilliantly expressed in a poem by a contemporary Indian poet (and mythologist), the late A. K. Ramanujan. The poem, entitled "Death and the Good Citizen," is well worth citing in full:

> I know, you told me,
>   your nightsoil and all
> your city's, goes still
>   warm every morning
> in a government
>   lorry, drippy (you said)
> but punctual, by special

arrangement to the municipal
gardens to make the grass
        grow tall for the cows
in the village, the rhino
        in the zoo: and the oranges
plump and glow, till
        they are a preternatural
orange.

Good animal yet perfect
        citizen, you, you are
biodegradable, you do
        return to nature: you will
your body to the nearest
        hospital, changing death into small
change and spare parts;
        dismantling, not de-
composing like the rest
        of us. Eyes in an eye bank
to blink some day for a stranger's
        brain, wait like mummy wheat
in the singular company
        of single eyes, pickled,
absolute.

Hearts,
        with your kind of temper
        may even take, make connection
with alien veins, and continue
        your struggle to be naturalized:
beat, and learn to miss a beat
        in a foreign body.
        But
you know my tribe, incarnate
        unbelievers in bodies,
they'll speak proverbs, contest
        my will, against such degradation.
Hidebound, even worms cannot
        have me: they'll cremate
me in Sanskrit and sandalwood,
        have me sterilized
to a scatter of ash.

        Or abroad,
they'll lay me out in a funeral
        parlour, embalm me in pesticide,

> bury me in a steel trap, lock
>   me out of nature
> till I'm oxidized by left-
>   over air, withered by my own
> vapours into grin and bone.
>   My tissue will never graft,
> will never know newsprint,
>   never grow in a culture,
> or be mould and compost
>   for jasmine, eggplant
> and the unearthly perfection
>   of municipal oranges.[9]

The Hindu poet regards the transplantation of eyes and heart as a Western phenomenon, in contrast with the Indian need to reduce the body to ashes, a religious imperative that, as we have seen, began three thousand years ago. And, as we shall see, the belief that a dead body is literally untouchable (except by Untouchables) prevented the development of anatomy and surgery in India and may still account for Hindus' disinclination to donate their organs.

Myths about Living Donors

Despite this ambiguous, or even negative, mythology of organ donation at death, however, Hindu mythology reveals a positive attitude toward donors who give up their entire lives, their entire bodies, in order that others may live.[10] But we may find a closer and more useful parallel to the ideologies of organ transplants in myths in which people donate one organ. Let us consider myths about four particularly popular organs: the eyes, the legs, the heart, and the head.

Eyes: King Shivi and the Sage Chyavana

Both Buddhism and Hinduism praise humans who give their eyes to others in a supreme act of generosity. The paradigmatic example of this occurs in both Buddhist and Hindu texts, and is the story of King Shivi. Here is the Buddhist version, from the *Shivi Jataka*:

Once upon a time, King Shivi sat on the royal throne, thinking of the gifts he had given: "This kind of external giving does not content me. I want to give something that is a part of myself. Today when I go to the alms-hall, I vow that if anyone asks for my own heart, I will cut open my breast with a spear, and as if I were pulling up a water-lily, stalk and all, from a calm lake, I will pull forth my heart dripping with blood-clots and give it to him; if he asks for the flesh of my body, I will cut it off and give it to him. If anyone should ask for my eyes, I will tear them out and give them."

Indra, the king of the gods, thought, "King Shivi has determined to give his eyes to anyone who asks for them. I will test him." So Indra took the form of an old, blind Brahmin and said, "I am blind, and you have two eyes; give me one of yours." King Shivi called for a surgeon named Shivaka and said, "Take out both of my eyes." Everyone tried to persuade him not to do this, but the king insisted. The surgeon did not want to pierce the king's eyes with a lancet, so he rubbed a strong powder into one eye, causing great pain; the eye came out of the socket and hung dangling at the end of the tendon. The king's garments were stained with blood, but he endured the pain and simply said, "My friend, be quick." The surgeon grasped the eyeball with his left hand, took a knife in his right hand, severed the tendon and laid the eye in Shivi's hand. The king gave the eye to the Brahmin, who put it in his own eye socket, where it remained. When Shivi saw this, with his remaining eye, he was full of joy, and he gave him the other eye as well. Indra took this one too, and went away. But after a while he came in his true form and restored the king's eyes.[11]

Here, as in most of the myths of organ donation, a final restoration occurs so that both the donor and the recipient end up having the organ in question.

The text dwells upon the gory details and physical pain, in part through a Buddhist tendency to denigrate the body, but in part to emphasize the king's courage as well as his generosity. To what extent do these details reflect actual knowledge of surgical possibilities? Ancient Indian texts speak of remarkable feats of deep surgery performed in the past by the semilegendary physician Jivaka, said to have lived at the time of the Buddha (in the sixth century B.C.E.).[12] Internal surgery was limited to "the removal of calculi from the bladder; the replacement of bowels exposed as a result of a wound; stitching the stomach wall; and Caesarean section in the case of mothers who died before giving birth."[13] As for external operations, there were said to be excellent plastic surgeons.[14]

The earliest classical medical text, that of Caraka (at the end of the first century C.E.), does not discuss surgery, since surgery was the domain of low-caste barbers, while Caraka regarded classical medicine as the work of *vaidyas*, or learned men, for whom surgery would be polluting. But later medical texts, such as that of Sushruta (c. sixth century C.E.), allow the *vaidya* to practice certain forms of surgery but not to dissect corpses, which severely limited the knowledge of anatomy in ancient India.

The story of King Shivi is told at far greater length in the Hindu epic, the *Mahabharata*, where it is not his eyes but his flesh that, Shylock-fashion, the king weighs against the need of another living creature.[15] And another Hindu tale similar to the Buddhist version of King Shivi is told in South India about a hunter who worshiped the god Shiva (no relation to King Shivi):

To prove the hunter's devotion, Shiva devised a test. . . . [The hunter] arrived to find the image of the god bleeding from the right eye. To stop the flow of blood, the hunter tore out his own eye and placed it on the [image of the god]. But then the left eye of the god began to bleed. The hunter placed his foot on the bleeding eye so that he would be able to find the spot; then he began to scoop out his remaining eye as a gift to the god. Shiva stretched out his hand from the [image] and stopped the devotee.[16]

Again, the myth tells us, it is good for a living donor to give an eye, even if the eye is not restored. The donor wins, in exchange, the grateful love of the god himself.

Eyes are equally prominent in the European mythology of organ transplant. A Czech story tells of a blind man who asked for the eyes of a young girl and was given instead, in secret substitution, the eyes of various animals. Each time, he saw what the animals saw: when he was given the eyes of fish, he saw fins and scales; when he was given the eyes of birds, he saw the sky and the clouds.[17] This story reflects the widespread folk belief that when you see with someone else's eyes, you see what that creature sees; more broadly, when you are given someone else's organs, you take on that person's personality in some way. This is a problem that continues to haunt many people who receive donated organs.

Another important Indian myth concerns the restoration of eyes, this time not by organ transplant but by a more general, and more vaguely miraculous, process of rejuvenation. It is significant for us in this context because it involves the first physicians, the divine twins known as the Ashvins. As physicians, the Ashvins hobnobbed with humans in ways that made the other gods refuse, at first, to let them join in the drinking of the Soma, the drink of immortality. But the Ashvins were able to ensure their own immortality in a very neat exchange, not of organs, but of powers:

The aged sage Chyavana was meditating in an anthill when the beautiful young princess Sukanya came along and saw his two eyes gleaming red out of the hill. He desired her and called to her, but his throat was dry and she did not hear him. Then, seeing the two eyes and wondering, "What is this?" in confusion and curiosity, she pierced the eyes of the old man with a thorn. The old sage became furious, and the king gave Sukanya to him in marriage in order to appease his fury.[18]

Sukanya served Chyavana happily for many years. Then, one day, the two Ashvins happened to be wandering about there. They came to Sukanya and said, "My dear girl, this is a blind old man, not whole, not fit to be a husband. Be our wife." "No," she said, "I will be the wife of the man to whom my father gave me." Pleased by her fidelity to her husband, they said, "We are the physicians of the gods; let us make your husband young and handsome. Then choose as your husband one from among the three of us when we have the same form and bodies." She was amazed and went to Chyavana and said, "My lord, the two Ashvins came to your hermitage and saw me, lovely in all of my body parts, and were overcome by lust. They said, 'We will make your husband an adolescent, with a divine body, and with sight. And we will give him the same limbs and form that we have, and you must choose your husband as one of the three of us.' So I came to ask you. The illusory magic of the gods is hard to recognize; I don't know if this is some trick of the two of them." He replied, "Let us do what they say quickly, without hesitation."

Chyavana and the Ashvins went into the pond and all came out similar. But Sukanya prayed to the Goddess, who put into her heart the knowledge of which was her husband, and she chose him. And by the grace of the Goddess the two gods were satisfied. Thus Chyavana obtained beauty, his two eyes, his wife, and youth. And he was so happy that he offered the Ashvins a boon, and they asked him to make them Soma-drinkers. And he did.[19]

The foolish young Sukanya blinds her future husband, but the wise, mature Sukanya unblinds him. (It is worth noting that the Ashvins themselves say nothing about restoring his sight, but she adds this essential embellishment when she reports to her husband what they had said, and in the end he does, in fact, get his sight back.) This is the first exchange, between the two stages of Sukanya. The second exchange takes place between the Ashvins and Chyavana: They give him his sight, youth, and good looks (through a kind of magical plastic surgery), and he gives them eternal youth, immortality. Again, the donation of the organ (in this case, eyes) is regarded as a barter, in which the donors lose nothing (for the Ashvins do not become blind) and indeed gain something (immortality). This is hardly a practical prescription for modern hospital practices, but it does demonstrate an underlying positive attitude toward the *idea* of organ donation.

Legs: Castor and Pollux; Cosmas and Damian

The rich mythology about identical twins (the ideal donors) includes many interesting variants on the theme of organ transplant. Indo-European texts tell us of twin mortals or twin gods who are associated with horses and with transferred life. In India, as we have seen, they are the Ashvins. In Greece, they are known as Castor and Polydeuces (Pollux, in Rome), who were half brothers of mixed birth (Leda bore Castor, the greatest of horsemen, to king Tyndareus, and she bore Polydeuces to Zeus). Thus, they share the same liminal immortality/mortality as the Ashvins.

It is said that, at death, one twin chose to be the donor of his entire body, his entire life, to the other: Polydeuces refused immortality unless Castor might share it, and Zeus therefore allowed them both to spend their days alternately in heaven and under the earth. At this time, Zeus also deified them and set them in heaven as the constellation of the twins, known as the Dioscuri (or, in Rome, the Gemini).[20] Like the Ashvins, who are half horses and whose name means horsemen, the Greek centaurs are also healers.

Now, one of the earliest recorded deeds of the Ashvins was to replace the amputated leg of a horse, a story told in the *Rig Veda*: "When the leg of the racing mare Vishpala was cut off like the wing of a bird, the Ashvins replaced it."[21] The myth of the divine twin physicians who replace a diseased leg surfaces again in Indo-European mythology two thousand years later. In this interesting transformation, Barry D. Kahan tells us of another set of twins known as "the Christian counterparts of the Greek gemini twin brothers, Castor and Pollux."[22] These Christian twins are Cosmas and Damian, born in the second half of the third century C.E. in Arabia to devout Christian parents. Cosmas and Damian were surgeons, and one of their many miraculous cures was the "Miracle of the Black Leg," allegedly performed c. 348 C.E. but first recorded in 1270.[23]

According to this legend, an elderly sacristan fell asleep near the altar and dreamt that Cosmas and Damian came to him and removed his gangrenous, cancerous leg with a saw, replacing it with the leg of a Moor buried that day in the Cemetery of Saint Peter, and attaching it at the thigh. Upon awakening, the old man felt no pain and discovered that his leg was whole, and black. He went to the cemetery and found his diseased leg lying in the grave beside the body of the Ethiopian. This is Barry Kahan's comment on the story:

The concept of transplantation was totally alien to the times in which the miracle took place. . . . Hieronymus Brunchwieg . . . stated that if someone tried to reattach a part of the body, it would be equivalent to "a monkey becoming a philosopher" or a man "trying to fly in the air." Sommering, in his 18th century treatise, pointed out that there were many discrepancies between reality and early artistic representation. But in art, nearly anything is possible; in science it is a rather different matter.[24]

Even in the art of the miracle story, we may see a shadow of racial bias that continues to haunt the contemporary science of organ transplants: that a black man's organ is used to heal a white man. The text seems to regard this operation as one in which, as in the myths of eye transplants we have seen, something is gained and nothing lost. The Christian gains a leg, and the Moor loses nothing, in part because he is already (and, conveniently, freshly) dead, but also in part because, being someone of another race and religion, he is a nonperson from the standpoint of the Christian text.

Hearts: The Monkey's Wife and the Crocodile

The mythology of heart transplants, throughout the world, occasionally bears the same message of generous self-sacrifice as the mythology of eye transplants that we have just glimpsed, but more often it is characterized by themes of greed and violence: People want to eat other people's hearts, and those whose hearts they want must find ways to trick them in order to survive. Unlike the mythology of eye transplants, and even more than the mythology of leg transplants, the mythology of heart transplants assumes that donors very definitely stand to lose something, indeed, their lives, and are therefore not willing donors at all.

One variant of this theme, which is attested in Swahili, Japanese, and Persian texts, is also known from ancient Buddhist and Hindu sources. This is the myth of the monkey's heart (in some cultures, a monkey's liver) that can cure diseases in human beings or other animals.[25] A version of the story was told in the Sanskrit text of the *Ocean of the Rivers of Story*, c. 1000 C.E.,[26] and then retold in the *Panchatantra*, which served in turn for the Persian compendium of *Kalila and Dimna*. Here is a summary of the *Panchatantra* version:

A monkey lived on the shore of the sea in a great rose-apple tree. One day he offered some of the apples to a crocodile, who brought them home to his wife. She tasted them and asked him where they came from, and when he told her about the monkey she said, "If anyone eats such nectar fruit every day, his heart must be turned to nectar. So, if you value your wife, give me his heart, and I will eat it. Then I shall never grow old or sick, but will be a delightful companion for you." The crocodile objected that the monkey was their adopted brother and their benefactor, but his wife complained, "You have never refused me before. You must be in love with the monkey, and it must be a she-monkey. That is why you stay away all day and do not hold me tight when you kiss me; and that is why you will not give me what I want: some other woman has stolen your heart." Still the crocodile begged her to desist, but she insisted, "If you don't love her, why don't you kill her when I ask you? And if it is really a he-monkey, why should you love him? Unless I eat his heart, I shall starve myself to death in your house."

Finally, the crocodile went to get the monkey, but as he was swimming with the monkey on his back he thought, "He is in my power, so I will tell him what I am going to do, and he will have a chance to pray to his god." When he told the monkey about his wife's desire for his sweet heart, the quick-witted monkey said, "I wish you had told me sooner. For I have a second heart, a very sweet heart that I keep in a hole in the rose-apple tree." The crocodile was delighted and swam back to the rose-apple tree, while the monkey murmured a hundred prayers to every sort of god. When they reached the shore, the monkey jumped up into the rose-apple tree and said, "You fool! You traitor! How can anyone have two hearts? Go home."[27]

The treatment of some animals in this story (crocodiles) as humans who marry and others (monkeys) as animals who are eaten makes it serve as a cautionary tale not only for heart transplants but also for vivisection. Myths of this sort may also becomes increasingly relevant to our considerations because the organs of baboons and pigs are now being transplanted into humans, raising new issues of human-animal relationships. (Kosher Jews, for instance, can receive pig parts as long as they don't eat them.) But the main moral for our purposes lies elsewhere. The folk wisdom of this story mocks the pious mythology of its own Hindu tradition, the idea that someone could give away an organ (an eye, for instance) and still, miraculously, keep it. The harsh world of the folktale takes a zero-sum view of such exchanges: If someone wins, someone else loses. If someone gets a heart and lives, someone else loses a heart and dies.

In this tale, the theme of the insatiable woman is cleverly conflated with the theme of the monkey's heart through the double entendre on *heart*, both as the organ that sustains life (in all folk beliefs until our quite recent criterion of brain death) and as the source of erotic attachment ("some other woman has stolen your heart"). The wife who sexually blackmails her husband to get her way (such as the pregnant woman who longs for exotic foods that her husband must procure at the risk of his life) often plays a part in the story of the monkey's heart; vampire women devour men in more ways than one.[28]

A wonderful story about a sexually voracious woman and a heart was told in a sermon in a Catholic seminary in the 1950s:

There was a man who was infatuated with a woman of ill repute. She said she would go to bed with him only if he gave her the heart of his mother. He went home and cut out his mother's heart, and as he was running to the house of ill repute to give it to the woman, he stumbled and fell. While he lay there sprawled on the ground, the heart spoke to him and said, "Did you hurt yourself, my son?"[29]

It is not entirely clear what the wicked woman will do with the heart, other than make sure that she has no rival for the love of her man. If she were a crocodile, she would eat it; if she were a certain sort of modern doctor, she would use it in a heart transplant operation. But we will return, below, to the modern mythology of sexually voracious women transplant surgeons.

The ambiguous status of the heart as the organ that is the key to both life and romantic love continues to trouble potential donors and recipients of hearts. In our great modern mythology of Oz, the Tin Woodman thought (wrongly) that he would not be able to love until the Wizard gave him a heart (transplant). People with artificial hearts sometimes wonder if they will still be able to love, though as one cynic remarked, "That's another organ." (The other organ in question is also transplanted from one male to another in mythologies that range from the ancient Egyptian myth of Osiris to contemporary Hindu myths of the god Shiva.[30])

Indeed, other organs besides the heart take on sexual connotations when the concept of putting one person's organ into another person's body is (often unconsciously) conflated with the sexual act. This mythology appears, for instance, in Bram Stoker's *Dracula*, where the men who give Lucy their blood in a transfusion feel that they have had sex with her and conceal the fact from her fiancé.

This same idea underlies the scene in the film *The Greatest Show on Earth*, in which the character played by Charlton Heston gets a blood transfusion from the character played by Cornel Wilde, his rival for the love of the character played by Betty Hutton. Wilde (a Frenchman) teases Heston that he will now be able to make love much better, and that he will see Wilde's features in the faces of his own children.

On the latent level (to return once more to Stuart Youngner's concerns), this mythological conflation of the two acts may make the donation of organs to a sexual partner appear vaguely analogous to some kind of nepotism, conflict of interest, or even incest, since one is simultaneously giving something to and entering the body of someone who is closely identified with oneself. It may make a wife hesitate to donate and organ to her husband, or, quite the reverse, within the framework of a patriarchal family system, it may compel a wife, often against her will, to donate a kidney to her husband. Mythologies, especially unconscious mythologies, are often double-edged scalpels.

Heads: Dadhyanch and Mariatale

The head (which Woody Allen, in *Sleeper*, referred to as "my second favorite organ") is by far the transplant organ of choice in myths. In fact, a transplanted head plays a crucial role in the sequel to a myth we have already encountered, the episode in which the divine physicians, the Ashvins, get to drink the Soma that Chyavana has promised them. Here, Indra, king of the gods, comes into conflict with a sage who, like Chyavana, has access to the Soma:

The Ashvins said to Chyavana, "Sage, we have granted your desire: you have become young again. Now teach us so that we may share the Soma." And he sent them to Dadhyanch.

Now, Indra had threatened to cut off the head of Dadhyanch if he told anyone the secret of the sacrifice: how the sacrificial animal is made whole when the head is cut off. The Ashvins gave Dadhyanch the head of a horse, through which he told them the secret of the sacrifice. Indra cut off the horse head, and then the Ashvins replaced Dadhyanch's head. Thus the Ashvins became sharers in the Soma.[31]

A number of Hindu gods lose their heads and receive, in return, the heads of animals (just as, in the Czech story, a man receives the eyes of various animals): Daksha gets a goat's head; Ganesha, an elephant's head; and so forth.[32] Closer to our theme, however, is the wide corpus of myths in which human beings receive the heads of other human beings. These stories are particularly relevant because they raise a problem that troubles many recipients of organ transplants, a problem we have already encountered in the Czech story of the transplanted eyes: Is the personality of the donor somehow encoded in the organ and transplanted into the recipient?

This question is dramatically addressed in an ancient Indian story, recorded from an oral Tamil tale, which Pierre Sonnerat retold in the eighteenth century:[33]

Mariatale, the wife of a great ascetic, could control the elements, but only as long as her heart remained pure. One day she was fetching water from a pool, and, following her usual custom, was rolling it up in a ball to carry it home. A lustful thought entered her heart. The water that she had already collected immediately turned to liquid and mingled back with the water of the pool. She could no longer carry it home without the help of a bowl. This impotence revealed to her husband that his wife had ceased to be pure, and in the excess of his anger, he commanded his son to drag her off to the place set aside for executions, and to cut off her head. This order was executed; but the son was so afflicted by the loss of his mother that his father told him to go and get her body, to join it to the head that he had cut off, and to whisper in its ear a prayer that the father taught him, which would immediately revive her. The son ran in haste, but by a singular oversight, he joined the head of his mother to the body of an Untouchable woman who had been executed for her crimes—a monstrous assemblage, which gave to this woman the virtues of a goddess and the vices of an unfortunate wretch. The goddess, having become impure through this mix, was chased out of her house and committed all sorts of cruelties; the gods, seeing the ravages that she was making, appeased her by giving her the power to cure smallpox. Only her head was placed in the inner sanctuary of the temple, to be worshiped by Hindus of good caste, while her [Untouchable] body was placed at the door of the temple, to be worshiped by Untouchables.[34]

As in the story of Cosmas and Damian, where someone of one race donated a leg to someone of another race (the race of the storyteller and, hence, the privileged race), here someone of a lower class supplies the organ to cure someone of a higher class: The body of the impure Untouchable is taken to cure the (head of the) pure Mariatale. But the body affects the head, or even defines the head; with the new body, Mariatale herself becomes a new person, a horrible and dangerous person. To deal with this problem, the gods make her quite literally half-caste: her head remains divine (and hence relatively pure), with the ability to heal smallpox, while her body becomes lower class (and hence relatively impure), with the ability to cause smallpox. From the standpoint of Mariatale, the operation is more of a body transplant than a head transplant, and the transplanted body of the Untouchable woman is at first assimilated to the receiving head of the upper-class woman and then rejected by it: The body saves the head, then changes it, and finally leaves it. This myth also reveals a highly ambivalent attitude toward the double-edged powers of healers, an attitude typical of many societies (including, I think, our own).

When the tale of transposed heads is told of men, it is used to make a rather different point, though still a point involving class conflict:

A young washerman named Dhavala married a girl named Madanasundari. After a while, Madanasundari's brother came to visit them, and the three of them went together to the festival of the goddess Durga. In the Durga temple, Dhavala was overcome with a desire to sacrifice himself to Durga, and he cut off his head; Madanasundari's brother followed him and did the same. When Madanasundari saw her husband and her brother beheaded, she resolved to commit suicide, but the goddess said, "Do not do anything rash, my daughter. Join the heads of your husband and brother to their bodies, and by my grace they will rise up alive." In her delight and confusion, Madanasundari stuck her husband's head to her brother's body, and her brother's head to her husband's body. They came to life, and Madanasundari did not at first know what to do. But the one who had her husband's head was her husband.[35]

The hero is a washerman, of a low caste, and since the parents consent to the match, we may assume that Madanasundari and her brother are of the same, or a comparable, low caste. But the two men are of different castes in another variant of this tale first brought to European attention by Sir Richard Burton.[36] In this variation, the two men are the woman's husband, with whom she is not particularly compatible, and the husband's best friend, whom the woman finds far more attractive. The great Indologist Heinrich Zimmer retold the story[37] and taught it to his friend Thomas Mann, in whose satirical retelling the transplanted heads develop in a most interesting way.[38]

In Mann's version, the woman thinks she has the best of both worlds when she chooses her husband's refined, intellectual, Brahmin head and the best friend's gorgeous, athletic, lower-caste body. In time, however, the Brahmin fails to care for the athletic body, and it becomes as puny as his own had been; meanwhile, the head takes on the coarseness of the new body, so that the wife ends up with the worst of both worlds. The athlete's head, on the other hand, soon develops the Brahmin's body into his own former Schwarzenegger physique, while his head somehow becomes more refined through the subtle influence of the Brahmin body, producing, in the end, precisely the configuration that the woman had hoped to have by choosing the *other* combination. In this myth, therefore, the heads at first prevail in conveying the dominant personality, but eventually the bodies exert strong counterinfluences, like the body of the Untouchable woman in the story of Mariatale.

The relevance of this myth to the metaphysical problems inherent in contemporary organ transplants need not be labored over. In many cases, the recipient feels that he or she has become a kind of double to the donor, implying a belief that the tissue itself has personality, especially when the organ in question is a heart. This idea is rooted in the mythological location of the person (soul) in the body rather than in the mind, or, more particularly, in the belief that, although the soul/brain/personality is in the head, the head is merely a part of the body, as transposable as anything else. This belief is necessarily explicit in the Hindu anatomy of the mind, which places in the head what Hindus call *manas*, a combination of what we would call mind (the rational function, the ability to do algebra) and heart (the emotional function, the ability to fall in love). Myths such as these, based upon different divisions of the turf of consciousness and personality, help us to become more aware of our own unconscious, arbitrary, and perhaps revisable divisions of the same turf.

The Great Transference: Karma

Often the dilemma of organ donation arises out of a boundary dispute, either about the boundaries of the body or about the boundary between life and death (the moment when death begins), two highly significant themes in most mythologies. The Hindu doctrine of karma carries with it a number of beliefs that suggest ways very different from our Western ways of regarding these boundaries, ways that might be useful in constructing new boundaries to replace those that the challenges of organ transplants have made obsolete.[39]

The theory of karma (action) argues that the actions a person commits in life, for better or worse, leave traces on the soul, and that the nature of these traces will determine the nature of that person's rebirth. After death, the reincarnating soul takes one of two paths: if good karma predominates over bad, the soul goes first to hell for a relatively brief period, where it works out or consumes its bad karma by being tormented, and then to heaven for a long period, where it enjoys the fruits of its good karma. If bad karma predominates, the soul goes first briefly to heaven and then for a longer sojourn in hell. In either case, after these two sorts of karma are consumed in heaven and hell, the soul is reborn in a station in life determined by the original balance of good and evil karma. (We have already encountered an earlier, more primitive version of this theory in the Upanishadic text about the dispersal of the body after death.)

The karma theory tells us that we are linked to all the other people in the world; they *are us*. This link applies not merely at death but also throughout life. Hindus believe that their souls and their bodies are changed by any intense contact with another person, particularly those involving food or sex (hence, the notorious Hindu fastidiousness about these contacts). If one person gives food to another, for instance, the donor takes away from the encounter some of the good karma of the recipient, and leaves behind with the recipient some of his own bad karma. In this sense it is very literally better to give than to receive.

The universe in which karma is exchanged is a closed one, which Hindus refer to as the *world-egg*. This means that it is a zero-sum system (except in those devotional cults in which *bhakti*, the love of and for god, blasts off the top of the world and makes possible infinite giving;[40] but let us confine ourselves for the moment to mainline Hinduism). If someone is to get more good karma, someone else must get either less good karma or more bad karma. (We have already encountered one aspect of this zero-sum world in the story of the monkey and the crocodile.) This belief led to certain exploitations of the karma system, such as those devised by the medieval sect called the Pashupatas. Members of this sect purposely pretended to be drunk and/or lecherous (when they were in fact sober and/or chaste) in order that passersby would (unfairly) accuse them of misbehaving, thus injuring them. In turn, this injury allowed the Pashupatas to siphon off onto themselves the good karma of the passersby and to jettison their own bad karma onto those same unwitting persons.[41]

Karma is encoded in both the body and the soul in what the anthropologist McKim Marriott has called "coded substance."[42] Evil deeds produce both immediate and long-term effects upon the body. The textbook of Hindu caste law, the *Laws of Manu*,[43] uses the law of karma to explain how, depending on their past actions, people are reborn as various classes of beings (book 12, verses 40–81), including bad people like lepers or blind men. In this context of the karma theory, any gift given or received is in a very real sense a gift of a part of one's own body. Marriott has coined the term *dividuals* to replace *individuals* in accounting for the fluid and shifting sense of ego in the karma theory.

It may well be, therefore, that the ways in which organ donations connect us with other people are more threatening to us in the West than they are to people who grow up with the idea of karmic transfer and, hence, with the idea of sharing other people's bodies. Would transplants make more sense in a society that has a less sharply defined boundary of the individual self? Yes and no. If the idea of the transfer of karma facilitates concepts of organ transfer, it is surely ironic that the Indian people, who have (in Bombay) the world's largest transplant center, where a thousand operations are performed every year, offer transplant organs only for payment; India has the worst record for cadaver donation.

We might adduce several reasons why Hindus do not feel inclined to donate organs. First, cremation is an essential part of Hindu funeral ritual, and we must recall the Vedic verses about preserving the corpse intact; if the funeral is not properly carried out, the ghosts will be angry. Second, as we learned from the history of Indian surgery, the story of King Shivi, Hindus believe that one must not touch a corpse. And third, as E. Valentine Daniel has pointed out,[44] the fluidity of bodies in India makes you more, rather than less, nervous about sharing body parts: other people's karma can get into you in all sorts of ways that you must guard against, including such intentional and aggressive transfers as those of the Pashupatas, which we have just seen.

In India, as everywhere (including America), people carry around within them a number of belief sets, and while one set (such as the belief in karma) might inspire belief in the value of organ donation (when asked on the street), another set (such as the belief in the importance of an intact corpse or, indeed, other aspects of the same belief in karma) might kick in at the moment of truth, when one is faced with the gruesome task of actually chopping up a beloved person who has just died. Both sets of ideas may function on the latent or on the manifest level. Just as many Christians do not in fact live by Christian principles, so many Hindus do not buy into Hinduism, and such people would not have karmic reasons for wanting to give, or not give, organs. In any case, strong personal reasons (such as love or money) often override and outvote myths and religious beliefs.

The Buddhist theory of karma, which argues for the endurance of the personality, might foster more positive attitudes toward organ donation. Whereas the Hindu view attaches the karmic accretions to the transmigrating soul, Buddhism maintains the same theory of rebirth while denying the existence of a transmigrating soul. The Buddhist texts explain this theory with several similes that are highly relevant to the questions about personal identity raised by organ transplants, particularly the survival of the personal identity of the donor in the organ within the body of the recipient. Specifically, the Buddhist answer might prove more useful than the Hindu answer in arguing against this deeply ingrained folk belief.

One of the most famous instances of this Buddhist argument occurs in *The Questions of Milinda,* which purports to record a conversation that took place between the Greek king Menander, who ruled in northwestern India about the middle of the second century B.C.E. (though the text is later by some centuries), and the Buddhist sage Nagasena, who converted the king to Buddhism. King Menander asks, "When a man is born does he remain the same [being] or become another?" to which Nagasena replies, "He neither remains the same nor becomes another." When the king asks for an example, Nagasena argues that, just as when a man lights one lamp from another, one lamp does not transmigrate to the other, so too "there is rebirth without anything transmigrating."[45]

This same Buddhist text provides us with another, more extended, image that argues for the purely conventional nature of the enduring personality:

King Menander asked, "How are you known, and what is your name?" and Nagasena replied, "I'm known as Nagasena, your Majesty; that's what my fellow monks call me. But though my parents may have given me such a name, it does not imply that there is a permanent individual." The king said, "If your fellow monks call you Nagasena, what is Nagasena? Is it your hair?" "No, your Majesty." "Or your nails, teeth, skin, or other parts of your body, or the outward form, or sensation, or perception, or the psychic constructions, or consciousness? Are any of these Nagasena?" "No, your Majesty." "Then for all my asking I find no Nagasena. Nagasena is a mere sound! Surely what your Reverence has said is false."

Then the Venerable Nagasena addressed the King. "Your Majesty, how did you come here—on foot, or in a vehicle?" "In a chariot." "Then tell me what is the chariot? Is the pole the chariot?" "No, your Reverence." "Or the axle, wheels, frame, reins, yoke, spokes, or goad?" "None of these things is the chariot." "Then all these separate parts taken together are the chariot?" "No, your Reverence." "Then is the chariot something other than the separate parts?" "No, your Reverence." "Then for all my asking, your Majesty, I can find no chariot. The chariot is a mere sound. What then is the chariot? Surely what your Majesty has said is false! There is no chariot!" "What I said was not false," replied the king. "It's on account of these various components, the pole, axle, wheels, and so on, that the vehicle is called a chariot. It's just a generally understood term, a practical designation." "Well said, your Majesty! You know what the word 'chariot' means! And it's just the same with me. It's on account of the various components of my being that I'm known by the generally understood term, the practical designation Nagasena!"[46]

David Hume invoked a closely related image (in this case, the construction of a ship rather than a chariot) to make the opposite case, the case *for* the continuing identity of one person in many forms:

A ship, of which a considerable part has been chang'd by frequent reparations, is still consider'd as the same; nor does the difference of the materials hinder us from ascribing an identity to it. The common end, in which the parts conspire, is the same under all their variations, and affords an easy transition of the imagination from one situation of the body to another.

But this is still more remarkable, when we add a *sympathy* of parts to their *common end,* and suppose that they bear to each other, the reciprocal relation of cause and effect in all their actions and operations. This is the case with all animals and vegetables; where not only the several parts have a reference to some general purpose, but also a mutual dependance on, and connexion with each other. The effect of so strong a relation is, that tho' every one must allow, that in a very few years both vegetables and animals endure a *total* change, yet we still attribute identity to them, while their form, size, and substance are entirely alter'd. An oak, that grows from a small plant to a large tree, is still the same oak; tho' there be not one particle of matter, or figure of its parts the same. An infant becomes a man, and is sometimes fat, sometimes lean, without any change in his identity.[47]

The Tin Woodman, after all, had replaced every part of his body, but still remained somehow human. This argument, too, might be adapted to argue for the predominance, and survival, of the original personality of the person who received even an organ so highly charged as a heart. And this is something that often needs to be powerfully affirmed, for transplant psychiatrists have noted that after the operation, the patient often really does become a different person (strong, healthy, independent), and this "crisis of good fortune" may pose problems leading to divorce or postoperative psychosis.

Yet most of us today would be willing to extend our selfhood to our children, and sometimes to a husband or wife. We might also extend our concept of selfhood through a loyalty to the group, though this extension often involves forms of racism and classism that produce the contrary effect—making people disinclined to accept the organs of people of other races. Despite the Enlightenment, pagan myths endure; and because of the Enlightenment, Enlightenment myths endure.

The moment of death, like personhood, is a boundary line that we must now newly construct. In order to deal with living donors, surgeons and nurses (and recipients) must be able to say that the donors are dead, so that it is permissible to take their organs; yet they are, by definition and by necessity, *living* donors. Moreover, modern medical technique has now given us the power to control the moment of death, to place the boundary line where we want it, like the movable partition between business class and tourist class in an airplane; this new power, too, requires us to find new mythologies to make meaningful unprecedented decisions about when that moment is to take place.

When we monkey about with the borders of the body or the moment of death, we are transgressing boundaries and shuffling the deck of our basic sense of order. Transgressing boundaries is what Mary Douglas has taught us to recognize as a basic threat to our sense of personal identity,[48] and the sense of order and disorder is what Claude Lévi-Strauss taught us, even earlier, to recognize as the basis of our entire cognitive world.[49] Very serious metaphysical battles are being fought on the operating-room tables these days.

Conclusion

Our own mythologies predispose us to certain unconscious attitudes regarding organ transplants. Generally, before the Enlightenment, people located human meaning outside the self (in God, or in society, as Durkheim would say), while after the Enlightenment, human meaning was thought to reside inside the self. I would hope that some of the insights preserved in other peoples' myths might open up the argument to other visions of the human body and of its situation within the fluctuating boundary line between life and death.

What is the reason for the enduring significance of these myths? Leslie Fiedler has rightly pointed out that there is horror at the heart (!) of this whole enterprise, that we cannot routinize it, but that we must confront it—both in the heart and in the head.[50] He reminds us that we must pay a psychological price for flying in the face of our myths, which now often lodge in nonreligious sources. His study of four great Gothic novels reveals that they constitute a living mythology, that they speak of our horror not of the ghosts of the past but of the ghosts of the future, of the medical science that is yet to come: about vivisection *(The Island of*

Dr. Moreau), chemotherapy *(Dr. Jekyll and Mr. Hyde)*, the use of cadavers *(Frankenstein)*, and blood transfusion *(Dracula)*. What I hoped to show in this chapter is that these old novels enhance the power of the new terrors by analogizing them to the even more ancient terrors expressed in myths. At the same time, they keep the old myths alive by giving them the transfusion, as it were, of new scientific terrors. Myths, like vampires, are undead.

Let me summarize the points that I intended to demonstrate in this brief survey. From other peoples' myths we learn that it is possible to resolve the wish to keep the body intact with the wish to recycle the parts. We learn that the idea of recycling organs after death has been conceived as a logical, natural process. Further, recycling from a living donor has been conceived as an extraordinary but possible and praiseworthy process in cultures that could not possibly have envisaged a scientifically contrived recycling. But we also learn that other cultures have ideas very different from ours about the "natural" way to dispose of a dead body or to appropriate a living organ. Negative attitudes toward re-memberment into the elements, together with the belief that a dead body is literally untouchable, may lead to a disinclination to harvest organs from dead donors.

Some myths about living donors of eyes and legs argue that the donor may attain valuable rewards in recompense for the gift, sometimes the restoration of the donated organ (a concept that we do not share) and sometimes some other, even more valuable, power. In contrast, other texts convey a far more hard-nosed attitude toward and acceptance of the likelihood that the person who gives an organ (such as a heart) will simply lose it, and gain nothing. Greed, too, may be seen as the driving motive of the recipient of an organ, particularly a heart. And other organs besides the heart take on sexual connotations when the concept of putting one person's organ into another person's body is (often unconsciously) conflated with the sexual act. Moreover, we also learn how deeply ingrained and widespread is the idea, often a racist or classist idea, that when you are given someone else's organs you take on the donor's personality in some way. Finally, the Hindu anatomy of the mind, based upon different divisions of the turf of consciousness and personality, may help us to become more aware of our own unconscious, arbitrary, and perhaps revisable divisions of the same turf.

The ancient metaphors of the body were often sacrificial (the human body was created by the sacrifice of a divine body, and in return humans offered parts of their bodies to the gods) or horticultural (the ancient Greeks and ancient Indians spoke of the body, particularly the female body, as a field that one could sow, a linguistic habit that continues in our contemporary talk of harvesting a body). Nowadays, these violent ancient images are often papered over with a Hallmark-card, superficially Christian discourse of "giving" and "sharing." But the submerged pagan metaphors of organ transplant resurface again and again to sabotage the Pollyanna propaganda.

I recently stumbled on a good example of these submerged pagan vestiges in the television episode "Dark Justice," thus described in the *TV Guide* for Friday, 1 May 1992: "Smooth operator Gibs poses as a patient to nab a black-market organ-stealing doctor." The villain is a woman who seduces her young male accomplice right on the operating room table. She progresses from just taking one kidney from a man (lured to a hotel room by a prostitute who works for the villain) to planning a murder so she can get a man's heart (what else?). When her accomplice begins to balk, she remarks, "The medical system is designed for this." The fact that the transplant doctor is a sexually voracious woman is a gratuitous touch that draws directly, though subliminally, upon *Dracula:* The transplant doctor is a vampire, whose presence in this story calls up ancient forces to indict the medical system.

A more positive, but equally mythological, attitude toward organ transplant is presented in the film *Jesus of Montreal.* In the film, when Jesus dies his eyes are given to a blind woman and his heart to a woman pronounced medically dead. To any Christian viewer, this action replicates, and imposes upon the medical process of organ transplant, Jesus's miracles of making the blind man see and raising Lazarus from the dead. To a student of Buddhist mythology, it replicates King Shivi's intention to donate his eyes and heart to the king of the gods. But even to a viewer with no formal religious training, the images call upon deeply submerged, widely shared, and often inaccessible beliefs about organ transplants.

A Personal Postscript about Organ Transplants

Let me conclude, as I began, with a family story. This time it is a story about organ transplants, a story that demonstrates one way in which participating in this project and experiencing certain events during the years of that participation revealed to me some of my own unconscious ideas about death and organ transplants.

As my involvement in the project deepened, I began to have serious misgivings about the wisdom of organ transplants, for all the reasons that are expressed throughout the chapters in this volume. I had more or less decided that I was against it all. Then, one evening, my older brother called me to say that his daughter was in the hospital, in the advanced stages of liver failure, and that they were hoping to find a donor in the next few days, for otherwise she would die. Instantly I began to pray that we would find a donor and kept closely in touch with my brother day by day until, just in time, one was found. My niece had the operation, survived, and is at the present very much alive, well, and happy. We celebrated the first anniversary of her transplant on the following Thanksgiving, at a gathering at which we all truly gave thanks.

It would be wrong to say that I had simply reversed all my opinions the moment the life of my own niece was at stake. Rather, the episode showed that I had, and (here is the point) had always had, unconscious feelings about organ transplants very different from those in my conscious mind. My chapter in this book is therefore a kind of attempt to formalize the bridge between those two sets of feelings in me and, I would hope, in the reader.

Notes

1.   See Wendy Doniger [O'Flaherty], *Other Peoples' Myths: The Cave of Echoes* (New York: Macmillan, 1988).

2.   *Rig Veda* 10.16.3. Wendy Doniger [O'Flaherty], trans., *The Rig Veda: An Anthology* (Harmondsworth, England: Penguin, 1981), 49.

3.   *Rig Veda* 10.14.7–8; Doniger, *The Rig Veda*, 44.

4.   *Rig Veda* 10.16.1; Doniger, *The Rig Veda*, 49. The great French translator of the *Rig Veda*, Louis Renou, translated the Sanskrit word that I have rendered here as *perfectly*, as *au point*.

5.   *Rig Veda* 10.16.6; Doniger, *The Rig Veda*, 50.

6.   See Wendy Doniger [O'Flaherty], *Dreams, Illusion, and Other Realities* (Chicago: University of Chicago Press, 1984).

7.   See below for a discussion of karma.

8.   Chandogya Upanishad 5.3.1–10. See Wendy Doniger [O'Flaherty], *Textual Sources for the Study of Hinduism* (Chicago: University of Chicago Press, 1990), 35–37. See also Brhadaranyaka Upanishad 4.4.

9.   A. K. Ramanujan, "Death and the Good Citizen," in *Second Sight* (Delhi: Oxford University Press, 1986), 25–26.

10.   See, for instance, the story of the sacrifice of Shunahshepha, in Doniger, *Textual Sources*, 19–24; and the story of Yayati, in Wendy Doniger [O'Flaherty], *The Origins of Evil in Hindu Mythology* (Berkeley: University of California Press, 1976), 237–43.

11.   E. B. Cowell et al., trans., *Jataka Stories, or Stories of the Buddha's Former Births*, vol. 4 (London: Pali Text Society, 1953), 250–56.

12.   *Vinaya Pitaka, Mahavagga*, trans., H. Oldenberg and T. W. Rhys Davids, vol. 13 of *Sacred Books of the East* (Oxford: Oxford University Press, 1881), viii. 4–5, cited by A. L. Basham, "The Practice of Medicine in Ancient and Medieval India," in Charles Leslie, ed., *Asian Medical Systems: A Comparative Study* (Berkely: University of California Press, 1974), 27.

13. Basham, "The Practice of Medicine."

14. P. Kutumbiah, *Ancient Indian Medicine* (Madras: Orient Longmans, 1962), 167–70, cited by Basham, "The Practice of Medicine."

15. *Mahabharata,* Critical Edition (Poona: Bhandarkar Oriental Research Institute, 1933–69), bk. 3, app. 1, no. 21, chap. 195 of the P. C. Roy translation. The *Ramayana* (Critical Edition [Baroda: Oriental Institute, 1960–75]) (2.12.5) also refers to the story of King Shibi [sic] and, immediately afterward (2.12.6), to a King Alarka, who plucked out his own eyes and gave them to a Brahmin, a myth not otherwise known to me.

16. Cited by David Shulman, *Tamil Temple Myths* (Princeton: Princeton University Press, 1980), 135.

17. Josef Baudis, *Czech Folk Tales* (London: George Allen and Unwin, 1917).

18. *Mahabharata* 3.12.1.

19. *Devi Purana* 7.2.3–65, 3.1–64, 4.1–56, 5.1–59, 7.2–53. For a much older version, see the *Jaiminiya Brahmana* 3.120–29, translated in Wendy Doniger [O'Flaherty], *Tales of Sex and Violence* (Chicago: University of Chicago Press, 1985), 64–66.

20. Pausanias 3.14.7; Apollodorus 3.11.2.

21. *Rig Veda* 1.117.6; 1.116.15.

22. Barry D. Kahan, "Cosmas and Damian Revisited," in *Transplantation Proceedings* 15, no. 4 (suppl. 1, no. 2, December 1983): 2211–16. Also see the chapter by Leonard Barkan in this volume.

23. Jacopo da Varagine, *Leggenda Aurea* (Libreria Editrice Fiorentina, 1952), 648–52.

24. Kahan, "Cosmas and Damian Revisited."

25. For a survey of the other variants, see C. H. Tawney, trans., *The Ocean of the Rivers of Story,* vol. 5, with notes by M. Penzer (London: Routledge, 1924), 127ff.

26. *Kathasaritsagara* 10.63.133; *Ocean of the Rivers of Story,* vol. 5, 127–29.

27. Arthur W. Ryder, trans., *The Panchatantra* (Chicago: University of Chicago Press, 1949). This story is at the beginning of book 4.

28. See Wendy Doniger [O'Flaherty], *Women, Androgynes, and Other Mythical Beasts* (Chicago: University of Chicago Press, 1981).

29. David Tracy told me this story on 4 April 1993.

30. See Wendy Doniger [O'Flaherty], *Siva: The Erotic Ascetic* (London and New York: Oxford University Press, 1973, reprinted 1981).

31. *Jaiminiya Brahmana* 3.120–29; Doniger, *Tales of Sex and Violence,* 64–66.

32. Wendy Doniger and Brian K. Smith, "Sacrifice and Substitution: Ritual Mystification and Mythical Demystification," *Numen* 36, no. 2 (December 1989): 189–224.

33. This text is several times removed from the original telling: It is my translation of the eighteenth-century Frenchman's translation from the oral Tamil.

34. Translated from Pierre Sonnerat, *Voyages aux Indes Orientales* (Paris, 1782), 245–47. The Tamil version was also translated into English by B. G.

Babington, *The Vedala Cadai, Being the Tamul Version of a Collection of Ancient Tales in the Sanscrit Language* (London, 1831).

35. *Kathasaritsagara* 12.130 (163) (Bombay: Nirnara Sagara Press, 1930); *Ocean of Story*, vol. 6, 204ff., notes on 276–77.

36. Sir Richard F. Burton, *Vikram and the Vampire, or Tales of Hindu Devilry*, illustrated by Ernest Griset (London, 1870; reprint, New York: Dover Books, 1969). Burton selected this story from the Marathi version of the *Vetalapancavimsati*, or *Twenty-Five Tales of a Vampire* and translated it *very* loosely.

37. Heinrich Zimmer, "Die Geschichte vom indischen König mit dem Leichnam," in the Festival Volume in honor of C. G. Jung, *Die kulturelle Bedeutung der komplexen Psychologie* (Berlin: Verlag Julius Springer, 1935).

38. Thomas Mann, *Die vertauschten Köpfe* (1940); H. T. Lowe-Porter, trans., *The Transposed Heads: A Legend of India* (New York: Alfred Knopf, 1941).

39. See Wendy Doniger [O'Flaherty], ed., *Karma and Rebirth in Classical Indian Traditions* (Berkeley: University of California Press, 1980).

40. See Wendy Doniger [O'Flaherty], "Ethical and Non-Ethical Implications of the Separation of Heaven and Earth in Indian Mythology," in Frank Reynolds and Robin Lovin, eds., *Cosmogony and Ethical Order: New Studies in Comparative Ethics* (Chicago: University of Chicago Press, 1985), 177–98. See also Doniger, *Origins of Evil*, 78–83.

41. See Daniel H. H. Ingalls, "Cynics and Pashupatas: The Seeking of Dishonor," *Harvard Theological Review* 55 (1962): 281–98.

42. McKim Marriott, "Hindu Transactions: Diversity without Dualism," in Bruce Kapferer, ed., *Transaction and Meaning* (Philadelphia: Institute for the Study of Human Issues, 1976); see also McKim Marriott and Ronald Inden, "Caste Systems," *Encyclopedia Britannica* (1973), vol. C, pp. 983ff.

43. See Wendy Doniger with Brian K. Smith, trans., *The Laws of Manu*, a new translation of the *Manavadharmasastra* (Harmondsworth, England: Penguin Classics, 1991).

44. E. Valentine Daniel, *Fluid Signs: Being a Person the Tamil Way* (Berkeley: University of California Press, 1984).

45. *The Questions of King Milinda (Milinda Panha)*, 2 vols., trans., T. W. Rhys Davids, *Sacred Books of the East* (Oxford: Oxford University Press, 1890–94).

46. *Questions of King Milinda*.

47. David Hume, *A Treatise of Human Nature* (1888; reprint, Oxford: Oxford University Press, 1951), bk. 1, pt. 4, sec. 6, 257.

48. See Mary Douglas, *Purity and Danger: An Analysis of Concepts of Pollution and Taboo* (London, 1966).

49. Claude Lévi-Strauss, "The Structural Study of Myth," in Claire Jacobson, trans., *Structural Anthropology* (New York, 1963).

50. See Fiedler's chapter in this volume.

11 *Leonard Barkan*

Cosmas and Damian: Of Medicine, Miracles, and the Economies of the Body

Personal Statement

Though others might dispute the title, I would insist on my qualifications as the person in the group with the least previous experience, knowledge, or interest in organ donation and transplant. My own professional activity has been concentrated in the literature and art of antiquity and the Renaissance, especially in the bridges across this multiple territory, that is, between words and images and between ancient and modern. It's true that quite a few of the materials that make for these relations have to do with notions of the human body; but the kind of body I have written books about is Leonardo's Vitruvian man in the circle of the universe, or Daphne's body when she is transformed into a laurel tree, or the body of the Laocoön statue dug up from the ground in 1506—not the late-twentieth-century body that is subject to advanced technological procedures and to the scholarly conversation that goes with those procedures.

We humanists are, of course, clever enough to cross these great distances of chronology, medium, and discipline by using the imaginative modes of analogy that constitute the very basis of our training. Perhaps I was asked to join the group so that I would furnish those analogies; if so, I will have proved a disappointment. Early on I came to the conclusion that more potential danger lay in bridging the gap between modern transplant and the history of culture as I knew it than in professing simple ignorance and irrelevance.

I can locate this discovery precisely during some after-dinner conversation at the first meeting. We had watched the great early Frankenstein *movie, and in the general discussion that followed—fueled by some very decent Meursault that was being generously poured—it emerged that everything in the story of the fabricated monster and in the way the film told that story was precisely relevant to organ transplant. Everybody responsible for that film, from Mary Shelley to Boris Karloff, seemed to have given their all so that we, sitting in Chicago in 1991, might glean some new insights into the problematics of donating and replacing body parts.*

This kind of reading makes me nervous. Each cultural representation, whether it comes from the ancient Near East, Romantic England, or 1930s Hollywood, is first of all embedded in the conditions of its own time and place. When we draw casual parallels, we learn only what we knew already, and we allow ourselves to believe that we have seen it confirmed. Not that the answer is to ignore the past. Far from it. But we must approach the past with the humility appropriate to visiting any country of which we are not natives. And we must ask ourselves through what systems of interpretation and translation we are operating while we visit that country.

All of which also applied to me as an alien visitor to the world of those who have studied the history of medicine, the ethics of modern technology, and the clinical or sociological practices of transplant in the modern hospital. I emerge from this splendid encounter without any confidence that I have learned to speak their language and even less confidence that they have an obligation to speak mine. After all, it takes years of constant practice to learn a foreign tongue; in the meantime, all each of us can do is enunciate clearly and listen carefully.

The past is the ultimate ghetto, and the people who lived and died a long time ago are perhaps the most disenfranchised minority of all. Even expert historians make the most sweeping claims about whole epochs and groups. For instance, medieval people's lives, according to Jacob Burckhardt, were "woven of faith, illusion, and childish prepossession,"[1] and they were aware of themselves not as individuals but only as members of a tribe, thus replicating a particularly versatile set of stereotypes. More to the present purpose is the fact that we shape the past on the basis of its present utility. Not that this is necessarily shameful—or, indeed, avoidable. There is, after all, no such thing as a past that is not exploited by the present. To call it a past is already to perform this act. To use the term *history* is to engage in a somewhat disingenuous double meaning, since the word claims to cover the aggregate of knowable and unknowable past events while in fact referring to the *account* of those events that is written in the present, that is, once the past was past.

A project that studies the humanistic and cultural significances of an especially up-to-date medical practice runs special risks in this highly fraught territory. With such a broad stretch of time at one's disposal and such an exceptional promise of social utility as is conveyed by the presence of doctors, lawyers, and theologians, the humanist-historian may perhaps be forgiven for a wholesale importation of the past into the present. But taking some narrative—an ancient myth about exchanging bodies or a nineteenth-century fiction about a monster fabricated in a laboratory—and declaring it relevant still risks a betrayal of serious historical method. As we all know or should know, each cultural representation is embedded in the language, the hermeneutics, the aesthetics, and the social and political conditions of its own historical moment and its own past.

But if it is all too easy to imagine relevant ancient myths, it is equally simplistic to declare with high professional snobbery that the past is itself a transplant that won't take. The question is really what the enterprise of the present moment wants out of history; and here I find a fruitful paradox, or even a contradiction, that may outline the appropriate terms for humanistic inquiry. An advanced scientific and technological discourse, especially when left to its own devices, depends in important ways on the assumption that its own temporal moment is unique. We are all familiar with these claims, whether they concern problems, like nuclear destruction, AIDS, and ecological disaster, or whether they concern solutions—and here, of course, the list is shorter, but it includes medical and scientific developments such as organ transplants. In short, nothing like this ever happened before.

Yet while such a self-description produces a set of easy satisfactions, in the end it also leads to a kind of historical loneliness. The past with all its apparent differences becomes the necessary field out of which to make the present—which we might in this case call the *ultra*present— signify something. How does the historian cooperate, or should I use the term *collaborate?* In the end all we can do is ask ourselves what qualifies us to speak for the disenfranchised past, how much we understand it in its own terms, and how fully we recognize what we bring along with us while we travel to this particular far country to do our fieldwork. This last element is the most important. We cannot claim to shed the baggage of our own time; for that very reason we should not imagine that the past is a set of raw materials to which we apply a scientific method of study that is itself outside the contingencies of history. Instead we must allow as free as possible a dialogue in which the past interrogates our methods as much as our methods interrogate the past.

Having said all that, I am going to begin by telling a story about two Christian saints. At the time of the Roman emperor Diocletian, there lived in Syria twin brothers named Cosmas and Damian, who, under the influence of their pious mother, had embraced the still-outlawed Christian religion.[2] They were great physicians who knew how to cure both human beings and animals, but unlike all their colleagues, they refused to take payment for their services, hence earning themselves the sobriquet ἀναργύροι, or fee-less. They lived in peace and love with each other except that on one occasion Damian was prevailed upon by a particularly grateful lady patient to take a small offering—three eggs to be exact—in return for curing her; when Cosmas heard about this, he was so furious that he declared he did not wish to be buried with his avaricious brother when their time came.

At all events, their fame brought them to the attention of the Roman proconsul in Syria, who demanded that they sacrifice to the gods. When they refused, he had them tortured, but they were indifferent to suffering. First, he had them thrown into a huge fire, but they suffered no pain while, instead, the flames engulfed a crowd of heathen spectators. Next, he had them crucified, but the stones flew back against those who were throwing them and wounded a great many of their tormentors. Then, he had four soldiers shoot arrows at them, but the arrows flew backward against the soldiers. Finally, he had them decapitated, and this time the martyrdom was irreversible. The Christians collected the remains and prepared the ordained, separate burial, when suddenly there arrived a camel who spoke in a human voice, ordering that the saints in fact be buried together.

This is relatively standard fare for the early Church, a composite myth with Roman elements (including references to Castor and Pollux and to physician-god Aesculapius) and Eastern elements, such as the camel and the eggs.[3] But the lives of saints never stop at their death and martyrdom. They are the original narratives that beget more narratives, while the faithful continue to have miraculous experiences under the protection of the various martyrs and, thus, continue to add more episodes to their (posthumous) lives. Cosmas and Damian lead a particularly full life after their death, from third-century Constantinople, to early Christian Rome, to medieval Spain and Germany, and to the High Renaissance in Florence, when they become the patrons of the Medici, owing to the fact that the name Medici itself means "doctors" (hence, too, the name Cosimo de' Medici). And the miracles keep pouring in—forty-seven or forty-eight of them in the canonical listings.[4] Over the centuries Cosmas and Damian develop a wide range of medical efficacies: against plague, scabs, scurvy, glandular problems, kidney stones, abdominal swelling, and bedwetting.[5]

The miracle of interest to us, which concerns none of the above diseases, appears to be quite a late one, not so much for the date at which it is supposed to have taken place (somewhere between 550 and 650 C.E.) as for the fact that we do not hear of it before the High Middle Ages—roughly the twelfth century. And that will come as no surprise, since both its concerns and its lifespan as a highly popular tale fit with a floruit of roughly the four centuries between the years 1200 and 1600. I offer the thirteenth-century version from the *Golden Legend*:

Pope Felix, who was an ancestor of Saint Gregory, erected a noble church in Rome in honour of Saints Cosmas and Damian. In this church a man whose leg was consumed by a cancer [we would probably say gangrene, which etymologically is the same word, as are *canker,* and *chancre*] devoted himself to the service of the holy martyrs. And one night as he slept, the saints appeared to him, bringing salves and instruments, and one said to the other: "Where shall we find new flesh, to replace the rotted flesh which we are to cut away?" The other replied: "This day an Ethiop was buried in the cemetery of Saint Peter in Chains; do thou fetch his leg, and we shall put it in place of the sick one!" Thereupon he hastened to the cemetery and brought back the Moor's leg, and they cut off the leg of the sick man and put the other in its stead. Then they anointed the leg which they had cut off, and attached it to the body of the dead Moor. When the man awoke and felt no pain, he put his hand to the leg, and discovered that the wound was no longer there. Wondering whether he was himself or another, he held a candle to the leg, and still found no ill in it. Then, overjoyed, he leapt from his bed, and narrated to all what he had seen in his dream and the manner of his curing. Speedily therefore they sent to the Moor's tomb, and found his leg cut off, and the sick man's leg laid in the tomb beside the Moor.[6]

What I am *not* going to do with this remarkable story is to assimilate it to either a transhistorical or an ahistorical world of analogy. I am not going to discuss Roman versus American race relations in regard to organ transplant. I am not going to compare sixth- with twentieth-century medical practice—or, for that matter, religious practice. I am not going to write a history of Cosmas and Damian iconography in the art and literature of the early modern period. I am not going to speculate on what really happened to the pious gangrene victim and give it a modern scientific name. Nor—and I suppose this is the most important thing I am not doing—will I find a place for this story in the universal matrices of folklore. I am thinking of the mentality beyond the famous, and in its way invaluable, Stith Thompson motif index of folk literature, from which I cite some relevant examples:

- Magic appearance of human limbs (Kaffir).
- Magic object transfers disease to another person or thing (Danish, Icelandic).
- Magic cure of broken limbs (Irish, Indian, Eskimo).

- Severed limbs replaced by Virgin Mary (Spanish).
- Limbs of dead voluntarily reassemble and revive (Jewish, North American Indian).
- Resuscitation with missing member (Danish, Greek, Indian, North and South American Indian).
- Resuscitation by sewing parts of body together (Indian).[7]

What I *am* going to do is try to place myself inside the narrative in its multiple versions and to ask a series of questions that follow what one might call the fault lines of the story, the places where the activity of inventing, or believing, or retelling these events seems at its most efficacious. These points of special importance often cluster around details that vary between one version and another, because those are the places where successive tale-tellers have revealed themselves and their own narrative needs.[8]

The first question I want to ask is best approached by citing a different version of the opening of the story, which comes from a Greek manuscript whose origins are more or less contemporaneous with the *Golden Legend:*

[The man suffering from gangrene] heard of the miracles of the glorious ἀναργύροι Cosmas and Damian. And after going to their house, he said to the saints, "I beg that you, saints, in the name of our Lord Jesus Christ take pity also on me, the sinner, that you may give me a cure of my right leg." On going out, the saints covered their noses, for he was already stinking because his bone was close to being corrupted. The saints said to him, "We cannot, ourselves, treat you for this wound, but our Lord Jesus Christ will give you the favor of a cure."[9]

They go on to tell him that he should ask his favor of God. Meanwhile the archangel Raphael appears to Cosmas and Damian and gives them the instructions about finding the dead man's leg. The sick man has a dream in which the operation is symbolically performed; then, in waking condition, the two doctor-saints go through the complete action of the transplant.

Expressed in hagiographic terms, the obvious difference here is that the miracle appears to be performed not by the mystic intercession of the saints after their martyrdom but by the two doctors in their lifetimes, as inspired by the Christian faith of all three protagonists. But whether they are alive or dead is not what really counts. The important issue is what we mean by a miracle. When the Virgin Mary regenerates the leg of Peter of Grenoble, which has been amputated owing to a grave bout of sacred fire, or when the aged Audomatus has his sight restored by touching the remains of Saint Vaast, or when Saint Benedict instantly cures a poor child's elephantiasis, none of these fortunate believers is made the object of a medical procedure.[10] These acts are simply miraculous; that is, they happen by instantaneous divine agency. The coordinates of Cosmas and Damian in all versions of the story are different: on the one hand, the two saints invariably do real and difficult surgical labor; on the other, they achieve a medical result that is as fantastic and improbable in the real world of the cultures telling this story as any of the saintly miracles involving the transport of whole cities or the resurrecting of the dead. While we observe the life of this story, then, we are in effect deconstructing what is to us the exceedingly banal expression *medical miracle;* in other words, we are reminding ourselves how that expression might be in rhetorical terms an oxymoron or in cultural terms a lived contradiction or paradox.

It is worth observing just how much of the real enters the world of Cosmas and Damian and in what way. When the two saints are rendered as living doctors, the medical situation is more down-to-earth, that is, Cosmas and Damian have to turn away from the stink. At the same time, it is more subject to inexplicable divine intervention; that is, the saints declare Christ, not themselves, to be the only author of miracles. In effect, then, telling the story the second way reveals the difficult split between the real and the miraculous that the legend insists upon. And the realistic details are everywhere and in all versions: not only the stinking of the leg but also the fact that the patient goes to Cosmas and Damian's "house" (οἰκός), which means their church if they are saints (especially dead saints) and their home office if they are practicing physicians. Even the *Golden Legend* version I began with, in which they are clearly martyred saints, has them fetching "salves and instruments" on their way to perform the miracle; elsewhere, we hear of *ferramenta* (iron instruments) and of *yrnis scharpe* (sharp irons), as well as details about the healing ointments.[11]

Even more to the point is the actual procedure: " 'Whence shall we get flesh, that, having cut away the rotten flesh, we may fill up the empty place?' " in one version;[12] or, in even greater detail, " 'Where could we get some flesh to fill the hole in this leg which has been eaten away by cancer?' . . . Having brought there the thigh of the Moor, they cut from it a piece of flesh and put it in the spreading sore on the man's leg; and then the man woke up fully cured."[13] In a way, it is the very opposite of a miracle: that is, a rigorously self-contained procedure with its own zero-sum-game economy (a concept we shall revert to). The cure does not come from any magical notion of heaven or the supernatural; when the doctors remove the diseased flesh, they must replace it with healthy flesh. Indeed, in most versions much is made of the fact that the donor (as we would call him) is newly deceased—"yet his flesche / Is caloure enucht & als fres" (his flesh is still cool enough and fresh)[14]—to arrive as closely as possible to a perfect interchange, which has its own poetic logic quite apart from the scientific plausibility we recognize in it.

Pictures will tell this story more fully. The disease is often rendered with grisly realism, which is quite in keeping with the canons of holy image making, especially outside Italy. More to the point, perhaps, is the realism of the miracle. In the operation as performed in an unattributed fifteenth-century German painting now in Stuttgart (figure 1),[15] one saint holds the leg carefully in place while the other binds it with a long strip of cloth. What are we to make of this gesture? Are they staunching the blood flow? Will the cloth actually hold the two pieces in place until they somehow grow together? We can hardly work by reference to real medical practice, since this is not a real medical practice. Perhaps the best way to read it is through the metaphor of botanical grafting, which was, after all, the only real procedure remotely resembling the operation being practiced here. (Amputation was possible but without anything to put in its place.)

Many other instances of medical precision appear in the images. A pair of painted reliquary doors, also fifteenth century, from the St. Michaelskirche in Munich (figure 2) include in one panel an amputation saw and in the other a tub of ointment about to be applied with a spatula;[16] in neither of the images do the two doctors even have haloes around their heads. Similarly unhallowed are the Cosmas and Damian of a sixteenth-century Flemish painting (figure 3), part of a diptych by Ambrosius Francken the Elder.[17] Once again, we see a kind of linen sleeve in readiness to attach the transplant (or possibly to serve as a tourniquet); there are also several appropriate tools, including the saw and the blood basin. Most striking of all are the attitudes of the two doctor-saints, which are so naturalistic that the saint on the left, who is attaching the black leg, has even rolled up his sleeves. And the context is certainly not the church, or even the house, of Cosmas and Damian, but a contemporary hospital with other bedridden patients, as well as that perfect tip-off of real-life medical activity, the examination of a urine specimen—here in the very light source that enables us to see the miracle performed.[18]

However, it would be quite wrong to ascribe all this to a simple desire to demystify the miracle. One observation of modern hermeneutic theory—I use Paul Ricoeur's elegant formulation—is that "enigma does not block understanding but provokes it."[19] Ricoeur's notion of enigmatic provocation is also congenial with Schütz's conception of shifting the accent of reality through "shock." Which is to say that symbolic

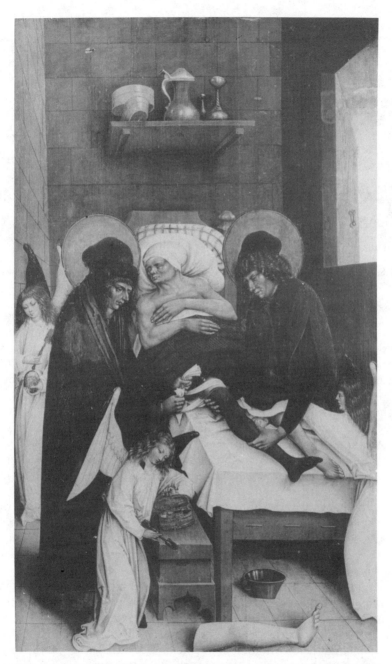

Figure 1. *Saints Cosmas and Damian Healing a Sick Leg*. Painting by anonymous fifteenth-century German artist. Württemberg Regional Museum, Stuttgart, Germany. Foto Marburg/Art Resource, N.Y.

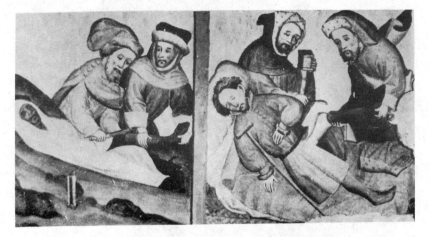

Figure 2. *Scenes from the Miracle Performed by Cosmas and Damian*. Painted door panels of a reliquary by anonymous fifteenth-century German artist. Saint Michaelskirche, Munich.

or enigmatic representations, like miracles, perpetually invite rational or experiential demystifications, which in the end serve to maintain the mystery as much as to explain it away. In the case of Cosmas and Damian, one could say that the real-life medical elements do not so much suppress the miraculous as become conflated with it.

This confusion becomes especially apparent with regard to the explanations of some pictorial representations proffered by "expert" observers—medical historians and hagiographers—from our own time. Of the two saints in a fifteenth-century Italian illumination (figure 4),[20] for instance, we are told that they are "cleaning their instruments."[21] And perhaps that *is* what they are doing. One might even say that the gestures were designed to be read by the then-contemporary viewer as professionally authentic, like the bone saw or the bedpan in other images we have considered. Yet this image was painted several centuries before the invention of the germ theory of disease; and the cleaning of surgical instruments would probably not have had anything like this prominence (or, indeed, have taken place at all) at the moment in history when this work was executed. What the gestures *do* resemble within fifteenth-century visual experience is the manner in which saints were identified by depicting them with their own emblems or attributes.[22] So the knife and the spatula (roughly coinciding with the two parts of Cosmas and Damian's miracle, that is, the cutting and the pasting) become signs at once of their sanctity and of their professional acumen.

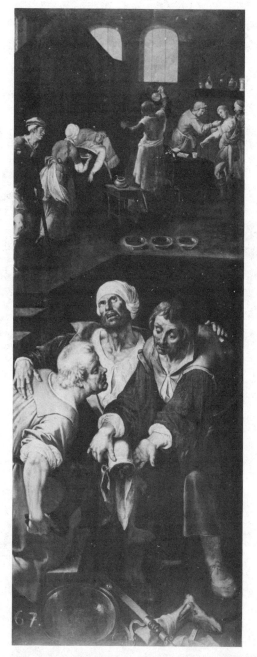

Figure 3. *Cosmas and Damian*. Painting by Ambrosius Francken the Elder. Koninklijk Museum voor Schone Kunsten, Antwerp, Belgium. Copyright A.C.L.-Brussel.

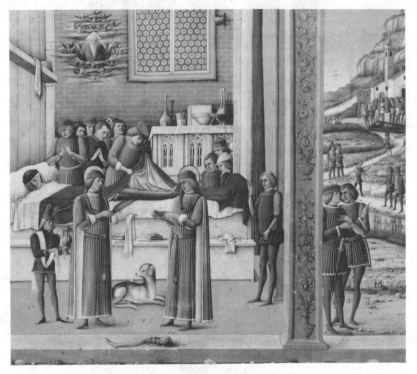

Figure 4. Illumination attributed to Girolamo da Cremona, from the fifteenth-century manuscript "The Brooke Antiphonal." Society of Antiquaries of London, London, England. Copyright Society of Antiquaries of London.

The conflation—to go back to my earlier terms—of *medical* and *miracle* may be even clearer in the persistent appearance of angels within the representations of this event, as in a fifteenth-century altarpiece by Jaume Huguet from a church near Barcelona (figure 5).[23] Once again, scientifically oriented historians refer to these figures as "surgical assistants."[24] Granted, it is certainly useful to have an extra pair of hands when doing an organ transplant. And if we go back to the Stuttgart painting (figure 1), we notice that one angel is helpfully holding back the covers while another is getting the ointment ready. But what shall one say of the angels in a fifteenth-century painting by Alonso de Sedano (figure 6)?[25] It is fortunate that one of them holds a candle so the operation need not be done in the dark. But this is a universal posture of angelic light, far removed from the specific exigencies of the Spanish Renaissance operating room, whereas the symmetrical manifestation

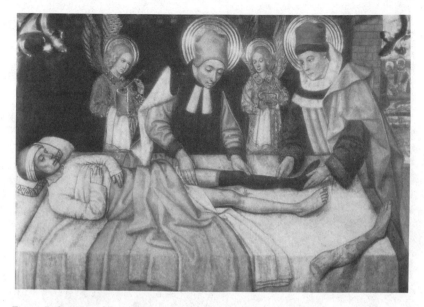

Figure 5. *Cosmas and Damian Performing the Miracle of the Leg.* Painting by Jaume Huguet. Church of Santa Maria, Tarrasa, Spain.

by another angel of the (slightly pock-marked) white leg can only be a hieratic manifestation of the miraculous. Not to mention the third angel, whose hands are clasped in prayer, or the liturgical garments in which all the figures appear. In fact—and I return to the Huguet altarpiece (figure 5)—what angels do to help out the saintly doctors, whether it involves bringing light or applying unguent, is remarkably similar to what angels perform in their purely heavenly rituals.

But to speak in the universal mode of the hermeneutic circle that joins all mysteries with all demystifications may be to ignore or undervalue the particulars of a miracle that is concerned specifically with medicine and the body. Obviously, not all Christian miracles are concerned with the human body, though a disproportionate number probably are; of those many, a minority set the events in a medical context (such as we might do). In part this corporeal focus has its origins in the story of Christ himself, whose double nature, both divine and human, meets in a corruptible and yet eternal body. For Catholics the sufferings on the cross are absolutely real and physical. And the developments in understanding the human body throughout the Middle Ages and the early modern period produce more ways to describe and represent the reality of Christ's (and Christians') corporeal experience.[26]

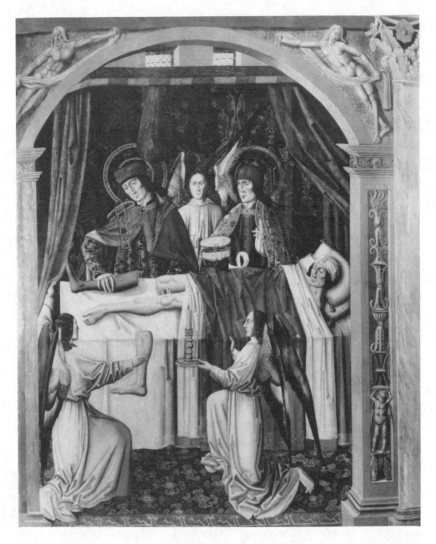

Figure 6. *Saints Cosmas and Damian Performing the Miracle of the Black Leg.* Painting by Alonso de Sedano. Wellcome Institute Library, London, England.

Thus, to return to Cosmas and Damian, the introduction of practical medical details into a miracle becomes a subcategory (like many other things) of what it means to have a human Christ. To understand the full significance of the operation they perform in the light of faith, I want to return to another element in its verbal and visual renderings. I choose the

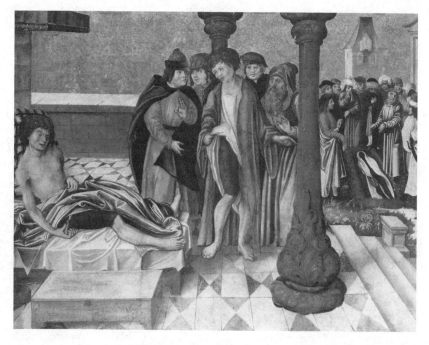

Figure 7. *Miraculous Cure of the Leg by Saints Cosmas and Damian.* Painting by anonymous sixteenth-century Austrian artist. Österreichische Galerie, Vienna, Austria.

early version from the Greek manuscript, though this element is present in almost all versions: "Then he returned to his home [cured] with great joy. Then his neighbors and acquaintances did not believe that his leg had been cut off until they had gone to the tomb and seen the leg."[27] To this we might add, once again, the fifteenth-century illumination (figure 4), which is almost entirely devoted to groups observing and confirming what has taken place, both at the sickbed and at the tomb, along with the interesting pair of figures in the right foreground, who seem to be making a connection between the events. Or else we might add a sixteenth-century Austrian altarpiece (figure 7),[28] in which the artist left out Cosmas and Damian altogether in favor of the two scenes of demonstration.

The lore of this miracle, in short, places exceptional emphasis on verification. In one sense this is rather surprising. The orthodox line on miracles, after all, is that they be believed without experiential test; indeed, the very definition of faith involves the acceptance of the impossible beyond or regardless of the evidence offered by the senses.

Why should this story be exceptional? If we go back to Christ's human body, we see the very exemplar of the verification problem. The apostle Thomas needed to touch the wounds of the risen Christ in order to believe in his divinity and resurrection; and while he thereby earned a rebuke and a somewhat dubious (forgive the pun) title, he not only kept his sacred status but also became the personification of a faith that *is* confirmed by the senses.[29] Of course, a faith remains that cannot be confirmed by the senses (presumably the highest form of faith), which also has its body story. For the mystery of the Eucharist, whereby the sanctified bread and wine become the body and blood of Christ, no one ever paints a fresco in which bakers produce a Jesus-shaped loaf or winegrowers plant a vineyard in the shape of God's circulatory system. But that is the mystical body. The body that human beings share with Christ—the body that can be stoned to death and can suffer gangrene or need a transplant—is the locus of a practical faith. Its miracles may need verification. Indeed, they may exist for the purpose of verification. In this way, just as (in certain respects) the transplant miracle symbolically prefigures modern medical practice, so the representation of the scene of verification prefigures an educational system for anatomy and medicine where, once again, the body becomes the locus of real demonstration and verification.[30] Nor are these prefigurings merely historical curiosities; they are also part of the cultural or epistemic context that makes scientific and technological change possible. So far as the particulars of Cosmas and Damian are concerned, the authentic sense experience of this act of faith is located not only in the tomb, where all those observers see the amputated limb, but also in the perpetual sign of the cured man with one white and one black leg. But that is a topic to which we shall return.

Another issue in the Cosmas and Damian story will bring us yet closer to the matter of transplant but may seem not to be an issue at all. The angel Raphael is telling the two doctors how to cure the suffering man: "Go to the church of the holy martyr cenobiarch. There is a dead man there. And go to his tomb, for he has been dead for four days. Take his right leg and put it on the man who has the splinter as your medical treatment for him. And on the day of resurrection let each one take his own limb, because they came to you with great faith in God."[31] With "on the day of resurrection let each one take his own limb," Raphael is rendering explicit one of the most powerful and difficult issues in the Christian understanding of the body. According to Christian doctrine— in this regard following Jewish belief quite closely—all the dead will be raised to life at the second coming of Christ, with everyone reassuming his or her original body.[32] Those of us who are relatively far from a living acceptance of this kind of grand eschatology can hardly gauge the significance of such a credo, not only as a literal tenet of faith but also as a point of origin for a whole attitude toward human bodies when viewed *sub specie aeternitatis*. In contrast, then, with the more familiar Christian tradition that glorifies the soul and declares of our physical housing "dust thou art, to dust thou shalt return," we encounter a critical article of belief according to which the body we live in will be as eternally ours as the soul is.

Perhaps the most important aspect of this credo is the difficulty of arriving at a precise understanding of what it means. How can we have bodies at the end of the world, and of what kind? The canonical source is in the New Testament, from Paul's first letter to the Corinthians:

But, you may ask, how are the dead raised? In what kind of body? A senseless question! The seed you sow does not come to life unless it has first died; and what you sow is not the body that shall be, but a naked grain, perhaps of wheat, or of some other kind; and God clothes it with the body of his choice, each seed with its own particular body. All flesh is not the same flesh: there is flesh of men, flesh of beasts, of birds, and of fishes—all different. There are heavenly bodies and earthly bodies; and the splendour of the heavenly bodies is one thing, the splendour of the earthly another. . . . So it is with the resurrection of the dead. What is sown in the earth as a perishable thing is raised imperishable. . . . What I mean, my brothers, is this: flesh and blood can never possess the kingdom of God, and the perishable cannot possess immortality. Listen! I will unfold a mystery.[33]

But Paul continues with a good deal more mystery than unfolding. This much is clear: the resurrected dead will have bodies—that is, will not be mere spirit—and they will have different bodies, each appropriate to the person whose soul inhabits it.

For a thousand years or more, the perplexities built into this all-important doctrine provoke the most insistent questionings about both the physical and the metaphysical nature of the human body. There are, of course, ways to tie this messy package together, as for instance, in the *Catholic Encyclopedia*:

All shall rise from the dead in their own, their entire, and in immortal bodies; but the good shall rise to the resurrection of the life, the wicked to the resurrection of judgment. It would destroy the very idea of resurrection if the dead were to rise in bodies not their own [which is the crucial gloss on some of Paul's evasions]. . . . These three characteristics, identity, entirety, and immortality, will be common to the risen bodies of the just and the wicked. But the bodies of the saints shall be distinguished by four transcendent endowments . . . "impassibility," . . . "brightness," . . . "agility," . . . "subtilty."[34]

But the history of reflection on the resurrected body is full of more questions than answers. I take the example of Saint Augustine, who, in the concluding pages of the *City of God*, grapples with the fact that Christians have been subject to ridicule on the grounds of this tenet.[35] He takes on all the most troubling possibilities. For instance, in what body are the victims of cannibalism resurrected—in their own, or in the bodies of those who ate them? Are aborted infants resurrected as half-grown fetuses? Are children resurrected as children, and nonagenarians as nonagenarians? He comes up with the general answer (more Platonic and Aristotelian than Christian) that all bodies are resurrected in their perfection, whether potential or achieved, and this perfection he associates with the body of Christ, who died in his ideal thirty-three years of manhood. But this answer merely raises more questions: Do individuals who were taller than Christ have something removed— which contradicts the scriptural claim that "not one hair shall perish" from the resurrected dead? And if all are raised in perfection, do women have to be resurrected as men, since, again according to Pauline prescription, the female gender is the imperfect form of the male?[36] (The tortuous answer to that one is no, for only in respect to sex and not to gender is woman imperfect, and sex will not be a property of resurrected bodies.)

I have rehearsed all this in order to establish some important subterranean issues in the miracle wrought by Cosmas and Damian. We are attached to our bodies for all eternity; indeed, eternity is in part structured and defined by the continuity of this attachment. This body is, even at the resurrection, a physical body, at least in the sense that its resemblance to our living body can be understood only through our physical individuality. Each body belongs to its owner in an absolute sense, which, considering that this doctrine was developed in the first few centuries of the common era, is more anomalous than we as moderns may think.

Historical thinking of our own time tends to define the concepts of self or individual subjectivity as related to notions of personal property, and although long postdating the epochs of Saints Paul or Augustine,[37] this absolute and unique identification was already attached to the living and resurrected bodies in those much earlier eras. Changes in the body, including the physical effects of aging or illness, along with grimmer possibilities like abortion or cannibalism, are mere accidents, wiped away by the eventual perfection of all things. But the transplant of someone else's limb is not a mere contingency in that sense, because it inhibits both individuals' abilities to be resurrected in their own bodies at the last trumpet. Miracles, whether saintly or medical, are all very well, but the possession of one's own body is an absolute that must be rectified in time for the end of the world.

My last set of interrogations relates to issues implicit in the resurrection problem but more directly focused on *this* world. I suppose that the leading question, in every sense of the term, is why the "donor" in the Cosmas and Damian story is a black man.[38] To address this matter, we need an appropriately historicized approach to the presence of racial and cultural aliens in the discourses of medieval and early modern Europe. The difference between a black man in the cemetery of Saint Peter in Chains and some parallel case in our own cultural practice is that the earlier, majoritarian cultures had much less real-life experience with such different racial or ethnic groups. They had *some* experience, of course: The Roman Empire did touch upon sub-Saharan Africa, and Africans are frequently represented in European art from late antiquity onward.[39] (One should, of course, note the important distinctions to be made between Moors and black Africans: Europeans of these periods sometimes understood these differences, sometimes didn't, and sometimes elided them deliberately.) The relative absence of these foreigners from the day-to-day life of Europeans means that they were marginalized in a different way from what we are familiar with, having to do more with instrumentalization and less with organized systems of oppression. Basically, Europeans knew very little about these aliens: in one version of the leg-transplant story, for instance, the donor is given the name Maurus, which is simply the Latin word for Moor, but apparently the teller of this version did not even recognize the expression as generic.[40]

What is *not* so different about the way Europeans viewed these aliens is that they were capable of being translated into an elaborately symbolic status. Indeed, precisely because the real presence of foreigners was minimal, they were mostly fitted into metaphoric categories, which in some ways resemble our modern stereotypes, except that they have less to do with supposed actual observation of behavior and more with abstract emblematics. Perhaps the best key to the ambiguities of our donor's racial status in this story is that he is often described as Ethiopian. It is a designation that removes him from the real-life experience of Europeans (to a far more distant location than, for instance, the geographic cues that surround Othello); it places him in the world of ancient myth and legend. Most important, it places him in the category of Christian, albeit of the most remote and legendary stamp, since Ethiopians represented a kind of distant lost tribe of Christianity.[41] After all, the whole business of exchanging limbs at the resurrection is meaningful only because *both* participants in the operation are redeemable as men of faith.

Visual representations of the scene will both demonstrate the need for all this tact and perhaps challenge it as well. A very simple predella

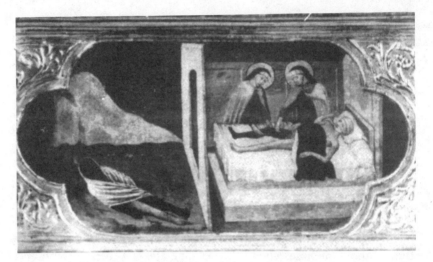

Figure 8. Altarpiece by Lorenzo di Bicci. Cathedral, Florence.

ascribed to the fifteenth-century Florentine Lorenzo di Bicci (figure 8)[42] divides the scene with exquisite directness: a brightly lit crowded interior where the saints are engaged in their operation upon the patient; the lonely landscape where the black man lies in his shroud. Perhaps the most striking feature is the remarkable perspective wall that separates the two figures, in notable contrast with the exchange of limbs that unites them. We could choose to read this image as dramatizing what we call race relations and even as a comment upon the good fortune of the white and the bad fortune of the black. But it seems at least equally appropriate to see the two sides of the wall for what they are: absolute opposition.

That vision appears more fully and clearly in a fifteenth-century painting by Fernando del Rincón (figure 9).[43] Once again, the white man is unquestionably fortunate and the black man unfortunate. The first is alive and brilliantly swathed; the second is dead and wretchedly laid out. What needs to be even more sharply observed here, though, is the way the two are mirror images of each other. The black man is almost literally the reflection of the white man, especially in regard to the position of the heads and arms. In more conceptual ways as well they are obviously mirror images: white, black; alive, dead; draped in brilliant color, covered in a plain shroud. They are, in short, placed in that curious territory where opposites are also identical.[44] This leads me to turn parenthetically to one of the most curious of all Cosmas and

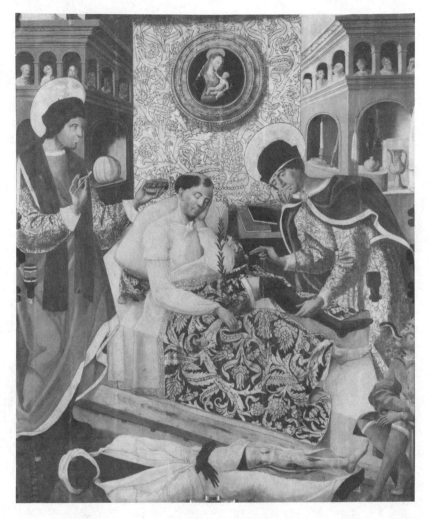

Figure 9. *The Miracles of the Doctor Saints Cosmas and Damian.* Painting by Fernando del Rincón. Prado Museum, Madrid, Spain.

Damian images (figure 10), a sixteenth-century Spanish wood carving now in Valladolid,[45] which makes a change in the narrative so radical and unprecedented that one wonders if the artist misunderstood the story: that is, the black man is alive. On the one hand, this creates a whole new story about the exploitation of the donor. On the other hand, it contributes to a kind of absolute equation between the two figures,

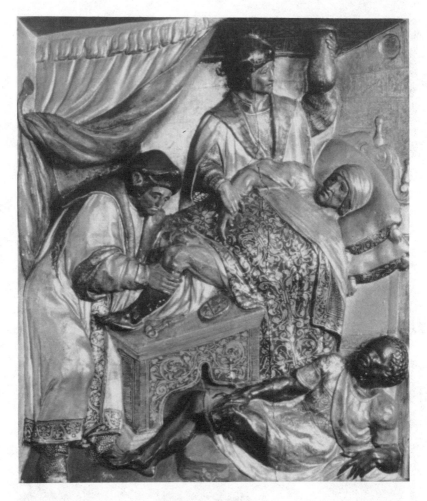

Figure 10. *The Miracle of Saints Cosmas and Damian.* Wood sculpture by anonymous sixteenth-century Spanish artist. National Museum of Sculpture, Valladolid, Spain.

who are in precisely the same recumbent position—their identity, of course, radically split by the transfer of the leg.

It is, of course, the transfer of the leg that most interests us. When we return to the Rincón painting (figure 9), we see that the most powerful parallel of all—not, incidentally, a mirror image in the literal sense— is the pair of legs, both so vividly extended on the right side of the painting. In the transplant, the issue of opposite and yet identical ceases to be a metaphor; it is literalized. Here, we touch upon the most powerful mystery in this legendary operation, more significant even than the race of the donor but, I think, closely related to it: that is, the fact that the gangrenous white leg gets attached to the corpse with the same logic as the healthy black leg gets attached to the living man. Sometimes this postmortem transplant is implicit in the written versions; sometimes it is explicit: "They put the leg of the man who had the splinter on to the leg of the dead man in the name of the Holy Trinity."[46] Sometimes, however, it is quite elaborately reasoned out in medical terms: "They went where the Moor had been buried and they found that the Moor had in his leg the disease that the devout man had had in his and the spreading sore was as fresh in the Moor's leg as if he were alive and had had the sore for a long time."[47] In the visual tradition, the corpse almost always has a white gangrenous leg. Even in the curious instance of the Austrian altarpiece (figure 7), where the transplanted part is literally the thigh, the parallel between the living patient's black thigh and the corpse's diseased white thigh is perfect.

But what are we to make of the perceived obligation to perform this second operation, which happens to conform so little to a twentieth-century view of the matter? It is not altogether frivolous to point out that the transplant onto the corpse removes us definitively from the world of medical efficacy. Despite the fact that one of our narrative versions reports the paradox of a living (but fatal) disease growing inside a corpse, the gesture of complete exchange establishes itself as transcending the utility of keeping either party alive. Nor, as we have seen, does it offer some sacred boon to the Ethiopian, who will have to engage in yet another exchange when Christ comes again.

One could speak of two alternative kinds of utility here. Let us call the first systemic. As the Pauline notion of the resurrection suggests, there is a grand economy in the universal matter of bodies. All the parts must be accounted for. Even when an organ is fatally diseased or not functioning, it cannot be thrown away. That is because the body is not only a mutable organic machine but also the most fundamental and enduring model of completeness: the microcosm, the miniature version of the universe, of all political and social structures, of geometry, and of all the man-made structures that arise out of geometry.[48] That metaphorical body is as real (though not in the same way) as the physical body, which can break down and become (or need to become) dismembered. In that sense, the body of the newly healthy recipient is complete only in the purely physical sense, not in the metaphysical sense so long as the donor's body has not been made whole, however temporary and however somatically ineffectual that wholeness may be.

The other kind of utility to the double transplant is more individual, or at least it is confined to the particular pair of individuals. I quote from an early version of the story in the *Acta Sanctorum:* "Waking up, when he felt himself without pain, he placed his hand on his leg, and found no lesion. Putting then a candle nearby, when he saw nothing wrong in the leg, he thought that he was himself not who he was, but that he was rather someone else."[49] The shock comes not from the disease or from the transplant or even from the different color of the leg; it comes from the absence of a boundary line. Whether one understands the body as the seat of the soul or of the psyche (which is, after all, just one of the Greek words for soul) or of some more modern entity like self or subjectivity, the awareness evinced here is that one's own body might become *other.* In that sense the donor is a black man because the black man is the radical other. Both the corpse and the living man must remain marked with this other for eternity, or at least until the coming of Christ.

This sense of being marked helps explain the visual fascination of the whole topic. The focal point of almost every Cosmas and Damian image is the difference between the two legs, often not only in color but also even in size. Indeed in yet another fifteenth-century Spanish version, by the artist Pedro Berruguete (figure 11),[50] the man is of no importance, but only the incongruously matched pair of limbs. Yet with the double transplant complete and the ligatures effaced, as in the Rincón painting (figure 9), the body becomes a site where the other is no longer so other. The economy of a complete exchange brings each body to some kind of new equilibrium. In fact, the world of exchange extends from this scene. Viewers of the scene as represented, say, by Fra Angelico (figure 12)[51]— where the amputated leg is not visible—have often thought that the black leg was the diseased leg rather than the new transplant:[52] an error, to be sure, but one that reminds us that the experience of the recipient includes another kind of exchange, according to which the new healthy leg retains some qualities of the old sick leg.

As an interesting converse, Rincón (figure 9) drapes the shroud around the black man's nontransplanted right leg so that the limb appears brilliantly white. And the outermost ring of these exchanges that become complementarities involves the two saints themselves. On the many pictorial representations where multiple panels illustrate the whole career of Cosmas and Damian, the miracle of the leg is directly juxtaposed with the saints' own martyrdom by decapitation; that is, Cosmas and Damian ultimately regain their glory when they offer a rejoining of bodies in exchange for their own mutilation. The economy of bodies is manifest over the widest expanse.

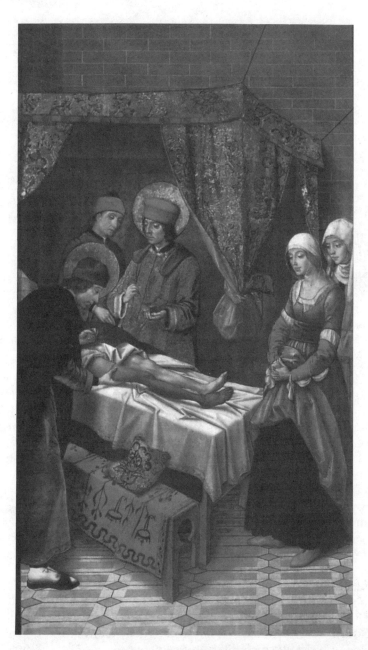

Figure 11. *Cosmas and Damian Performing Leg Transplant*. Painting by Pedro Berruguete. Sacristy of the College of Cosmas and Damian, Covarrubias, Spain.

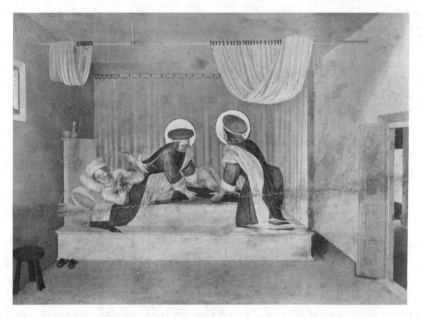

Figure 12. *A Miracle of Saints Cosmas and Damian.* Painting by Fra Angelico. Museum of San Marco, Florence, Italy. Alinari/Art Resource, N.Y. Copyright 1994 Fratelli Alinari.

Having sworn off the making of facile transhistorical parallels, I have chosen a story that represents, after all, a late medieval organ transplant (as it happens, of an organ beyond our present capacity to transfer). I have studiously refrained from elaborating the obvious parallels. And yet I have rather coyly led the topic around to issues of demonstrable contemporary relevance, such as the relations between medicine and the miraculous and the various ways in which the presence of an alien organ serves to call into question profound and enduring beliefs concerning flesh and spirit, both in individual experience and in the constituting of human beings as a society. By way of setting these relevances in a proper methodological frame, I would propose that the matter of organ transplant, whether in the church of Saints Cosmas and Damian or in a Pittsburgh hospital, needs to be glimpsed in historical terms as an *epi*phenomenon.

The phenomenon proper is the history of cultural and individual attitudes toward the body—physical and metaphysical, human and divine, physically corruptible and symbolically perfect, the first and last thing in any culture that individuals can call their own. One thing (at least) that transhistorical parallels *do* make clear is that human beings could experience a fearful challenge to this final certainty long before they could perform the physical operation. In the space between the imaginative projection of such anxieties in the early modern period and the twentieth-century experience of recipient and donor lie all the nuanced particularities of history.

Notes

1. S. G. C. Middlemore and Irene Gordon, trans., *The Civilization of the Renaissance in Italy*, pt. 2 "The Development of the Individual" (New York: Harper, 1958), 121.

2. Lives of saints, like other mythological materials, find their beginnings in separate narratives, often with diverse local origins, that are then collected and canonized as though they proceeded from a single source. When retelling and interpreting any of these stories, it is important to recollect the discontinuous and accretive nature of their narrative constituents and not to assimilate them to the more organic forms of modern single-author storytelling. In the present case, for instance, students of hagiography have distinguished several Cosmas and Damian pairs. In the Eastern tradition, which is the source of these stories though they long predate the actual separation of the churches, there appear to be three distinct pairs of brothers who go under these names and to whom miraculous experiences are ascribed: one pair from Asia, one from Rome, one from Arabia—each pair, in fact, with its own saint's day. The Western church conflated them, concentrating on the Arabian pair, and gave them yet a different feast day (27 September).

The argument of this chapter focuses largely on materials from the Western tradition, because it is concerned with a miracle known almost exclusively in the West. The canonical source in the Western church for Cosmas and Damian, as for most saints' lives, is the thirteenth-century collection by Jacobus de Voragine known as *The Golden Legend*. For collections of other primary materials on this pair of saints, see Ludwig Deubner, *Kosmas und Damian: Texte und Einleitung* (Leipzig: B. G. Teubner, 1907); Ernst Rupprecht, *Cosmoe et Damiani, sanctorum medicorum, vita et miracula* (Berlin: Junker und Dünnhaupt, 1935); A. J. Festugière, *Sainte Thècle, Saints Côme et Damien* (Paris: A. et J. Picard, 1971). See also the excellent overview by Walter Artelt in *Lexikon der christlichen Ikonographie* (Rome: Herder, 1968), s. v. "Kosmas und Damian." An extremely useful collection of texts relevant to the miracle under discussion in this chapter is offered both in their original languages and in translation in Douglas B. Price and Neil J. Twombley, *The Phantom Limb Phenomenon: A Medical, Folkloric, and Historical Study* (Washington, D.C.: Georgetown University Press, 1978).

3. The elements of Western mythology in the Cosmas and Damian story are probably more than casual parallels. It has been argued that elements in the story of Castor and Pollux were directly transferred to the Christian saints. See Ernst Lucius, *Die Anfänge des heiligen Kultes in der christlichen Kirche* (Tübingen: Mohr,

1904), 202; Ludwig Deubner, *De Incubatio* (Leipzig: B. G. Teubner, 1900), 77–80; and Hippolyte Delehaye, *Les légendes hagiographiques* (Brussels: Bureaux de la Société des Bollandistes, 1905), 195–96. Louis Réau, *L'iconographie de l'art chrétien* (Paris: Presses Universitaires de France, 1958), 3.1.333, points out that several temples of Aesculapius were transformed into churches consecrated to Cosmas and Damian. As for elements of Eastern mythology, see Michel van Esbroeck, "La diffusion orientale de la légende des saints Cosme et Damien," in *Hagiographie, cultures et sociétés* (Paris: Etudes augustiniennes, 1981), 61–77; Deubner, *Kosmas und Damian*, 40–52; and W. E. Crum, "Place Names in Deubner's *Kosmas und Damian*," *Proceedings of the Society of Biblical Archeology* 30 (1908): 45–52.

4.   See, for instance, Hippolyte Delehaye, "Les recueils antiques des miracles des saints," *Analecta Bollandiana* 43 (1925): 8–18. Fourteen more are added by François Halkin in "Publications récentes de textes hagiographiques grecs," *Analecta Bollandiana* 53 (1935): 374–81.

5.   See Réau, *L'iconographie*, 3.1.334.

6.   Jacobus de Voragine, *The Golden Legend*, trans., Granger Ryan and Helmut Ripperger (Salem Ayer, N. H., 1941), 577–78.

7.   Stith Thompson, *Motif Index of Folk Literature*, 6 vols. (Bloomington: Indiana University Press, 1955–58). For the motifs listed, see his entries D61, D2161.4, D2161.33, D2161.5.2.4, E31, E33, and E35.1.

8.   My principal indebtedness in this kind of study is to the structuralist view of myth. In particular, I would cite the introduction to Claude Lévi-Strauss, *The Raw and the Cooked* (New York: Harper and Row, 1969), as, for instance, "Mythological analysis has not, and cannot have, as its aim to show how men think. . . . I therefore claim to show, not how men think in myths, but how myths operate in men's minds without their being aware of the fact" (12). Also of interest is the same author's *Structural Anthropology* (New York: Basic Books, 1963), 206–31; and V. I. Propp, *The Morphology of the Folktale*, 2d ed. (Austin: University of Texas Press, 1968).

9.   Price and Twombley, *The Phantom Limb Phenomenon*, 402. Price and Twombley date this version as the oldest of those they reprint, though the manuscript itself (F16, Rome, Biblioteca Vallicelliana) goes back only to the fifteenth century.

10.   For Peter of Grenoble, see Price and Twombley, *The Phantom Limb Phenomenon*, 9–87. The "Life of St. Vaast," whose feast day is 6 February, can be found in the *Golden Legend*, 161–62, and the story of St. Benedict and the infant suffering from elephantiasis appears in the *Golden Legend*, 202, under 21 March.

11.   *Ferramenta* comes from the twelfth-century *Acta Sanctorum* (Price and Twombley, *The Phantom Limb Phenomenon*, 404), and *yrnis scharpe* appears in the *Legends of the Saints in the Scottish Dialect of the Fourteenth Century* (Edinburgh: W. Blackwood and Sons, 1896), 301. Caxton's version of *The Golden Legend* (Price and Twombley, *The Phantom Limb Phenomenon*, 412) speaks of ointments.

12.   *Acta Sanctorum*, Price and Twombley, *The Phantom Limb Phenomenon*, 404.

13.   Price and Twombley, *The Phantom Limb Phenomenon*, 412. From a lengthy Catalan compilation of stories, miracles, and saints' lives, published as *Recull de eximplis e miracles in Biblioteca catalana*, ed. Mariano Aguiló y Fuster (Barcelona:

C. Verdaguer, 1873). The manuscript on which that edition is based dates from the fifteenth century, but the materials themselves appear to be much older.

14. Price and Twombley, *The Phantom Limb Phenomenon*, 406.

15. Originally found in the town of Ditzingen. See Marie-Louise David-Danel, *Inconographie des saints médecins Côme et Damien* (Lille: Morel et Corduant, 1958), 46.

16. On this important reliquary and its connections with local worship, see Anneliese Wittmann, *Kosmas und Damian: Kultausbreitung und Volksdevotion* (Berlin: E. Schmidt, 1967), 192–207; and David-Danel, *Iconographie*, 67–68.

17. On the Corporation of Barber Surgeons of Antwerp, which commissioned this piece for their Confraternity of Cosmas and Damian, see David-Danel, *Iconographie*, 136–39; and J. Pieters, "L'image offrande de la corporation des chirurgiens-barbiers d' Anvers," *Æsculape* 27 (1934): 170–89.

18. This image affords a glimpse into the enormous utility of Cosmas and Damian throughout the Middle Ages and the Renaissance as patrons of medical and charitable institutions. See the excellent treatment of these materials in Wittmann, *Kosmos und Damian*, esp. 133–51; and David-Danel, *Iconographie*, esp. 103–54, 191–206.

19. Paul Ricoeur, *Freud and Philosophy*, trans. Denis Savage (New Haven: Yale University Press, 1970), 18.

20. See J. J. Alexander, "The Provenance of the Brooke Antiphonal," *Antiquaries Journal* 69 (1969): 385–87.

21. Price and Twombley, *The Phantom Limb Phenomenon*, xxxiv.

22. On this quality of self-exhibition, see Réau, *L'iconographie*, 1.416, who speaks of saints' attributes as "a language of signs, a sort of code somewhat analogous to the hieroglyphic alphabet of the Egyptians or to modern rebuses, with this difference that there is nothing secret, cryptographic or esoteric about it and that it aspires on the contrary to be as intelligible as possible."

23. On this piece, of somewhat disputed and/or multiple authorship, see David-Danel, *Iconographie*, 37–38, 46.

24. Price and Twombley, *The Phantom Limb Phenomenon*, xxxiv.

25. Alonso de Sedano's painting was originally housed in the Church of SS. Cosmas and Damian at Burgos. See C. R. Post, *A History of Spanish Painting*, 14 vols. (Cambridge, Mass.: Harvard University Press, 1930–66), 4.1.211.

26. See (from very different perspectives) Edgar de Bruyne, *Corpus mysticum: L'eucharistie et l'eglise au moyen age* (Paris: Aubier, 1949); Piero Camporesi, *The Incorruptible Flesh: Body Mutation and Mortification in Religion and Folklore* (Cambridge: Cambridge University Press, 1988); and Leo Steinberg, *The Sexuality of Christ in Renaissance Art and Modern Oblivion* (New York: Pantheon Books, 1983).

27. Price and Twombley, *The Phantom Limb Phenomenon*, 403.

28. See David-Danel, *Iconographie*, 48–49.

29. See John 20:24–29. Thomas is the only doubter among those apostles who witness the Resurrection, but he is also the only voice in the gospels that directly asserts Christ's divinity, in response to which Jesus says, " 'Because you have seen me you have found faith. Happy are they who never saw me and yet have found faith' " (New English Bible).

30. On this tradition, see the admirable work by Andrea Carlino, *La fabbrica del corpo: Libri e dissezione nel Rinascimento* (Turin: Einaudi, 1994).

31. Greek manuscript, Price and Twombley, *The Phantom Limb Phenomenon*, 402.

32. On the complex questions surrounding this theological subject, see M. J. Harris, "Resurrection and Immortality: Eight Theses," *Themelios* 1 (1976): 50–55; Gisbert Greshake and Jacob Kremer, *Resurrection mortuorum: Zum theologischen Verständnis der leiblichen Auferstehung* (Darmstadt: Wissenschaftliche Buchgesellschaft, 1986); Hermann J. Weber, *Die Lehre von der Auferstehung der Toten in den Haupttraktaten der scholastischen Theologie* (Freiburg: Herder, 1973); Caroline Bynum, "Bodily Miracles and the Resurrection of the Body in the High Middle Ages," in Thomas Kselman, *Belief in History: Innovative Approaches to European and American Religion* (South Bend, Ind.: University of Notre Dame Press, 1991), 68–106; and, particularly important to my own thinking, Caroline Bynum, "Material Continuity, Personal Survival and the Resurrection of the Body: A Scholastic Discussion in its Medieval and Modern Contexts," in her *Fragmentation and Redemption: Essays on Gender and the Human Body in Medieval Religion* (New York: Zone Books, 1991), 239–97.

33. New English Bible, I Corinthians 15:35–51.

34. *Catholic Encyclopedia* (New York: Appleton, 1911), 12:793.

35. See *City of God*, bk. 22, chaps. 12–21. Compare the extensive, if helter-skelter, treatment by Peter Lombard, *Sententiae*, bk. 4, distinctions 43–50; and Aquinas, *Summa contra Gentiles*, bk. 4, chaps. 83–84, both discussed illuminatingly in Bynum, *Fragmentation and Redemption*, 241–43.

36. See especially I Corinthians 11:3–12, where Paul asserts both the secondary status of women and the necessity of both sexes to the communion of Christ.

37. See, for instance, the classic statements in Michel Foucault, *The Order of Things* (New York: Vintage Books, 1973), preface (xv–xxiv) and "Exchanging" (166–214).

38. Judith-Danielle Jacquet, in her very interesting essay on Cosmas and Damian ("Le miracle de la jambe noire," in Jacques Gélis and Odile Redon, eds., *Les miracles, miroirs des corps* [Paris: Presses et publications de l'Université de Paris, 1983], 23–52), offers some powerful arguments about the relations between the blackness of the donor and the medical practices to which his body (as well as that of the recipient) is submitted. Jacquet sees the choice of the Ethiopian as a reference to the practice whereby anatomists were permitted the occasional privilege of dissection if they confined themselves to the corpses of criminals or other marginalized persons. Though that practice long postdates the origins of the story, it may well have helped to give this aspect of the narrative its continuing significance. I am in general much indebted to the provocative arguments of this fine essay.

39. See the essays in L. A. Thompson and J. Ferguson, *Africa in Classical Antiquity* (Ibadan, Nigeria: Ibadan University Press, 1969); see also the invaluable Jean Vercoutter et al., *The Image of the Black in Western Art* (Cambridge, Mass.: Menill Foundation, Inc., 1976), especially, Frank M. Snowden, Jr., "Iconographical

Evidence on the Black Populations in Greco-Roman Antiquity," (vol. 1, 133–245), and Jean Devisse and Michel Mollat, "Africans in the Christian Ordinance of the World," (vol. 2, pt. 2).

40.   From "An Alphabet of Tales" (British Library Additional MS 25,719), an English translation of a late-thirteenth-century compilation probably written by Arnolf of Liège: " 'This day was ther a man of Ynde new berid; and therefor go feche vs of that, at we may fill the hole with.' & this man of Ynd hight Maurus" (Price and Twombley, *The Phantom Limb Phenomenon*, 408). India ("Ynde") is yet another element in the confusion/conflation among exotic places where the inhabitants have dark skin.

41.   See E. Denison Ross, "Prester John and the Empire of Ethiopia," in Arthur Percival Newton, ed., *Travel and Travellers of the Middle Ages* (New York: A. A. Knopf, 1926), 174–94; and Jean-Marie Courtès, "The Theme of 'Ethiopia' and 'Ethiopians' in Patristic Literature," in Vercoutter et al., *The Image of the Black*, 1976, vol. 2, pt. 1, 9–32.

42.   Vasari, in his life of Lorenzo di Bicci, seems to have conflated several generations of the family; it has been difficult to disentangle these attributions ever since (nor does Vasari actually mention the *Cosmas and Damian*). See *Le vite de' più eccellenti pittori scultori ed architettori*, ed., G. Milanesi (Florence: G. C. Sansoni, 1906), 2:49–90.

43.   See David-Danel, *Iconographie*, 48–49.

44.   In regard to such oppositions as these, Devisse and Mollat (in "Africans," in Vercoutter et al., *The Image of the Black*) offer the suggestion that they are more than merely logical or aesthetic; they are also related to the Galenic system of medicine in which one cures by contraries (75). See also their excellent treatment of later Cosmas and Damian iconography, 204–8.

45.   See M. Genevrier, "Un miracle de S. Côme et de S. Damien," *Bulletin de la Société de l'histoire de la médecine* 18 (1923): 16–18.

46.   Greek manuscript, Price and Twombley, *The Phantom Limb Phenomenon*, 403.

47.   Catalan compilation, ibid., 412.

48.   On this tradition, see Rudolf Allers, "Microcosmus: From Anaximander to Paracelsus," *Traditio* 2 (1944): 319–407; Marian Kurdzialek, "Der Mensch als Abbild des Kosmos," *Miscellanea medievalia* 86 (1971): 35–93; and my *Nature's Work of Art: The Human Body as Image of the World* (New Haven, Conn.: Yale University Press, 1975).

49.   Price and Twombley, *The Phantom Limb Phenomenon*, 404.

50.   See David-Danel, *Iconographie*, 45–46.

51.   For the considerable work by Fra Angelico on various materials relating to Cosmas and Damian, see David-Danel, *Iconographie*, 80–101. The principal work is the retable at the Convent of San Marco in Florence with twelve predella scenes from the life of Cosmas and Damian. See William Hood, *Fra Angelico at San Marco* (New Haven, Conn.: Yale University Press, 1993).

52.   See, for instance, Paul Richer, *L'art et la médecine* (Paris, 1901), 396, cited in David-Danel, *Iconographie*, 44.

12 *Renée C. Fox*

Afterthoughts: Continuing Reflections on Organ Transplantation

Personal Statement

In the concluding pages of our book, Spare Parts,[1] *Judith Swazey and I announced our departure from the field of organ replacement after some forty years of intensive involvement in it as firsthand researchers. Our decision to disengage ourselves entailed more than "participant-observer burnout," we said; it was also "a value statement."[2] By our leave-taking, we declared, we were "intentionally separating ourselves from what we believe is an overly zealous medical and societal commitment to the endless perpetuation of life and to repairing and rebuilding people through organ replacement—and from the human suffering and the social, cultural, and spiritual harm we believe such unexamined excess can, and already has, brought in its wake."[3] What we questioned particularly are some of the premises on which organ transplantation in the United States is currently proceeding: the "not-totally rational beliefs that transplantation is an unequivocally and unconditionally good way of sustaining lives, [and] that the more organs proffered, procured, and transplanted the better",[4] the "death is the enemy" to be "overcome" outlook that energizes these medical-surgical acts; and the hubris-ridden unwillingness to recognize and consent to our human finitude that this perspective implies.*

This chapter is an epilogue to that statement. It is a retrospective attempt to examine on a more philosophical and personal level what drew me toward this

sphere of inquiry and engrossed me for so long. In addition, it contains follow-up
observations and reflections on what I regard as the progressive routinization
and profanation of organ transplantation that have been occurring during the
1990s—developments that have reinforced my decision to leave the field, and
my resolve to give moral testimony about what has driven me out of it.

The Sublimity and Tyranny of the Gift

The deepest significance of organ transplantation lies in its gift-exchange
dimensions—in the nature and magnitude of what is given, taken, and
received. The living parts of persons, offered in life or death to known or
unknown others, are implanted in the bodies of individuals who have
reached the end stages of grave illnesses. This corporeal act of giving,
and the surgical process of amputation and transferral through which it
is effected, is carried out for the life-sustaining benefit of others. It is what
philosopher Hans Jonas has termed a "supererogatory" gift, "beyond
duty and claim . . . reckoning and rule."[5] Although such a gift of self
epitomizes one of my highest values, organ transplantation has always
confronted me with the question of how willing and able I would be
to give to strangers as well as intimates in this flesh-of-my-flesh way.
(Since for medical reasons I am eligible to donate only my corneas, I will
never be able to answer this question definitively.)

Some of the phenomena associated with who offers and who is
permitted to be a live donor have continually preoccupied me. For
example, I have given much thought to the biologically deterministic
and circumscribed conception of the family that underlies transplanters'
refusal until recently to consider as live donors anyone other than
parents, children, or siblings of prospective recipients. Is this the most
basic and fullest definition of family? I have doubtingly wondered. The
transplanters' outlook has emanated chiefly from the matching of tissue
and blood-type, which they consider integral to managing the rejection
reaction triggered by the body's "recognition" of "foreign" tissue, and
also by their wariness, on other than biological grounds, about what
might motivate persons who are not members of a prospective recipient's nuclear family of origin to make such a sacrificial gift. Irrespective
of its sources, this is a very narrow notion of kinship and family, one
that I find too psychologically and morally restrictive. The more recent
willingness of the transplant community to expand the notion of familial
relatedness by considering not only spouses and second-degree relatives
but also certain kinlike friends as possible donors is more in keeping
with my own philosophical conceptions of a less biologically defined
and exclusive view of human relationships and connectedness.

I have given much thought, as well, to the fact that cadaveric organ donations go to, and become part of, individuals whom we do not know—strangers, and perhaps even persons who might have been our enemies. This is a supreme expression of the universalistic values and convictions by which I try to lead my life. It is the antithesis of the particularism that I continually try to surmount. The universalism on which it is premised, however, is somewhat qualified by the strong interest that most recipients of cadaver organs and their kin express in knowing what kind of person the donor was and what type of life he or she lived. The needs of recipients and their families to associate such a lifesaving gift with a human image and to express gratitude to a never-encountered other are involved here. But the desire to learn specific details about the donor also derives from recipients' anxiety about the individual and social attributes that may have been transposed into their bodies along with the transplanted organ. On some level below consciousness, recipients experience anthropomorphic concern about whom they have become so closely associated with in this more-than-anatomic way—about the gender, ethnicity, race, religion, education, and social class of the donor, along with his or her moral character and way of life.

One of the most chastening insights that years of contemplating the gift dimensions of organ transplantation have afforded me derives from what Judith Swazey and I have called "the tyranny of the gift."[6] The gift that the recipient receives from the organ donor is so extraordinary that it is intrinsically unreciprocal. It has no physical or symbolic equivalent. As a consequence, the giver, the receiver, and their families may find themselves locked in a creditor-debtor vise that binds them painfully to one another. I was raised by my family to be generous to others, particularly to help those in need, in a Jewish subculture in which giving gifts of money and time, concern and care, was regarded as both a moral obligation and a spiritual blessing.[7] Witnessing firsthand the heavy burden and new forms of suffering that being the recipient of an inherently unrepayable gift of an organ can cause has been a soberly edifying experience for me. It has enabled me to qualify and desentimentalize the goodness of the gift without depreciating or belittling it.

Self and Other

Closely connected with the "theme of the gift" (to use sociologist Marcel Mauss's phrase) are the ways in which thinking about the medical-surgical act of transplanting parts of one person into another has contributed to my reflection on the self, its definition and boundaries, and its relationship to others.[8] Growing up American means that I have been raised in my family, through my education, and by immersion in the cultural tradition of the society to value individualism. In many respects, mine is an old-fashioned individualism, one that emphasizes individual responsibilities as much as individual rights and that opens onto a larger sense of solidarity and community. Even so, this Western- and American-shaped notion of self is much more individuated, bounded, and atomized than the relational sense of self, anchored in kinship, that is integral to the non-Western societies of the world, their cultural outlooks, and their cosmic views. This comparative perspective is more than academic for me. I have experienced it directly as a participant-observer doing sociological research in both Zaire and China. The very different, but mutually relational, definitions of self in these two cultures have challenged me—all the more so as I have come to realize how idiosyncratic the highly individuated Western conception of self is when viewed in a global framework.

The messages that organ transplantation conveys about the individuality of persons, their differences, and their apartness, on the one hand, and about their commonality and connectedness, on the other, are enigmatic. The rejection reaction—"the innate and unrelenting intolerance of individuals to grafts of other people's tissues and organs"[9]—is a strong biological expression of our individual uniqueness and separateness. The language of immunology used to describe this reaction, beginning with the concept of rejection itself, interprets it as the capacity of the body to distinguish between "self" and "not-self." What is more, this "recognition" is depicted as the precursor to aggressive, even violent, actions by the body to rid itself of the "foreign" tissue implanted into it from an alien, threatening not-self. "Killer" cells come into play, combating "helper" cells in trying to rid the body of this menacing tissue. Eventually, even if the transplantation is clinically successful and the immunosuppressive therapy used to prevent a rejection reaction is effective, the transplanted organ or tissue will be rejected, unless it is donated by a genetically identical twin. Such a twin, though not-self, comes as close to replicating self as another can. The current immunological approaches to dealing with the rejection reaction include methods not only to avert, postpone, and moderate this response but also to "trick" the body into defining the implanted tissue as self, or as compatible with it.

In this connection, transplant surgeon Thomas E. Starzl and his colleagues have become progressively convinced that the capacity of the immunosuppressive, antirejection drugs to induce the recipient's body to "tolerate" and retain whole-organ grafts rests on a process of cell migration and systemic *chimerism*. In Greek mythology, the Chimera is a fire-breathing monster with the head of a lion, the body of a goat, and the tail of a serpent. Modern biology has adopted this term to refer to an organism containing tissues from at least two genetically distinct parents. What Starzl and his associates have observed in cases of successful solid organ transplants is that a population of donor cells (leukocytes) from the transplanted organ migrates to and "seeds" other tissues of the recipient's body; simultaneously, a "reverse traffic" of similar recipient cells flows into the graft. Starzl believes that this microchimeric interchange of self and not-self is fundamental to the recipient's long-term "acceptance" of a transplanted organ.[10]

The responses of donors, recipients, and their families to the experience of organ transplantation suggest that, on preconscious and unconscious levels, they feel that something akin to the transfer of psychic and social as well as biological qualities of self to the other has taken place. Partly because of the import of the "gift of life" that has been exchanged, a blurring of boundaries between donors, recipients, and their families often occurs. In a Western (American and European) cultural setting, this blending of self and other can be both uplifting and anxiety provoking. In some cases, for example, a sense of being haunted by those who have given of themselves or their loved one in this way besets recipients; and donor family members often feel a strong need to search for the person in whom a part of their close relative continues to function and to sustain life. The symbolism of the organ that is transplanted plays an important role in this regard. For example, the meaning of the heart in our society and culture is such that donor families and recipients are especially likely to feel that an essence of the donor has been transferred along with the still-beating heart.

In other societies (for instance, in certain Asian and central African countries), the line of demarcation between self and one's family members is less sharply defined than in the United States. Moreover, in these societies a person may view those who are not members of the same family, kinship network, or ethnic group as "unlike us," ritually impure, dangerously alien, or even as "nonpersons." I do not know what kinds of feelings organ transplantation might release in such cultures. Whereas the giving and receiving of organs between related persons who are known to one another might be less threatening to one's sense of self and identity in these societies, the exchange of organs between strangers might be more magico-religiously as well as psychosocially frightening. We have no cross-cultural studies that explore these aspects of transplantation.[11]

What, then, does transplantation metaphorically teach about how absolute or relative, inborn or "man-made," the differences that distinguish us and separate us from one another are? How individuatedly individual are we, and ought we to be? To what extent and in what ways can we break through the barriers between self and others and transmute the otherness of the other without unduly tampering with the integrity and identity of the individual person? The answers to these questions are by no means clear-cut. Organ transplantation has not provided them for me, but it has given me an arena in which I can see these issues about self and other, autonomy and relatedness, particularism and universalism, enacted in a powerfully evocative fashion.

The Entwining of the Scientific and the Nonscientific

As the foregoing suggests, the immunological concepts and vocabulary associated with organ transplantation and the rejection reaction have richly illustrated for me how much more than strictly scientific material is coded into the precepts and the language of modern Western medicine. This would not be a revelatory insight were it not for one of the positivistic assumptions on which our medicine is based, namely, that because it is so highly developed scientifically and technologically it is *not* imprinted with cultural beliefs and values the way traditional and folk medicine systems are. We have a rational tendency to suppose that, although our medicine emanates from our empirical and theoretical knowledge, our techniques, and our mode of thought, it is relatively uninfluenced by our worldview. And yet, underneath its technical veneer, the language of immunology, with its warfare-infused terms concerning the body's battle with disease-bearing microorganisms and with invasive foreign tissue, its neo-individualistic terms about problematic encounters between self and not-self, and its allusions to Greek mythology, vividly expresses ideas about disease, the human body, and the person that are distinctively Western.

Organ transplantation has also uncovered emotionally charged symbolic and anthropomorphic meanings that we attach to our bodies and their parts. What is psychologically and interpersonally involved in receiving the organs of a donor into one's body has brought closer to the surface the qualities of mind, personality, character, spirit, and soul that we identify with our corporeal selves.

Transplantation alone has not converted me to a belief in the existence and import of the symbolic and the unconscious in our lives. Through religion, literature and art, and my training in clinical psychology, psychiatry, anthropology, and sociology, this dimension of reality has long been an acknowledged sphere of my awareness. However, the willingness of donors, recipients, their families, and also transplant physicians and nurses to share their subterranean feelings about organ transplantation with me has reinforced my conviction that scientific and medical progress does not catapult us beyond the reach of those areas of our being where nonlogical perceptions, compelling images, reified symbols, and tenacious myths reside. Quite to the contrary, such progress may even generate new forms of scientifically shaped magic.[12]

Origins and Consequences of How Transplant Physicians Cope

The opportunity to be a participant-observer among transplant physicians has also contributed to my long-standing interest in the shared defenses that medical professionals develop to deal with the emotional demands of their work. In the organ transplantation context—with its high level of uncertainty and risk, its relationship to end-stage disease, its closeness to death, its daring involvement in removing vital organs and transferring them from one human body to another, and its continual wrestling with the rejection reaction—medical professionals (especially transplant surgeons) seem to rely heavily on a particular set of coping mechanisms. These are what Judith Swazey and I have variously described as a "courage to fail," "dare greatly," "climb every mountain," "we shall overcome," "accentuate the positive," "limitless progress," "you've got to believe," and "desperate optimism" outlook.[13] Seen in a Freudian framework, this purview could be characterized as a professionally structured form of collective denial. For the anthropologist Bronislaw Malinowski, it would have exemplified the "ritualization of optimism" that he regarded as an essence of magic.[14] And from a moral and spiritual perspective, it might be considered a professionally rationalized form of hubris. In any case, this profile is a flamboyant version of some basic American values.

Reflecting on transplant surgeons' ways of coming to terms with what their work asks of them has made me more pensive about the double-edged nature of their coping mechanisms and the dilemmas they pose. The same ideology and psychological mechanisms that motivate physicians to transplant human organs, that reinforce their medical and moral rationale for doing so, and that provide them with effective coping strategies make it difficult for them to recognize the harmful, along with the beneficial, concomitants of transplantation and to set limits on their determination to prolong lives through these means. As a consequence, the professional defenses that facilitate their work and enhance the conviction and competence with which they carry it out can contribute to dangerous dauntlessness on their part. Because the "limitless progress" and "we shall overcome" aspects of transplanters' outlook and commitment epitomize highly esteemed American values, they also raise unsettling questions for me about the potential vices that dwell within some of the virtues we societally celebrate.[15]

As organ transplantation has developed over the forty years that I have followed its unfolding, it has become increasingly unrestrained. From transplanting the kidney, the field has grown to encompass the transplantation of virtually every solid organ in the human body other than the brain, and many sorts of tissues and bones as well. A growing number of multiple-organ transplants are being performed. In addition, many physicians seem willing to carry out a boundless series of retransplants on patients who have undergone an initial one. And as the number of patients on transplant waiting lists continues to outweigh the number of organs available for transplant, physicians have been giving serious consideration to expanding the donor pool by using so-called marginal organ donors (persons over the age of fifty and those with certain illnesses) as sources. In my view, this has brought us to the brink of the "totally replaceable body," enunciated by Dr. William J. Kolff, the inventor of the artificial kidney, and of the very thing the late Protestant theologian Paul Ramsey warned against in his commentary on earlier phases of organ transplantation—"our triumphalist temptation to slash and suture our way to eternal life."[16]

The Technical and Moral
Routinization of Organ Transplantation

The transplantation of organs is now frequently described as a common surgical procedure, and it has been performed on more than a hundred thousand patients since the first successful human kidney transplant was carried out in 1954. Many of the surgical and immunological problems by which it was once beset, it is claimed, have been solved or ameliorated. Transplantation is no longer a heroic feat, it is contended, or an extraordinary intervention. Rather, it has taken its place within a repertoire of equally impressive, proven, and efficacious forms of advanced modern therapy.

On the surface, this portrayal of transplantation appears to be a straightforward, objectively accurate statement about the evolution it has undergone over the course of the four decades of its clinical history. But the insistence on the commonplaceness of transplantation deflects attention from its most distinctive and *un*ordinary features: the unparalleled nature of what is still involved when physicians remove the gift of organs entrusted to them from one person's body and place them inside the body and life of another person.

The routinization of transplantation is being pushed close to banalization while awed respect for what is offered and taken, given and received, and accepted and rejected through this medical-surgical act is progressively eroded.

Does the physician have the moral right to accept from a healthy individual who desires to amputate a vital portion of his body, such a gift, so as to prevent the death of one of his fellow men? Does the surgeon have the right to remove a liver, a heart, a kidney from a cadaver in order to practice what Elkinton has termed "cannibalizing," in reminiscence of the wartime art of recreating new cars with spare parts obtained from two useless vehicles? . . . The very individuals who, not without hesitation, have committed themselves to the adventure of renal transplantation in man are the first to admit how difficult it is to be certain that one is following the proper road in this regard.[17]

This is what physicians Jean Hamburger and Jean Crosnier, pioneers in the field of organ transplantation, wrote in the mid-1960s about the "moral and ethical" concomitants of "these amazing new developments in medical science." The passage of time, increased clinical experience, and further medical and surgical progress, it would seem, have diminished physicians' astonishment and marvel about organ transplantation, resolved their questions about its justification, and quenched their moral anxiety about "how far and how fast to venture on the transplant voyage."[18]

Gone, for example, is the moral frisson that the implications of organ transplantation once elicited in the medical community—the mixture of "wonder and dread"[19] that it evoked throughout the 1950s and 1960s. No longer do we hear or read statements like these: "In rejecting the conception of man's isolation, John Donne was more prophetic than he realized. The collective ownership of human spare parts should prove that man is indeed 'involved in mankind'—to the literal extent of hearts and kidneys and livers . . . in an awesome immortality of tissues. . . . these tissues merit the careful scrutiny of all prospective participants in the life-diminishing, death-denying process of transplantation."[20]

During the 1950s and 1960s, and in the first half of the 1970s as well, transplant surgeons and physicians, and the jurists, theologians, and philosophers with whom they conferred about "the social and moral problems raised by the use of borrowed organs," were intensely aware of the unique nature, in all the history of medicine, of what transplantation entailed.[21] Concern focused especially on live kidney transplants and the harm to which the surgeon deliberately subjected the healthy donor, who was usually a close, tissue-matched relative of the severely ill recipient. They described it as "the invasion," "injuring," and "maiming" of a person's body in a "major surgical operation" that involved the removal of a vital organ "for the good of somebody else." Was it or was it not "covered by the principle of totality," they worriedly discussed, "whereby a part of the body may be sacrificed to the good of the whole"? Might organ donation be justified on the grounds that "a spiritual good is better for an individual than a material good, and even though the donor has lost something materially he has gained something spiritually which is greater?" For ideally, they agreed, not only was the action of the donor "extremely meritorious"; it also "transcend[ed] any moral system of rights and duties."[22]

When they adopted new, brain-oriented criteria for pronouncing death that would facilitate the use of organs from cadaveric donors, transplanters of this era agonized over what death was, as well as when it occurred; over the relationship between cellular, physiological, intellectual, social, and spiritual death (and life); over the fact that no matter what criteria are used, the precise moment of human death can only be approximated; over the "live cadaver" status of the person declared dead whose heartbeat continues; and over removing organs from individuals in this twilight zone between life and death.[23]

From the time that the first human organ transplants were performed in the 1950s, and all during the 1960s and 1970s, transplant groups treated the "give and take"[24] of exchanging organs as such an extraordinary gift of life that, in certain respects, it was likely to be as "strange"[25] and stressful an experience for donors, recipients, their families, and members of the medical team as it was lifesaving and ennobling. Transplant teams clinically observed and actively grappled with the "gift-exchange dimensions" of organ transplantation: its more-than-biomedical meaning, and the psychic and social effects of the symbolic power of giving and receiving an organ.[26] They were concerned about what truly motivated living organ donors to give of themselves in this way ("Does such willingness to be a donor reflect psychopathology, or could it reflect healthy altruism derived from general moral concern?"),[27] and about the undue emotional and familial pressure to which potential live, related donors might be subject. They were also troubled by how both cadaveric and live transplantations could enmesh donors, recipients, and their kin in relationships that were painfully complicated by the creditor-debtor aspects of this unrepayable gift of life, and by the animistic feelings that were evoked about some of the psychic and social qualities of the donor being transferred along with the organ into the body and being of the recipient.

Not only did transplanters discuss among themselves these phenomena that "in some respects [they considered] unique to the transplant situation";[28] they also took active steps to help donors, recipients, and their families deal with them, often with the consultant help of psychiatrists and psychiatrically trained medical social workers. Out of these practitioners' firsthand clinical experiences, interventions, and study, a rich literature describing and analyzing the impact of organ transplants on donors, recipients, their families, and their medical caretakers developed. These writings were published during the 1960s and 1970s in journals like *Seminars in Psychiatry*, the *American Journal of Psychiatry*, the *British Journal of Psychiatry*, the *Journal of the American Medical Association*, and the *New England Journal of Medicine*.[29] But since then, such articles rarely appear in the literature; psychiatrists and social workers play a more peripheral role on transplant teams; and little mention is made of the distinctive experiences, reactions, and problems of transplant donors, recipients, and their families that arise from the significance of what is given and received in the process of organ transplantation.[30]

Does all this simply mean that, because, over time, transplantation has been done more proficiently and has become a more common procedure, involving a much larger number and range of donors, recipients, organs, medical teams, and hospitals than in earlier phases of its development, it has become "but another example of the instrumental approach to disease and illness that characterizes our highly technological medical care system"?[31] Or is something occurring that is potentially more ominous than such institutionalization and routinization of organ transplantation? Certain events that have taken place in the transplant field during the first years of the 1900s incline me toward the latter view. The combined impact of the expansion of transplantation, the ardor that has fostered this expansion, the shortage of donated organs that is felt to exist, and the sense of urgency about alleviating the shortage seem to me to be leading to the profanation of the meaning of giving, taking, and receiving human organs, and of the reverent respect for the dignity of human life and death that ought to undergird these acts.

Indicators of the Profanation of Organ Transplantation

What I regard as profanation is observable, for example, in the movement away from the conception of human organ transplantation as a gift of life, the movement toward the commodification of organs that is taking place, and the reduction of the body to "only a thing-in-theworld"[32] that this commodification implies.

"Regulated Commercialism of Vital Organ Donation: A Necessity?"—
one of the plenary sessions at the Fourteenth International Congress of
the Transplantation Society held in Paris in August 1992—demonstrated
how much serious interest in this option currently exists in transplant
milieux. It also laid bare the narrowly materialistic character of assumptions about the human body, our existence within it, and our willingness
to give of its parts on which such a commercialized view of organ transplantation is premised. Jurist Lloyd Cohen was invited to present the
"pro" position at this session on the creation of a "futures market" that
would give healthy individuals a chance to contract for the sale of their
organs for transplantation, to be retrieved, delivered, and utilized after
their death.[33] Cohen based his argument on his strongly held conviction
(what he termed a "moral canon") that people's bodies are their own
"private property," which they have the right to dispose of as they see
fit. He acknowledged that in life the body incarnates "the human spirit,"
and that in death it should not be "treated as mere carrion"—that some
"symbolic recognition of the sanctity of the human body" should be
maintained. But he contended that what he variously termed religious,
ethical, aesthetic, and psychological "barriers" to organ donation that
are associated with a view of the human body as "so precious and sacred
a thing" are "not very powerful." Nor, he claimed, was "the uneasiness
generated over organ transplantation . . . operationally [different] from
a host of other activities in which people engage despite deep-seated
antipathies to the contrary." Those who are reluctant to donate organs,
he stated, feel this way primarily because they are being asked to assume "the psychic costs [of their "aversions"] without being offered
a sufficient compensating benefit." Thus, he concluded, "the simplest,
most direct, most efficient, and least expensive way to induce them [to
donate their organs] is to pay them" through the mechanism of a futures
market in cadaveric organs.[34]

I am not suggesting that Lloyd Cohen's perspective represented the
majority opinion of the members of the Transplantation Society who
were assembled. I was given equal time on the program to present
the "con" position on financial compensation for organ donation.[35] But
the fact remains that the economically deterministic, utilitarian, profit-
oriented, desacralized outlook on the human body and psyche, and the
meaning of life and death on which Cohen's advocacy of an organs
futures market rests, was accorded a respectful hearing by the Grand
Auditorium audience of transplanters.

If this presentation were a singular occurrence, it would have ephem-
eral significance. What gives it import, however, is its relationship
to the morally questionable features of the protocols and policies for

obtaining organs from so-called non-heart-beating cadaver donors that an increasing number of transplant groups, medical centers, and organ procurement organizations in the United States are in the process of developing or are already implementing.[36] In their determination to increase the number of donated organs, they are reintroducing the traditional cardiopulmonary criteria used to pronounce death during the early years of solid organ transplants, until the concept of brain death and criteria for it were established over the course of the 1970s and 1980s, and "heart-beating cadaver donors" became the norm. To date, two non-heart-beating cadaver donor protocols have received the most attention: the one devised and elaborated by the University of Pittsburgh Medical Center and the other originating from the Regional Organ Bank of Illinois.

The University of Pittsburgh's primary interest is focused on patients from whom viable organs might be procured and who die according to cardiopulmonary criteria because they or their families have decided that life-support measures should be withdrawn and resuscitative efforts forgone.[37] Under its protocol, after the decision has been reached to withdraw life-sustaining therapy from a potential non-heart-beating donor, he or she is sped to the operating room, where, to keep warm ischemic time to a minimum, surgical skin preparations and sterile draping for organ procurement take place, and a femoral arterial line is inserted in the patient's body. The prospective donor-patient receives comfort medication but only for demonstrated need. Despite the fact that the patient has been put on "comfort measures only," the protocol allows (with family consent) for him or her to be returned to "full-code status" during the time leading up to the procurement of organs. This means that the patient may be subjected to invasive, potentially distressing and harmful procedures in order to "save" the organs to be removed for donation. Death is pronounced by cardiopulmonary criteria after a mere two minutes' duration of electrocardiographic indicators (ventricular fibrillation, electrical asystole, or electromechanical dissociation) instead of the six to seven minutes that physicians usually observe in other medical centers under nontransplantation circumstances. Immediately after the certification of death, the removal of vital organs proceeds. Totally isolated from his or her family, the patient dies a "desolate, . . . 'high tech' death" in a surgical suite, "beneath operating room lights, amidst masked, gowned, and gloved strangers," who have previously readied his or her body for "eviscerating surgery," that may have begun when he or she was only equivocally dead.[38]

The kind of "death by protocol"[39] that is involved here goes beyond the trivialization and commodification of what is sacred about the human body and the life and death within it that Lloyd Cohen's proposal for a futures market in transplantable organs implies. In my view, the conditions of death that the Pittsburgh protocol requires are not only undignified. They are also indecent in a way that brings them close to the foreboding image once invoked by theologian Paul Ramsey: the reduction of persons to "an ensemble of . . . interchangeable . . . spare parts" in which "everyone [becomes] a useful precadaver."[40]

In their account of the history of the University of Pittsburgh Medical Center's policy of non-heart-beating organ donation, Michael A. DeVita and James V. Snyder state that more that a hundred individuals participated in its development, which took place over a four-year period of time.[41] However searching the discussion of "psychological, political, practical and ethical concerns" about this policy may have been before it was "approved according to university and hospital procedures,"[42] and whatever reservations and objections may have been expressed about it in the process, the fact remains that it was ratified and put into motion, seemingly without collective insight into what was inherently wrong about asking patients and their families to accept such a way of dying.

Since the publication of this article, the Pittsburgh protocol has been revised to make it possible for a prospective donor's family to stay with the patient in a nonsurgical setting until death is pronounced, if they wish to do so. This modification in procedure resulted from the medical center's experience with a family that was strongly committed to having their relative become a non-heart-beating organ donor, but who insisted on remaining with the patient until death occurred, as a precondition. In a recent article, DeVita, Snyder, and their coauthors report, "After careful discussion, we moved the patient to a quiet area near the OR [operating room] and allowed the family to remain at the bedside until after death was pronounced. The patient was then brought to the waiting OR."[43] It was because of what was deemed to be "this favorable experience," which was not unduly "stressful" for the family or the team of health care professionals involved, that the protocol was changed. What is disquieting about the Pittsburgh group's decision is that it grew more out of their post hoc, pragmatic realization that they could make these changes and still obtain the organs they sought, than from their discernment of what might have been morally wrong with the way they had previously organized the patient-donor's death.

The Regional Organ Bank of Illinois (ROBI) protocol is even more troubling, because of its disregard for the principle of informed consent and because of the deceitful strategy that was used in the effort to have it adopted by the Loyola University Medical Center of Chicago. The ROBI protocol sets forth a research plan to study the feasibility of transplanting kidneys from recently deceased non-heart-beating patients who die in the emergency room or shortly before arriving there. It entails attempting to preserve their kidneys inside their bodies by inserting catheters into their femoral and arterial systems and perfusing their organs with cold preservative solutions. The protocol was introduced to Loyola's institutional review board (IRB) by a trauma surgeon on the medical center's staff who agreed to act as its principal investigator. There were intimations that ROBI was interested in beginning to perfuse the kidneys in the deceased person's body while still in the process of locating the nearest of kin and getting their permission to remove the organs for transplantation. After considerable discussion, the Loyola IRB decided to approve the study, but only under conditions of prospective informed consent by the family for starting the procedure to preserve the kidneys as well as to use them for transplantation.

Subsequently, on 21 June 1993, a newspaper article was published in the *Chicago Tribune* suggesting that, under what was referred to as the Loyola rather than the ROBI protocol, the organ preservation procedure was being performed without family consent. Loyola's IRB acted swiftly and aggressively to inquire into the matter, immediately contacting the primary investigators and asking them for an explanation. To their consternation, the IRB discovered that, in fact, the protocol being used was not the one they had approved. What had been substituted for it was a changed version drafted by ROBI that made it unnecessary to have family consent to initiate cold perfusion of the kidneys or to tell the deceased person's relatives that this procedure had been done if they did not agree to organ donation. The IRB was outraged; lawyers were consulted; a cease-and-desist letter was sent by legal counsel to the investigators and ROBI; and this experiment with non-heart-beating organ donation was terminated at Loyola (after nine pairs of kidneys had been procured in this way).

In September 1993, at a meeting of the Society for Bioethics Consultation, a member of the Loyola IRB learned from two physicians who are nationally involved in ethical debates about organ transplantation that ROBI had distributed to persons around the country a packet of material containing their research protocol to initiate preservation of organs in non-heart-beating donors without obtaining family permission, accompanied by a letter from the chair of Loyola's IRB indicating conditional approval of it. The chair's letter had *not* been written in response to the protocol included in the packet. Rather, it concerned the protocol that the Loyola IRB had ratified, which required family consent. The material that ROBI had circulated suggested otherwise. The IRB member quickly contacted the IRB chair; legal counsel was consulted once more, along with Loyola's associate dean of research; and a letter was sent by the

Loyola lawyers to the director of operations of ROBI requesting that all persons and institutions to whom the packet had been circulated be informed of ROBI's "error." It was not until April 1994 that Loyola's legal counsel received a copy of *The Bridge*, a magazine published by ROBI four times a year "for [its] employees, staff and friends," which included perfunctory mention of the fact that "a document showing IRB approval from Loyola University Medical Center was mistakenly included" in the information "about the non-heart-beating study here at ROBI" that had been sent out. "This letter related to an earlier proposal we had submitted," the notice stated. "We regret the error and any confusion or embarrassment it may have caused."[44]

The "story" of the ROBI protocol dramatically and disturbingly illustrates how an evangelical attitude toward transplantation, combined with zealotry about procuring organs and unwillingness to accept limits, can result in grave violations of the moral practice of medicine and medical research, in ways that desecrate the bodies and deaths of patients, disregard the rights and needs of patients' families, and undermine the collegial trust and integrity of relations between health professionals. The Loyola episode was further complicated by the guile of the regional organ procurement organization involved (ROBI) and its seeming willingness to use any means to fulfill its sense of mission about obtaining organs for transplantation. In the end, the social control mechanisms operating inside Loyola worked well enough to call a halt to the inadvertent misconduct into which the medical center had been drawn. The action they took was carried out quietly and with restraint. Thus far, no serious punitive sanctions have been leveled against the Loyola physicians who used the ROBI protocol without informing the IRB.

Especially when viewed in historical perspective, some of the concomitants of the current drive to obtain organs from non-heart-beating donors and of the movement to "de-gift" the donation of organs and recast it in a market framework point to what I regard as the very slippery slope down which transplantation has begun to slide as a consequence of the routinization, the fervor, and the frantic search for organs that now characterize it.[45]

I end here, as I began—with gratitude for all that observing and reflecting upon organ transplantation have taught me over the years and with mounting concern about the medical, moral, and spiritual profanation that I see it undergoing.

Notes

1. Renée C. Fox and Judith P. Swazey, *Spare Parts: Organ Replacement in American Society* (New York: Oxford University Press, 1992), 197–210.

2. Ibid., 199.
3. Ibid., 210.
4. Renée C. Fox, "Regulated Commercialism of Vital Organ Donation: A Necessity? Con," *Transplantation Proceedings* 25, no. 1 (February 1993): 55.
5. Hans Jonas, "Philosophical Reflections on Experimenting with Subjects," in Paul A. Freund, ed., *Experimentation with Human Subjects* (New York: George Braziller, 1970), 16.
6. See especially Renée C. Fox, "Organ Transplantation: Sociocultural Aspects," in Warren T. Reich, ed., *Encyclopedia of Bioethics*, vol. 3 (New York: Free Press, 1978), 168–69; Renée C. Fox and Judith P. Swazey, *The Courage to Fail: A Social View of Organ Transplantation and Dialysis* (Chicago: University of Chicago Press, 1974), 20–32, 133; Renée C. Fox and Judith P. Swazey, *The Courage to Fail: A Social View of Organ Transplants and Dialysis*, 2d ed. rev. (Chicago: University of Chicago Press, 1978), 812–13; Renée C. Fox, Judith P. Swazey, and Elizabeth M. Cameron, "Social and Ethical Problems in the Treatment of End-Stage Renal Disease Patients," in Robert G. Narins, ed., *Controversies in Nephrology and Hypertension* (New York: Churchill Livingstone, 1984), 56–57; Fox and Swazey, *Spare Parts*, 39–42. For additional conceptual and substantive insights into the gift-exchange dynamics of transplantation (with specific reference to blood), see Thomas H. Murray, "Gifts of the Body and the Needs of Strangers," *Hastings Center Report* 328 (April 1987): 30–38.
7. For a discussion of the concepts in Jewish religious and moral tradition underlying this aspect of my upbringing, see the chapter in this volume by Elliot N. Dorff.
8. Marcel Mauss, *The Gift: Forms and Functions of Exchange in Archaic Societies*, trans. Ian Cunnison (Glencoe, Ill.: Free Press, 1954), 66.
9. R. E. Billingham, "Basic Genetical and Immunological Considerations," in *Symposium on Organ Transplantation in Man, Proceedings of the National Academy of Sciences, U.S.A.*, vol. 63 (Washington, D.C.: National Academy of Sciences, 1969), 1020.
10. See Thomas E. Starzl, Anthony J. Demetris, Noriko Murase, Suzanne Ildstad, Camillo Ricordi, and Massimo Trucco, "Cell Migration, Chimerism, and Graft Acceptance," *Lancet* 339 (27 June 1992): 1579–82; Thomas E. Starzl, Anthony J. Demetris, Massimo Trucco, Camillo Ricordi, Suzanne Ildstad, Paul I. Terasaki, Noriko Murase, Ross S. Kendall, Mirjana Kocova, William A. Rudert, Adriana Zeevi, and David Van Thiel, "Chimerism after Liver Transplantation for Type IV Glycogen Storage Disease and Type I Gaucher's Disease," *New England Journal of Medicine* 328 (18 March 1993): 745–49; Thomas E. Starzl, Anthony J. Demetris, Massimo Trucco, Adriana Zeevi, Hector Ramos, Paul Terasaki, William A. Rudert, Mirjana Kocova, Camillo Ricordi, Suzanne Ildstad, and Noriko Murase, "Chimerism and Donor-specific Non-reactivity 27 to 29 Years after Kidney Allotransplantation," *Transplantation* 55, no. 6 (June 1993): 1272–77; Thomas E. Starzl, Anthony J. Demetris, Massimo Trucco, Noriko Murase, Camillo Ricordi, Suzanne Ildstad, Hector Ramos, Satoru Todo, Andreas Tzakis, John J. Fung, Michael Nalesnik, Adriana Zeevi, William A. Rudert, and Mirjana Kocova, "Cell Migration and Chimerism after Whole-Organ Trans-

plantation: The Basis of Graft Acceptance," *Hepatology* 17 (June 1993): 1127–52; Thomas E. Starzl, Anthony J. Demetris, Noriko Murase, Angus W. Thomson, Massimo Trucco, and Camillo Ricordi, "Donor Cell Chimerism Permitted by Immunosuppressive Drugs: A New View of Organ Transplantation," *Immunology Today* 14, no. 6 (June 1993): 326–32.

11. In her chapter in this volume, Wendy Doniger sets forth some interesting speculative ideas about the implications of the Hindu doctrine of karma—especially beliefs about karmic links and transfers between people's bodies and souls—for attitudes toward organ transplantation.

12. I refer here to "scientific magic," a concept that I coined to refer to essentially magical ways of thinking and acting that simulate medical-scientific attitudes and behaviors or lie burrowed within them, and that help physicians engaged in practice and in research to face problems of uncertainty, limitation, and meaning by "ritualizing [their] optimism," as anthropologist Bronislaw Malinowski would have put it. See Renée C. Fox, *The Human Condition of Health Professionals* (pamphlet), Distinguished Lecturer Series, School of Health Studies (Durham: University of New Hampshire, 1980), 26; Renée C. Fox, "The Sociology of Medical Research," in Charles Leslie, ed., *Asian Medical Systems: A Comparative Study* (Berkeley: University of California Press, 1976), 106–7; Renée C. Fox, *The Sociology of Medicine: A Participant Observer's View* (Englewood Cliffs, N.J.: Prentice-Hall, 1989), 194–98.

13. See especially Fox and Swazey, *Courage to Fail*, 109–21 (chap. 5: "A Sociological Portrait of the Transplant Surgeon"); and Fox and Swazey, *Spare Parts*, 154–69 (chap. 6: " 'Made in the U.S.A.': American Features in the Rise and Fall of the Jarvik-7 Artificial Heart").

14. Bronislaw Malinowski, *Magic, Science, and Religion, and Other Essays* (Glencoe, Ill.: Free Press, 1948), 70.

15. See transplant surgeon Barry D. Kahan's chapter in this volume for observations on what he considers to be some of the undesirable side effects this outlook has had on the field of transplantation.

16. Paul Ramsey, *The Patient as Person: Explorations in Medical Ethics* (New Haven, Conn.: Yale University Press, 1970), 238.

17. Jean Hamburger and Jean Crosnier, "Moral and Ethical Problems in Transplantation," in Felix T. Rappaport and Jean Dausset, eds., *Human Transplantation* (New York: Grune and Stratton, 1968), 37. The citation of Elkinton's concept of cannibalizing refers to an editorial titled "Moral Problems in the Use of Borrowed Organs, Artificial and Transplanted" that J. R. Elkinton wrote in *Annals of Internal Medicine* 60, no. 2 (February 1964), 309–13, of which he was then editor, and that he signed J.R.E.

18. Francis D. Moore, *Give and Take: The Development of Tissue Transplantation* (Philadelphia and London: W. B. Saunders, 1964), 165. (The quoted phrase in the text is the subtitle of chap. 11, "The Doctor's Dilemma," 165–70.)

19. David Daube, "Transplantation: Acceptability of Procedures and the Required Legal Sanctions," in G. E. W. Wolstenholme and Maeve O'Connor, eds., *Ethics in Medical Progress: With Special Reference to Transplantation* (Boston: Little, Brown, 1966), 200.

20. " 'Any Man's Death Diminishes Me' " (unsigned editorial), *New England Journal of Medicine* 278, no. 26 (27 June 1968): 1455.

21. Elkinton, "Moral Problems in the Use of Borrowed Organs, Artificial and Transplanted," 313.

22. Francis D. Moore, "Medical Responsibility for the Prolongation of Life," *Journal of the American Medical Association* 206, no. 2 (7 October 1968): 385; G. B. Bentley, discussion of R. Cortesini's "Outlines of a Legislation on Transplantation," in Wolstenholme and O'Connor, eds., *Ethics in Medical Progress*, 185; and G. B. Bentley and Joseph E. Murray, quoted in the final discussion of David Daube's "Transplantation: Acceptability of Procedures and the Required Legal Sanctions," in Wolstenholme and O'Connor, eds., *Ethics in Medical Progress*, 207–8.

23. Henry K. Beecher, "Ethical Problems Created by the Hopelessly Unconscious Patient" (special article), *New England Journal of Medicine* 278, no. 26 (27 June 1968): 1429; David W. Louisell, "Transplantation: Existing Legal Constraints," and discussion, in Wolstenholme and O'Connor, eds., *Ethics in Medical Progress*, 78–103.

24. Moore, "Medical Responsibility for the Prolongation of Life," 385–86.

25. John P. Kemph, "Psychotherapy with Donors and Recipients of Kidney Transplants," *Seminars in Psychiatry* 3, no. 1 (February 1971): 158.

26. John P. Kemph, "Renal Failure, Artificial Kidney and Kidney Transplant," *American Journal of Psychiatry* 122 (1966): 1270–74; W. A. Crammond, "Renal Homotransplantation—Some Observations on Recipients and Donors," *British Journal of Psychiatry* 113 (1967): 1223–30.

27. Harry S. Abram, "Psychological Dilemmas of Medical Progress," *Psychiatry in Medicine* 3 (1972): 55. Here, Abram refers to the way that this question is raised in Carl H. Fellner and Shalom H. Schwartz, "Altruism in Disrepute: Medical Versus Public Attitudes toward the Living Organ Donor" (special article), *New England Journal of Medicine* 284, no. 11 (18 March 1971): 582–85.

28. Donald T. Lunde, "Psychiatric Complications of Heart Transplants," *American Journal of Psychiatry* 126, no. 3 (September 1969): 373.

29. For a representative cross-section of these articles, see the references in Fox and Swazey, "Gift Exchange and Gate Keeping," chap. 1 of *Courage to Fail*, 5–39.

30. In contradistinction to this pattern, Stuart J. Youngner's chapter in this volume draws on his in-depth psychiatric interviews with patients waiting for transplants and with transplant recipients.

31. John A. Robertson, "Medical Excesses" (review of *Spare Parts* by Renée C. Fox and Judith P. Swazey), *Science* 259, no. 5091 (1 January 1993): 111.

32. This is theologian Paul Ramsey's concept. See Ramsey, *Patient as Person*, 209.

33. Lloyd Cohen's presentation, "A Futures Market in Cadaveric Organs: Would It Work?" delivered on 19 August 1992 at the "Controversies" plenary session was subsequently published in *Transplantation Proceedings* 25, no. 1 (February 1993): 60–61. I have not only drawn from his presentation but also

consulted a much longer law review article that he wrote on the same subject. See Lloyd R. Cohen, "Increasing the Supply of Transplant Organs: The Virtues of a Futures Market," *George Washington Law Review* 58, no. 1 (November 1989): 1–51.

34. For a more extensive discussion of Lloyd Cohen's notion of a futures market in transplantable organs and the assumptions underlying it, see the chapter by Thomas H. Murray in this volume.

35. My presentation was published as "Regulated Commercialism of Vital Organ Donation: A Necessity? Con," *Transplantation Proceedings* 25, no. 1 (February 1993): 55–57.

36. United Network for Organ Sharing, "Non-Heartbeating Donation on the Rise: Transplant Community Turning to Original Source of Organs to Meet Demand," *UNOS Update* 10 (November 1994): 3–5. According to the United Network for Organ Sharing survey data presented in this article, 20 of the 66 active organ procurement organizations (OPOs) in the United States in 1994 (30 percent) had policies on the use of non-heart-beating donors, and another 10 were developing them; 25 OPOs (42 percent) had procured organs from this type of donor; and 23 OPOs had transplanted non-heart-beating donor organs.

37. The University of Pittsburgh Medical Center protocol is reprinted in *Kennedy Institute of Ethics Journal* 3, no. 2 (June 1993): A-1–A-15, a special issue called "Ethical, Psychosocial, and Public Policy Implications of Procuring Organs from Non-Heart-Beating Cadavers." Its guest editors are Robert M. Arnold and Stuart J. Youngner. See also the article with the same title that Youngner and Arnold wrote for the Working Group on Ethical, Psychosocial, and Public Policy Implications of Procuring Organs from Non-Heart-Beating Cadaver Donors, published in the *Journal of the American Medical Association* 269, no. 21 (2 June 1993): 2769–74. This article draws on the papers presented at a conference that examined the University of Pittsburgh Medical Center's policy on procuring organs after death from patients who choose to forgo life-sustaining treatment, with special emphasis on the broad range of issues raised by the Pittsburgh protocol for the renewed use of non-heart-beating cadaver donors. Some of these papers were subsequently published in the June 1993 issue of the *Kennedy Institute of Ethics Journal*.

38. Renée C. Fox, " 'An Ignoble Form of Cannibalism': Reflections on the University of Pittsburgh Medical Center Protocol for Procuring Organs from Non-Heart-Beating Cadavers," *Kennedy Institute of Ethics Journal* 3, no. 2 (June 1993): 231–39.

39. I am indebted to Albert Yan, M.D., for this insightful image.

40. Paul Ramsey, *The Patient as Person: Explorations in Medical Ethics* (New Haven, Conn.: Yale University Press, 1970), 208–9.

41. Michael A. DeVita and James V. Snyder, "Development of the University of Pittsburgh Medical Center Policy for the Care of Terminally Ill Patients Who May Become Organ Donors after Death Following the Removal of Life Support," *Kennedy Institute of Ethics Journal* 3, no. 2 (June 1993): 141.

42. Ibid.

43.   Michael A. DeVita, Rade Vukmir, James V. Snyder, and Cheryl Graziano, "Non-Heart-Beating Organ Donation: A Reply to Campbell and Weber," *Kennedy Institute of Ethics Journal* 5, no. 1 (March 1995): 43–49, quotation from p. 47.

44.   The foregoing account of the development and content of the ROBI protocol for non-heart-beating organ donation and the way that the Loyola University Medical Center of Chicago became involved in its implementation is largely based on personal communications from anthropologist and bioethicist Patricia Marshall, who is a member of Loyola's institutional review board, and physician Ken Micetich, who is the chair of that IRB. I am very grateful to them for their generosity and candor in telling me about these events and for their willingness to let me recount these happenings in this chapter.

45.   In her chapter in this volume, Ruth Richardson draws disquieting parallels between some of the methods currently being used or proposed to deal with the problem of the shortage of organs for transplantation and the morally dubious means through which human corpses were obtained for dissection in the United Kingdom during the sixteenth, seventeenth, eighteenth, and early nineteenth centuries.

Contributors
Index

Contributors

LEONARD BARKAN, Ph.D., is the Samuel Rudin University Professor of the Humanities at New York University, where he teaches English and fine arts. He is the author of *Nature's Work of Art: The Human Body as Image of the World* (1975), *The Gods Made Flesh: Metamorphosis and the Pursuit of Paganism* (for which he won the Christian Gauss Prize for 1986), and *Transuming Passion: Ganymede and the Erotics of Humanism* (1991).

WENDY DONIGER (formerly Wendy Doniger O'Flaherty), Ph.D., D. Phil., is the Mircea Eliade Professor of the History of Religions at the University of Chicago. She has completed two doctorates in Sanskrit and Indian Studies (from Harvard and Oxford). She currently serves on the international editorial board of the *Encyclopaedia Britannica* and on the board of *Daedalus*.

Among her many books are *Hindu Myths: A Sourcebook*, translated from the Sanskrit, 1975; *The Rig Veda: An Anthology, 108 Hymns Translated from the Sanskrit*, 1981; *The Laws of Manu*, 1991 (with Brian K. Smith); *Women, Androgynes, and Other Mythical Beasts*, 1980; *Mythologies*, an English-language edition of Yves Bonnefoy's thirteen hundred–page *Dictionnaire des mythologies*, 1991; and *Other Peoples' Myths: The Cave of Echoes*, 1988.

ELLIOT N. DORFF, M.H.L., Ph.D., is the rector and the Sol and Anne Dorff Professor of Philosophy at the University of Judaism, Los Angeles, California. He was ordained a Conservative rabbi by the Jewish Theological Seminary of

America in 1970 and earned his Ph.D. in philosophy from Columbia University in 1971.

Dorff is a member of the Conservative movement's Committee on Jewish Law and Standards, and its commission to write a new Torah commentary. His papers, written in 1991 and 1992, formulated what came to be the validated stance of the Conservative movement on end-of-life issues and on human sexuality. He currently serves as chair of the Academy of Jewish Philosophy and the Jewish Law Association. In the spring of 1993 he served on the ethics working group of the President's Task Force on National Health Care Reform in Washington, D.C.

Dorff has published some sixty articles on Jewish thought, law, and ethics, together with five books: *Jewish Law and Modern Ideology; Conservative Judaism: Our Ancestors to Our Descendants; A Living Tree: The Roots and Growth of Jewish Law; Mitzvah Means Commandment;* and *Knowing God: Jewish Journeys to the Unknowable.*

LESLIE A. FIEDLER, Ph.D., is the Samuel Clemens Professor and a SUNY Distinguished Professor of English at the State University of New York, Buffalo. His two major studies of American fiction, *An End to Innocence: Essays on Culture and Politics* (1955) and *Love and Death in the American Novel* (1960), assert that racism, repressed homosexual emotion, and misogyny are primary influences in American art and life. His literary study *Freaks: Myths and Images of the Secret Self* (1978) explains how grotesque deformity can become the norm and ideal in literature. *What Was Literature? Class Culture and Mass Society* (1982) advances the argument that great writing comes not from a cultural elite but out of popular culture.

RENÉE C. FOX, Ph.D., is the Annenberg Professor of the Social Sciences at the University of Pennsylvania, Philadelphia, where she is a professor of sociology with joint appointments in the Department of Sociology, the Department of Psychiatry, the Department of Medicine, and the School of Nursing.

Fox's major teaching and research interests—sociology of medicine, medical research, medical education, and medical ethics—have involved her in first-hand studies in continental Europe (particularly in Belgium), in Central Africa (especially Zaire), and in the People's Republic of China, as well as in the United States.

Fox is the author of seven books, among them *Experiment Perilous: Physicians and Patients Facing the Unknown; The Courage to Fail: A Social View of Organ Transplants and Dialysis* (with Judith P. Swazey); *Essays in Medical Sociology: Journeys into the Field; Spare Parts: Organ Replacement in American Society* (with Judith P. Swazey); and *In the Belgian Château: The Spirit and Culture of a European Society in an Age of Change.*

BARRY D. KAHAN, Ph.D., M.D., is a professor of surgery and the director of the Division of Immunology and Organ Transplantation at the University of Texas Medical School at Houston; the chief surgeon of renal transplantation at Hermann Hospital, Houston, Texas; and the director of the Hermann Organ Transplant Center. He has served as president of the American Society of Transplant Surgeons, treasurer of the International Transplantation Society, and treasurer of the International Society for Organ Sharing. Dr. Kahan's bibliography currently includes over 580 published works, including 86 book chapters. Kahan's publications span the past three decades of the modern application of transplantation, representing a chronicle of the surgical development and immunological evolution of organ transplantation.

MARGARET LOCK, Ph.D., is a professor in the Department of Social Studies of Medicine and the Department of Anthropology at McGill University, Montreal, Quebec, Canada. She is the author of *East Asian Medicine in Urban Japan: Varieties of Medical Experience* (1980), translated into Japanese as *Tophi Bunka to Toyoigaku* (1990), and *Encounters with Aging: Mythologies of Menopause in Japan and North America* (1993), which won the Eileen Basker Memorial Prize and the Canada-Japan Book Award.

Much of Lock's research has been conducted in Japan; her particular interest is the interrelationships of culture, modernization, and health and illness. She has done research on the revival of the traditional medical system in Japan and on life-cycle transitions, including adolescence, the elderly, and female midlife. Her present research is a comparative study in Japan and North America on changing conceptualization about life and death as a result of new medical technologies.

THOMAS H. MURRAY, Ph.D., is a professor of biomedical ethics and the director of the Center of Biomedical Ethics in the School of Medicine, Case Western Reserve University, Cleveland, Ohio. Murray's research interests cover a wide range of ethical issues in medicine and science, including genetics, aging, children, and health policy. He is a founding editor of the journal *Medical Humanities Review,* and is a past member and founder of the Working Group on Ethical, Legal and Social Issues to the National Institutes of Health Center for Human Genome Research.

LAURENCE J. O'CONNELL, Ph.D., S.T.D., is the president and chief executive officer of the Park Ridge Center for the Study of Health, Faith, and Ethics, Chicago, Illinois. He also holds an adjunct appointment in the Department of Medicine at the Stritch School of Medicine at Loyola University of Chicago in Maywood, Illinois. O'Connell earned a Ph.D. in religious studies and an S.T.D. from the University of Louvain, Belgium. He serves on the boards and committees of several health care and ethics organizations in the United States and Europe and has participated in policy development at the state and national levels. In 1993 he was part of the ethics working group of the President's Task Force on National Health Care Reform in Washington, D.C.

O'Connell is a frequent presenter at conferences concerning faith, ethics, and public policy issues related to such health care issues as AIDS, abortion, care for the aged and dying, euthanasia, imperiled newborns, and health care reform.

RUTH RICHARDSON, D.Phil., is Wellcome Research Fellow in the History of Medicine, Department of Anatomy and Developmental Biology at University College in London. Her doctoral thesis focused on the procurement of corpses for dissection in British anatomy schools between the Renaissance and the present day. Her book *Death, Dissection and the Destitute* was published in 1989. In her current work at University College she is examining the cultural impact of sanitary legislation concerning the disposal of the dead, with a particular focus upon the dead of London. Richardson has published numerous articles in medical and historical journals and has lectured in the United Kingdom, Europe, the United States, and Canada.

STUART J. YOUNGNER, M.D., is a professor of medicine, psychiatry, and biomedical ethics at Case Western Reserve University School of Medicine in Cleveland, Ohio, and the director of the Clinical Ethics Program at University Hospitals of Cleveland. He serves on the editorial advisory boards of the *Kennedy Institute of Ethics Journal* and the *Journal of Medicine and Philosophy*. He is currently serving as president of the Society of Bioethics Consultation. Youngner has written and spoken extensively about organ transplantation, defining death, and end-of-life decision making.

Index